eating well,
living better

THE
GRASSROOTS
GOURMET
GUIDE TO
GOOD HEALTH
AND **GREAT FOOD**

eating well, living better

MICHAEL S. FENSTER, MD

ROWMAN & LITTLEFIELD PUBLISHERS, INC.
Lanham • Boulder • New York • Toronto • Plymouth, UK

Grassroots Gourmet is a registered trademark of Red Tail Productions, LLC.

Published by Rowman & Littlefield Publishers, Inc.
A wholly owned subsidary of The Rowman & Littlefield Publishing Group, Inc.
4501 Forbes Boulevard, Suite 200, Lanham, Maryland 20706
www.rowman.com

10 Thornbury Road, Plymouth PL6 7PP, United Kingdom

Distributed by National Book Network

British Library Cataloguing in Publication Information Available

Library of Congress Cataloging-in-Publication Data

Fenster, Michael S., 1964-
 Eating well, living better : the grassroots gourmet guide to good health and great food /
Michael S. Fenster.
     p. cm.
   Includes bibliographical references and indexes.
   ISBN 978-1-4422-1340-1 (pbk. : alk. paper) — ISBN 978-1-4422-1341-8 (ebook)
   1. Nutrition—Popular works. 2. Diet—Psychological aspects—Popular works. 3. Health—
Popular works. 4. Food preferences—Popular works. 5. Cookbooks. I. Title.
 RA784.F46 2012
 613.2—dc23   2011024308

∞™ The paper used in this publication meets the minimum requirements of American National
Standard for Information Sciences—Permanence of Paper for Printed Library Materials,
ANSI/NISO Z39.48-1992.

Printed in the United States of America

This work is humbly dedicated to:

My mother, who shared her passion for cooking and never hesitated to let me know when I messed up in the kitchen or anywhere else;

My father, who was always there and helped me to "keep going" even though he warned me not to do it;

Lindsey, Davis, and Cheyenne, the best test kitchen ever; and

Jennifer, who makes all things possible and without whom there is no light.

contents

acknowledgments

THERE ARE so many people to thank for helping bring this crazy idea to full fruition. If anyone reading thinks that they should have been mentioned here but aren't, you are probably right. I apologize, and any omissions are accidental and solely my fault.

I have to thank my mother. She gave me her love of food and passion for excellence. The days I played hooky from school to watch Julia Child and the Galloping Gourmet with her and then cook from their cookbooks in the kitchen were some of my best-spent days, a priceless education. I also need to thank my dad for being there to pick me up and help me keep going. Even though he warned me about my harebrained schemes, he never made me feel too bad about them. I hope I have finally learned something so I can be done with all the "learning experiences" and perhaps save him further embarrassment. I need to thank Drs. Ragosta, Powers, and Sarembock. They gave me the best cardiology training any fellow could ask for, and they demonstrated what being a true physician and healer is all about. Whenever I try to decide what the right thing to do is, I hear their voices, and they still make me laugh. I also need to thank my martial arts instructors and friends: Soke Masaaki Hatsumi, who saved me from myself by sharing his martial art with the world; Shihan Kevin Millis, who took on a grubby student from across the country and helped him achieve a dream; Shihan Wild Bill Johnson, my friend and training partner for decades without whom I could never have progressed; and Lindsey,

Davis, and Cheyenne, who were always there to taste the food, whether they wanted to or not. I appreciate your honesty, even if it's not always what I wanted to hear. Spending time with you in the kitchen are memories I shall always treasure. I must also thank my literary agent, Leticia Gomez, who worked tirelessly to find a home for this book. I also need to thank my editor, Suzanne Staszak-Silva, who gave this book a home and helped edit it into an even better read, which I thought impossible. I still do not like the Oxford comma, though.

And finally but certainly not in the least, I must thank Jennifer. Without her love and support, none of this would be. Indeed, I would not be. You are my love and my light.

foreword

THERE'S A LOVE affair going on with food. You can see it everywhere you look. The grocery stores are filled with food that we all think we love, but in reality it's just an illicit affair (with junk)! We are carrying on with food that just isn't good for us. From dyes to pesticides and artificial ingredients, we're overindulging on food that makes us feel empty and alone, much like that one-night stand that we *wish* would garner the true love of our life. We're searching for meaning, sustenance, and satiation from Frankenfoods that are no good for us. The good news, my friends, is the search is over. Within the pages of this book, Dr. Mike Fenster shows us how to truly savor and enjoy real food—the food we were meant to spend our lives with—forever. As an interventional cardiologist and professional chef, he knows the human body inside and out and knows the right foods that will tickle your fancy—and help kick-start a love affair of the marrying kind!

Dr. Mike's recipes and tips encourage the reader to put flavor back into food and restore the true essence of your body and soul in a gastronomic way. Dr. Mike helps you walk the line between too much and too little with his Zen-like approach to eating: pure, fresh, balanced, and loaded with nutrition and taste without overdoing it. This book is a how-to for anyone interested in learning his or her way around the kitchen without all of the hype and bologna. His candid, charismatic voice is ever present among the pages as if he is standing over your shoulder, coaching you through your kitchen, grocery lists, and recipe cards. He tells it like it is—from personal experiences to current research—while leaving you with useful information, tips, and ideas that you can put to use during your next meal preparation. Consider Dr. Mike your Sherpa in the kitchen, an intelligent, charming guide taking you on an adventure and food love affair to remember.

Beth Aldrich, author, *Real Moms Love to Eat: How to Conduct a Love Affair with Food, Lose Weight, and Feel Fabulous* (2012)

why this book?

SO, YOU'VE taken a gander at the front cover and this book's title, and now I have your undivided attention.

Dr. Mike?

Doctor?

Really?

Then you peeked at the back cover to see if the guy calling himself "Doc" is truly, by some strange coincidence, a real, honest-to-goodness medical doctor, an M.D. Lo and behold, he is, and to top it off, he has actually worked in the food and restaurant industry, cooking in kitchens and along the way obtaining a culinary degree. At this point, you may feel inclined to ask, "Is this really a medical professional who actually practices what he preaches?" While that may seem a bit schizophrenic on the surface, please don't tune me out just yet because it will eventually make perfect sense to you. If you've come this far, dear reader (and even if you were to put this book down now this very instant and walk away, you are still a dear reader), sooner or later you are bound to ask yourself, Why this book? Why another cookbook? Why another program? Doesn't the world have enough of them already? I think that is a bloody brilliant series of questions because I asked myself the same things.

Now that your curiosity has been piqued, you are probably wondering: "How can these two seemingly disparate paths, medicine and cooking, possibly converge?" As presented in the media today, cooking seems to revolve around a purely supersized, hedonistic approach to forbidden gustatory pleasures. On the other side of the road stands current medical advice, goose-stepping gurus decrying these very pleasures as a speedy ticket to a painful and slow death, with much gnashing of teeth and wailing along the way. What seemingly insane, freakish twist of fate could have produced an individual who seems to be the offspring of Julia Child and Marcus Welby? Well, it is actually not two distinctly different paths but more like two ends of a circle. "But wait," you say. "A circle actually has no distinct ends." Exactly, Grasshopper.

Let's look a little closer at these two territories: the medical arts and the culinary arts. The commonly shared border between the two becomes clear—the Arts. And the finest Art of any form is one that follows the form of Nature. And Nature is all about Balance. Thus like any artistic endeavor that swings too widely and delves too deeply into one area of focus, it can lose that connection to Nature and become unbalanced. It can become a caricature of itself. Without the face of compassion, the medical arts becomes a cold, calculated, scientific, and sterile process. It may fix and cure but most certainly does not heal. It is a bit of an irony that this character trait seems to play such a miniscule role in selecting those to lead in the deployment of health care. Despite its profundity of scientific achievement and success in treating a vast array of pathologies, Western medicine is often delivered so impersonally and leaves so many patients feeling unsatisfied—cured but not whole and well.

Likewise, without a passion for excellence, the culinary arts yields consumables but does not nurture. It provides nutrition but not nourishment. An Eastern concept to food preparation suggests that a great chef puts some of his own essence, his own *chi*, into each creation. This gives it that indescribable, that *je ne sais pas*, that makes it delicious in a way that a mass-produced product—even using the finest ingredients—can never achieve. It is the reason an original work of art shines above the copies, why a live performance has something that the recording never will. Food prepared without this passion, for lack of a better word, yields gluttons, not gourmets. Regardless of the artistic endeavor, the approach must be one of balance. We need only look at political and religious extremism for other examples of the consequences of unstable pursuits. My more than thirty years of practicing the martial arts has taught me to keep balance and perspective in all endeavors; more on that later.

Sometimes it is easier to define a thing that is new or difficult to conceptualize by what it is not. Think of Sesame Street's "Which of these things is not like the others?" And no, the answer is not Bert and Ernie's sleeping arrangement. Is this another celebrity cookbook? No, because I am not a celebrity, neither by Hollywood standards nor by culinary standards. The "cookbooks" by Hollywood celebrities are read by the same people who actually give a damn about what Paris Hilton is doing today. They follow celebrity for celebrity's sake. Celebrity chef offerings do often contain, however, great information. I read a lot of them. These folks are master craftsmen and craftswomen, and you can garner a lot of great techniques, information and ideas from getting a glimpse inside their noggins. I encourage perusing these (see the list of resources at the back of this book). Yet, you need to understand that these offerings are written by restaurant chefs creating restaurant meals. A restaurant meal is a product sold to you, hopefully with a taste so delicious that you come back for more. It is a product in a business plan. It is not intended, nor should it be, as a diet to sustain your health and well-being. It doesn't mean it can't be, but *caveat emptor*, that's not its purpose.

This is also not a weight-loss book. It is a sad sign of the times that every time we say the word *diet* it is taken not as the noun referring to what we consume but as the verb form of trying to achieve weight loss, as in "to diet." If you currently consume the average American or Western diet and follow this program, I guarantee you will shed some pounds. You will shed even more if you add a little exercise. However, this is not a program about weight loss only. If you need to call Jenny to achieve some poundage reduction, fine. If you need to lose weight, do it and achieve it by whatever means necessary. This is the lifeline of sanity once you've gotten to where you need to be; you need not be a prisoner ordering meals only from "the system" for the rest of your days like a captive in *The Matrix.* A majority of these programs focus on short-term solutions and snake-oil sales pitches. They prey upon our innate desire for a magical cure that gives us what we want with no effort or work. Delicious, healthful food takes effort. I find it incredibly fun and satisfying to create, and I think you will, too—but it most definitely requires effort.

This is not a companion book to some crazy exercise program, either. There is no infomercial, catalogue of exercise products, nutritional supplements, cookware, videos, or other very expensive paperweights to purchase. This book is based on sound medical principles and data, but it is not a penance program in nutrition perdition. Many of the health/dieting/cooking books written from the medical perspective are a lot like a book teaching you how to walk on your hands. It is interesting, but the novelty quickly wears off and eventually everybody returns to walking on their feet; we simply were not meant to go through life ambulating that way. No one has ever completed a meaningful journey walking on his or her hands.

These days, I practice interventional cardiology and international cuisine. They are both part science, part art, part technique and a damn lot of work. Come to think of it, they are not much different from the martial arts. These disciplines all require the accumulation, assimilation and application of a great deal of information. We now live in the Information Age. If you have no idea how to prepare a beef Wellington to die for, you can go on the Internet and read about how to pull it off. You can also download videos and print recipes. There are a lot of books with information and step-by-step procedures. Heck, you can even go out and buy a piece of meat, some puff pastry, and practice your beef Wellington–making technique until you've gotten it perfect. The same just-practice-until-you-get-it-right algorithm is generally frowned upon in current medical circles (although I have always wondered why it was called a "practice"). Between the Internet, television, books, and DVDs, one can almost acquire a culinary expertise just by immersion. Just like in college, however, there are some "professors" who ought to be avoided like the plague.

This book was born out of a functional need. While practicing medicine I continued to cook and cater, help manage a restaurant and eventually took some time and earned my culinary degree. One day it hit me like a bolt from the blue. My muses merged together at lightning speed at a general cardiology talk I was presenting to the community to help educate the public. I had spent my usual twelve to twenty hours getting things together for the talk, a run-of-the-mill cardiology lecture designed to encourage compliance with all the things doctors tell patients they should do (most of which doctors themselves don't do). I researched data and statistics until I was blue in the face, made an outline, prepared PowerPoint slides and even created graphics and pasted pictures. All this was done, of course, in my "spare time." I spoke eloquently and entertainingly for about forty-five minutes and then opened up the floor for questions. "Surely," I thought, "the wisdom I have imparted to the audience must have sparked some sort of self-realization for them." Would there be a heartfelt confession perhaps? Or maybe a penetratingly sharp observation of the data I had painstakingly presented? Was I in for a question so deep and insightful that it not only demonstrated a complete grasp of the knowledge I had meticulously laid before them but also would inspire a publication-worthy hypothesis?

No.

The people just wanted to know what they could eat.

Right then and there, my two muses hit me on either side of the head with twin two-by-fours. All this lecturing—complete with charts and graphs of death and disease, pictures of the damnation that was sure to follow if the rules of conduct as espoused by we Lords of Medicine were not heeded—all this mumbo jumbo turned out to be fear mongering and intimidation in the first degree. Sure we had an important message to relay. We were trying to convey things that had been shown to help people live longer and healthier lives. Yet, the message was a bit draconian. There was no room for the variances life inevitably throws your way. Like so many Hail Marys to expiate our sins, we tell people, "You must follow this prescription, you must exercise, you must not smoke, and you cannot eat this and must eat that." This "one and only" path of salvation seemed a bit Inquisitionesque. Forget the data and the biochemistry. Forget patting ourselves on the back with the study-derived algorithms we were using. The simple fact remains. People like to eat. People do not eat nowadays simply for nutrition alone and haven't done so for millennia. It is part hard-wired cravings, part instinct driven, part emotional experience, part societal custom, and a whole lot of joy and pleasure. It is a pursuit second only to sex (and for some that's arguable). It is a pure and simple pursuit of happiness, end of story. It makes us feel good to eat, drink and enjoy food. Like with alcohol, we need to do this responsibly, not go all Prohibition. I believe they repealed that bit of temperance because it is so contrary to human nature, and as the Roman emperors learned in the end, it is always mob rule; Rome *is* the mob. Like it has been said: We need to teach them to fish, not cram omega-3–rich salmon down their gullets while telling them how good it is for them. Once they catch that fish, we need to teach them how to make it so damn tasty that they'll *want* to eat it time and time again, not because it is good for you, but because it simply tastes delicious.

So the public cooking demonstrations began and progressed and evolved into blogs and articles and a television show. Therefore, dear reader (and you are very near and dear to this chef's heart if you've come this far), for several reasons this is not just another cookbook like all the others. No one really needs another cookbook, I know. No one needs empty promises from the meal-in-a-minute messiahs hawking "delicious" desserts and such that taste like frozen and then microwaved pig turds. No one needs some soul-sucking stranger treating you like a dietary heretic for wanting to enjoy your food (soul sucking is strictly the purview of ex-spouses). It does take some basic skills, some minimal effort, and a large infusion of passion.

The time has come for a Metallica pearl of wisdom (MPOW): "My lifestyle determines my death style." And like the guys from Metallica, I know of what I speak. This program is a way to control an area of your life (and the lives of those close to you) in a positive manner. This is a way to end a death style and initiate a true lifestyle change. This is a culinary survival guide *and* a prescription for happiness, complete with occasional *pommes frites*. Food is fuel, and most people can appreciate that fact. Yet, we must also appreciate that food is more than just fuel; it supplies all the raw materials from which we construct the infrastructure of our bodies. Cells, cell parts, organs, bones, and tissue are constantly being broken down and replaced—replaced with what we ingest. We need healthful food for the body. For like the infrastructure of America itself, the infrastructure of the average American is crumbling into disrepair.

The purpose of this book is to provide a basis upon which you can develop an absolutely delicious food program in a sustainable manner, sustainable in that it is good for the Earth, for your locale and most importantly for you and your loved ones because you follow it every day (willingly) and it sustains your good health. It is to provide food that tastes good first and foremost because that is what nourishes our souls.

So why buy another self-indulgent cookbook?

Don't.

So, why buy a lifetime of denial?

Don't.

Buy into a solution to a problem created by these extremes that is plaguing so many: how to eat things that make you healthy *and* taste good at the same time. Become a Grassroots Gourmet. Why? Because becoming a Grassroots Gourmet is the first step on the path to becoming your own culinary Buddha. A Grassroots Gourmet is an acolyte of Nature's wisdom in the kitchen temple, to be sure, but so much more. With a foundation in food and health knowledge, you will learn why we crave certain foods and seek out poor eating behaviors. You will follow the Threefold Path of the "Bes," and you will learn proper principles for maintaining good health and eating great-tasting food that is great for you. You will move beyond simply counting calories and understand what healthful eating is really about and how and why it can include a variety of choices, including fat, sugar and salt—in moderation, of course. You will apply the appropriate technique where and when you need it. You will get to eat the delicious food you want and learn how to select local foods; how to read labels; how to make better food choices; and how to live joyfully, hopefully, and healthily. The path of the Grassroots Gourmet leads to culinary nirvana and epicurean enlightenment. In the following chapters, I lead you down that path and at the end you will be able to determine your own gastronomic reality, one grounded in reason.

how i achieved culinary buddhahood (and you can, too)

GREAT CHANGES and significant occurrences often seem to hinge on, at the time, small events or decisions: a contaminated petri dish leads to the discovery of penicillin; a battlefield decision defeats the Persian Empire, preserving ancient Greece and birthing Western civilization; a misplaced order fallen into enemy hands prevents the Confederate invasion of the North; and the list goes on. As Tolkien notes in *The Lord of the Rings*, "even the smallest person can change the course of the future," and seemingly so can the smallest event or decision.

On a personal level, we can often recount occurrences like this that have shaped large territories of our lives: the chance encounter that becomes a lifetime romance, the strange happenstance that shapes a career, a seeming failure that pushes us in the direction of ultimate personal victory. These are the types of occurrences that have us wondering whether we are captains of our own destiny or merely fated to sail passively the winds of predetermined fate, our self-determination but an illusion.

My own path started out in incredibly disparate and seemingly contradictory ways. I grew up with a love of food, not unlike many who in later years find themselves in some food-related vocation. My mother was a good and avid home cook. I remember playing hooky from school (and my mom knew perfectly well that I wasn't sick at all) to watch Graham Kerr (the Galloping Gourmet) and Julia Child with her on television. I can remember helping my mother make the recipes from those cookbooks. I also recall getting in trouble between six and eight years old when, in an effort to fully imitate the Galloping Gourmet, I also poured myself a little libation in the kitchen. The fact that I had prepared a glass of rye whisky (having no idea what it was) with a little cola and found it so delicious that I offered my mom a sip (while she was fixing the weekend breakfast) should really have portended things to come. In fact, I enjoyed food so much that despite participating in sports year round, I had to get my clothes in the husky boys' section of Sears. Nowadays I am sure that name would be banned for causing irreparable psychic injury and making a young person like me too self-conscious of his or her personal shortcomings. But if that weren't enough, the Sears people made sure everyone knew you were a fat little porker by putting not just length and waist on the non-removable tag sewn at the back of the pants but also in large lettering a sign proclaiming "husky." It was the butt billboard telling the world, "I have a fat ass." All this angst before you even hit the teenage years. As for my delicate psyche, it just made me embarrassed because I *was* fat. Eventually that inspired me to lose the weight (although I still struggle), but the love of food has always remained.

This love of food is not just eating but also exploring the wild taste sensations, creative preparations and thrill of the hunt within the protective confines of the market. All through these childhood years, I can remember cooking at the stove with my mom. I can recall helping her prepare, cook, and serve for dinner parties back in the day when people actually had dinner parties in their homes and not just the catered or prepared food of today. Back then you couldn't log onto the Internet to look things up. It was watch some TV and get the book or magazine. Despite the rye whiskey incident (or maybe because of it), I was the designated bartender for these *soirées* by the tender age of twelve. I was reading and memorizing *Mr. Boston's Bar Guide* and making drinks by jigger measures (as I wasn't allowed to taste the drinks). I can still picture the shocked adult faces when I'd pour out a really nice Tom Collins or whiskey sour. Even though they were delighted with the results and I was quite the professional, my tip jar was always pretty empty at the end of the evening. Cheap bastards are a rather ubiquitous food service phenomenon at all levels.

Growing up, my family moved and traveled frequently. In some places it was difficult to be the new and chunky kid. But the positive of that occurrence was that I got to experience many diverse food cultures firsthand. There was New York City with Little Italy and Chinatown, the Boston waterfront, New Jersey delis, and fresh Maine lobster at the end of a pier in Boothbay Harbor, just to name a few. And no matter where we went, or what the situation, the kitchen always provided sanctuary.

Perhaps that is why, no matter how often or where we moved, my love of food and cooking never left me. While attending college I had my first professional food experience. In our college dormitory, my roommate, Randy, and I set up a late-night snack business for our fellow students. It turned out to be a gold mine for us. Late at night as a famished college student, you either try to order some takeout food or ransack the mini-fridge your parents had bought you. Although I was armed only with a hot pot and a sandwich maker, Randy and I were able to offer grilled ham and cheese sandwiches, hot soups, and the like. Randy took care of the business end of the enterprise and set the menu prices. I was the designated cook. The students loved the food but were continually pissed at Randy for his exorbitant "convenience" charge. I have to hand it to Randy: he was a very clever businessman.

After our first year in the food industry, Randy and I went our separate ways and I engaged in the more mainstream commercial food service. Like every other college student out there, I always needed to earn a little money on the side, especially as spring break approached. As a newbie in the restaurant world, I first stepped through the fast food doors. At a particular fast food enterprise, my culinary prowess was instantly recognized when I started on the grill. I'm proud to say there was no lengthy working up from the very bottom rungs of this ladder for me. Due to my innate talent, I had easily exempted out of Fryolator 101 and was put directly to work at the grill. I did not need multimillion dollar double-blind, placebo-controlled, randomized studies or a Morgan Spurlock movie to give me the (lack of a) skinny on consuming a predominately fast food diet. I was back shopping for some of those "husky" pants. My high school acne, having cleared upon entering the college scene, kept reappearing like a *Saw* sequel—with just as much gore. Leaving my grill spatula behind, I started working at some local restaurants of the less-toxic variety. I worked my way up from dishwasher to line cook to running the back of the house at several local establishments. While never Michelin-star, fine-dining places, they were fine local restaurants that used fresh regional ingredients and original recipes. In these kitchens I learned to cook: basic techniques, how to prep, how to properly shuck an oyster and cook a fish, how to touch a steak and gauge doneness, how to plate, how to curse nonstop until I was out of the weeds and how to unwind after work until 4 or 5 a.m. I worked my way up and loved every minute of it. Culinary survival skills, indeed.

Over the years I continued to refine my techniques and expand my knowledge base. I even got my culinary degree and helped manage a fine dining restaurant and wine bar. The degree filled great gaps in my knowledge and added a few refinements, but my cooking skills were forged nights and weekends in the hot, cramped kitchens of a college town. The management experience just proved that I knew about running kitchens, cooking food, drinking wine and not a damn thing about business. I later went back to school and got an M.B.A. because I was not a good businessman at that time. I *über* sucked at it.

They did not teach you anything about business in medical school, either. When you are going through medical school, it is hard enough just to continue to keep up with the massive amounts of material you must master before you ever see a patient. Then in your third year, you start seeing and treating real patients and still have to learn reams of data. After medical school you get your M.D. and enter your residency program as an indentured servant. For me, that was three years in an internal medicine program. The second verse is the same as the first as you repeat the indentured servitude doing a fellowship. That was another four years as I spent time doing National Institutes of Health (NIH)–sponsored research in microvascular physiology, part of which was spent doing unspeakable things to small rodents. Some things you can never be proud of, no matter what the ultimate outcome. My final year of training was doing a subspecialty fellowship in interventional cardiology. From there you are aborted from the warm, wine-scented sacred womb of academia onto the beach of reality like a baby sea turtle running for the ocean, with approximately the same survival odds.

Medicine, they forget to mention in the brochure, is big business. You either learn quickly or get picked off and swallowed up. You learn the business ropes in the school of hard knocks or not at all. After getting my ass kicked so many times, I had to face the fact that my own ignorance on the business side was killing me. Consequently I went back as a student to learn those lessons. A lot of my colleagues never do. As physicians, as experts expected to know everything, they cannot bring themselves to admit they do not know. I have seen more good physicians, partnerships and programs ruined by ego and greed than by any other malady.

What saved me from that fate was karma, a special karma known as a two-by-four. For those not in the know, that is when karma must hit you in the head with a two-by-four before you begin to pay attention. This karmic gift was the result of my martial arts training. I had been taught during my training that the day you are so consumed by your ego that you cannot move freely because you are afraid you may not look the expert is the day you die.

I had always had an interest in the martial arts. In college, because other injuries had prevented me from doing certain athletics, I followed up on that interest. Martial arts is like ice cream: The different styles contain the same basic ingredients but come in many flavors and toppings. You need to pick the one that you like. After a little trial and error, obtaining a belt rank here and a belt rank there, I found the style that clicked with me and I've been an avid practitioner of that style for almost thirty years now.

I have learned and continue to learn much from my study of martial arts. One of the earliest concepts I was exposed to was that of *sanshin*, the three hearts, or three spirits, practice. It consists, among other things, of a methodology of analysis by which constructs are broken down into their three essential components. In many cultures throughout the world, both contemporary and ancient, the concept of understanding fundamental principles as a trinity of aspects is not a unique concept. What was unique at the time, I remember, was our *soke*, or grandmaster, remarking that no one could even begin to conceptualize understanding and integrating the *sanshin* as a single concept until he or she was at least forty years of age and had studied and practiced diligently for many years. As a brash twenty-something, I was sure I got it right away. What I did get right away was an ongoing lesson in humility as I was routinely whipped by what appeared to be frail old men; wispy, weak-looking women; and geeky guys. Now, many years and many beatings later, I have begun to understand.

As I studied the demanding physical techniques, I also studied meticulously the spiritual and intellectual accoutrements. As any student of the Japanese martial arts, I eventually came across Miyomoto Musashi. He was arguably the greatest swordsman who ever lived. Musashi lived in the brutal period of seventeenth-century Japan. He fought in large-scale battles as well as individual duels. In his more than sixty single-combat duels, he never lost and allegedly fought to a draw only once and even that is disputed. He is best known today for his writings, especially his *Book of Five Rings*. While ostensibly a training manual on sword techniques, it is widely regarded today as an indispensible martial and business guide on strategy as well as a life-lesson commentary. It is held in the same esteem as Sun Tzu's Chinese classic *The Art of War*.

What is fascinating about Musashi's journey is how he uses the techniques and lessons learned on the razor's edge of life and death single combat to carve a path to enlightenment. Such was his insight that, when he achieved understanding at the top of his game, he refused to duel anymore. He replied that he had obtained what he sought, thus there was no further need for potential bloodshed. He did give unarmed demonstrations against armed opponents. Reportedly he left them cowering in the corner, unable to move or strike. Musashi then began to write and pursue other activities. With no formal training other than swordsmanship, he became an author whose works are still best-sellers centuries after his death, an artist whose paintings hang in museums, a sculptor whose works are likewise on display and a forger of *tsubas*, or sword guards, which are insanely valuable. In his works Musashi recorded his response when asked how he can master all these endeavors, as each one could easily consume a lifetime of study. He answered that once you understood one, in his case the Art of the Sword, you could understand them all. Your insight, he remarked, had to take you to that single place, that empty space where there is nothing yet everything. It is a very oriental concept that is difficult to translate, but it refers to a place where all Art resides and no particular Art. In the English translation, it is often referred to as the Void. But it is not a void as we might think of it, meaning an empty space. It is a place that is undefined and unlimited in potential and therein cannot contain any one thing. It is a totipotent and undifferentiated space of potential. It is like that description of time and space before the big bang when the universe was in this small dot of nothingness. But that dot of nothingness contained everything the universe would become. This confusion is the source of much misinformation. Musashi observed that from this place the process of creation was the same, whether it was a sword stroke or a paintbrush stroke. It was the small details of execution that differed. All Art, and thus all Life, springs from the same godhead.

Cooking for me had always been an artistic expression. However, there is a certain amount of science involved in cooking. In the execution of all things artistic, there are certain principles that must be followed. Medicine I always approached as my science had taught me. My decisions were based on rational thought, testable hypotheses, reason and outcomes data. Yet for each patient, the regimen needed to be handcrafted, adjusted and tempered; a lot like baking, where things can be individualized but you better follow the basic recipe. In martial arts there was an obvious mix of science and art. Interactions of human beings, limbs, joints, vital organs, and weapons followed very scientific principles. Yet in the arrangement, combination and application of these principles was unlimited artistic license. The scientific principles are like musical notes: simply sound vibrations at a certain frequency and amplitude. It takes the application of Art to transform these notes from a cacophony to a symphony.

For many years I drew upon these activities as very separate endeavors, my somewhat related but distinctly separate *sanshin*. When I had done my basic science bench research, the working environment was tough. I was surrounded by folks who viewed themselves as "real" scientists who ran "proper" experiments by controlling for all the variables save the experimental one, not "pseudoscientists" like me who did "applied" and imprecise experiments and protocols working with people. But my most hard-core (and critical) scientific mentor also opened a Pandora's box of possibilities. One day he had us present our research to our fellow students. He then proceeded to rip everyone a brand new and shiny excremental orifice. He ultimately exposed that the "facts" upon which we based things, including the very measurements we were using, were at some level taken on faith. Ultimately the existence and interaction of very tiny things were mathematical probabilities and possibilities. They existed outside the realm of direct experience. As Ken Wilbur has commented, there comes a time in our understanding of the universe when you can no longer separate the observer from observed, the mapmaker from the map. If you doubt this lesson, just read some quantum mechanics and theoretical physics. This field attempts to describe how the universe really and truly functions. It reads more like a Buddhist koan than any scientific treatise.

So like several-days'-old chili, over the last several years, these seemingly disjointed elements blended together in a kind of harmony. I began to see the Art in each: culinary arts, medical arts, and martial arts. And while they all had their artistic expression drawn from the same well, it was their unique science that gave each its individual face. Yet at their core, they were the same; my cooking could heal, my martial art could nourish and my medicine could protect. By doing so, for me, they became a singular and proactive (as opposed to reactive) venture. They became *Ichi-ryu*, one spirit.

Hence it was without any sense of coincidence but a sense of fortune that I entered a bookstore not so long ago for nothing in particular; just a need for a coffee compelled me inward. Then I was drawn to wander sections I usually do not tread for fear of finding something I must read and thus procrastinate further finishing my "to do" list. My list was already too long. But enter and wander I did. Already having appropriated the culinary Buddha moniker and scribbled out the Grassroots Gourmet theory and three-fold path commentary, I espied *The Middle Way* by the Dalai Lama, one of my favorite authors and speakers. As always, his prose was inspired and inspiring and his *Middle Way* led me to my middle path. So I walked into a bookstore one day for a coffee and here we are; I hope in some small way this inspires you to find your middle path.

And if you meet the culinary Buddha on your middle path, kill him, for any outer Buddha that you meet is a creature of external construct like your ego. Kill him because the culinary Buddha who traverses *your* middle path must come from inside *you*, from your own innate culinary Buddha nature. Anything else is a false icon of shadow and lies.

understanding extremes

A **COIN CAN** be described as having heads on one side and tails on the other. To comprehend the coin, we must understand heads, tails, and the space in between. The space between heads and tails exists as neither precisely heads nor precisely tails and as a form of both heads and tails. Life can be described as having both happiness and suffering. It is the natural inclination of all living things to seek happiness and avoid suffering. Watch any group of animals; they pursue those things that make them happy and actively avoid those things that would bring suffering. Human beings are no different. As we seek happiness or move away from suffering, we move toward more extreme positions. These extreme positions are the natural consequence of this movement. When it comes to our food, these positions form the borders of hedonism and asceticism.

Hedonism can be described as the pursuit of pleasure as the result of the "seeking of happiness" instinct. William Blake wrote that the "road to excess leads to the palace of wisdom . . . for we never know what is enough until we know what is more than enough." This embodies the learning principle when we find ourselves at the hedonistic border. If we find X pleasurable or activity Y brings us happiness, then we tend to seek 2X or try to enjoy Y twice as long. If that is without adverse consequence, then we increase the multiplier. At some point we reach a zone or boundary of excess. At that position, as Blake intimates, we should understand that we have crossed into some form of excess. A slice of chocolate cake was delicious, but the whole cake made us sick; a night of carousal with the boys (or girls) was a good time, but do it every night, and you endanger your reputation, not to mention your overall health and well-being . . . well just ask Tiger where you wind up after all that night putting. Sometimes we experience the effects of crossing the boundary personally; sometimes we learn from the mistakes of others; sometimes we intuitively understand the consequences and determine that it is not right. If life is a game, then we need to know where the out-of-bounds are located. That, I believe, is why God invented hangovers; that and the fact that hangovers have probably generated more prayer than any preacher's Sunday sermon.

The lure of excess is alive and well within the foodie world. Within the media overindulgence is everywhere apparent and proselytizing. Television is rife with shows demonstrating not just a hedonistic approach but also a flat-out homage to gluttony. The biggest this, the most that—there is an unspoken nod toward an attitude that equates quantity with value. *Man vs. Food*? Since when did what we eat become a competitive opponent? I must admit, though, that Adam Richman is a personal hero because I don't know how he isn't 750 pounds and cruising in a Jazzy from eatery to eatery. He must have a metabolism that is the equivalent of a hummingbird, weight adjusted of course. Overabundance has become so commonplace that "to supersize" is an accepted verb.

In the cardiac catheterization laboratory, we use the phrase "bigger is better." It represents the principle that, when fixing the arteries by placing metal tubes, or stents, in them, the larger the caliber that we can safely make the arteries, the better both the short- and long-term prognosis for that patient. Yet the "bigger is better" philosophy does not equate to more quantity is better. For example, more stents in an artery is not necessarily a better thing. The more stents that are placed, the higher the likelihood of some long-term complications. In fact, one could argue that a "more is better" attitude is at the root of many of a patient's problems. When looking at responses to wants or needs, it is possible to evaluate it as a combination of two different kinds of variables: quality (Q_l) and quantity (Q_n). Not always but often the economies of reality prohibit unlimited amounts of both variables. When we make a decision about wants or needs, we are making a value assessment. We often measure that value in terms of currency; it is or is not worth a certain amount of dollars. In essence the equation could be rewritten such that for any *x* amount of dollars, one could receive some response represented by a combination of *n* quantity and *l* level of quality: $X_s = Q_l + Q_n$. We, as a nation when it comes to food, seem to be obsessed with the *n* variable. More of whatever, bigger portions, and so on, is deemed to be the better value. So like Beldar Conehead from France, we consume mass quantities. If you continue to put down layer upon layer of food-like stuff in your arterial pipes, you will eventually upgrade to your own shiny new metallic stent or even a whole new set of bypasses. You can consider the swill you've ingested as the primer coat for that new $2,500 coronary stent or the $25,000 worth of bypasses that were placed in your arteries. Yet we *can* differentiate value in terms of quantity and quality. If I offered the same person who slams down twenty-two one-dollar Big 'N Hearty value meals (which become juicy and loosey on the way out) twenty-two black-and-white 6" TVs or one 60" HDTV LED flat screen, I am sure the one flat screen wins, even though there is less in quantity, hands down. This type of example proves people can recognize when quality is more important than quantity in the determination of value.

That is an important concept because more can be fatal. We have another saying in the cardiac catheterization laboratory: "Better is the enemy of Good." Like everything else in America, we tend to think more is better, which makes it the enemy of Good if you're following along. For example, a Japanese study looking at more than 23,000 men and more than 35,000 women between ages forty and seventy-nine who completed questionnaires about dietary habits was published in 2010 in the journal *Stroke: Journal of the American Heart Association* as part of the Japan Collaborative Cohort Study.[1] The people in the study were examined and grouped according to their intake of folate (vitamin B_9), vitamin B_6 (also known as pyridoxal, pyridoxine, or pyridoxamine), and vitamin B_{12}. The researchers followed these groups for several years, and at a median of fourteen years followup, 986 people had died from stroke, 424 from heart disease, and 2,087 from all diseases related to the cardiovascular system. Vitamin B_{12} was not found to be associated with a reduced risk of mortality. However, it was found that higher consumption of folate and B_6 was associated with significantly fewer deaths from heart failure in men. In women, they detected significantly fewer deaths from stroke, heart disease, and total cardiovascular deaths. To avoid confounding variables, anyone taking supplements was eliminated from the analysis, thus the findings reflected intake from diet. The protective effects of folate and vitamin B_6 did not change even when researchers made adjustments for the presence of cardiovascular risk factors. They concluded that both men and women may benefit from consuming foods rich in B vitamins and folate and that these foods may help reduce the risk of heart failure in men and the risk of death from stroke and heart disease in women. The researchers suggested that a diet rich in these compounds may help offset dietary intake of other compounds like homocysteine or offset genetic predispositions to disease states. While the study was performed in Japan, the researchers say their findings are consistent with other studies in North America and Europe.

So while a diet rich in folate and B vitamins is clearly beneficial, in the following case of diabetics with any kidney disease, *more* is not only *not* better; it is fatal. In a study also published in 2010 in the *Journal of the American Medical Association*, it was revealed that high-dose vitamin B therapy is dangerous for diabetics with kidney disease.[2] Of people with diabetes, about 40 percent develop kidney disease. The original hypothesis was that high-dose vitamin B therapy (folic acid, vitamin B_6, and vitamin B_{12} supplementation) would improve patients' kidney function and reduce their risk of heart attack and stroke, as the previously described Japanese study where diets rich in these compounds suggested this to be true. So by way of typical Western thinking, if a little in the diet is good, a whole lot more (in quantities only available by supplementation) must be better. However, this study found that high-dose vitamin B therapy was associated with a significant worsening of kidney function, and twice as many patients taking supplementation had heart attacks and strokes as compared to patients not taking the high-dose supplementation. Dr. David Spence of the University of Western Ontario, one of the authors of the study, states, "Vitamin B therapy may still be beneficial in people with normal kidney function, but this is clear evidence that high doses of vitamin B should not be given to those with kidney problems."[3]

A similar result was reported on calcium supplementation. An article in the *British Medical Journal* in 2010 suggested calcium supplementation may increase the risk of a heart attack in women taking the supplement.[4] The trial was a meta-analysis that looked at data from eleven smaller trials comprising about twelve thousand older female patients. The data showed that, although the total number of women having heart attacks was small (around 1 to 2 percent), among those taking calcium supplements, there was a 31 percent increased risk of having a heart attack. Of import, it is critical to realize that supplements with vitamin D were excluded from the analysis. It is also important to note that this type of result is correlative not necessarily causative. However, a very interesting sidebar is that studies that have looked at diets rich in calcium have not shown any increased cardiac risk.

Even things encouraged because of their many health benefits appear to have boundaries. Exercise is good and not enough Americans actively engage in this activity. But can there be too much exercise? The conventional wisdom would say no, yet we have recorded that extremes of exercise can have detrimental consequences. For example, for women who do some extreme marathon running, it can cause amenorrhea. When it comes to cardiovascular health, however, the thought was that you cannot really overwork the heart muscle.

A study by marathon runner and Canadian cardiologist Dr. Eric Larose suggests differently. First and foremost, please note that any cardiac muscle damage appears transient and completely reversible. That being said, it appears that the stress of marathon running does cause some heart muscle damage. The study was presented at the 2010 Canadian Cardiovascular Congress.[5] It involved analyzing twenty marathon runners of varying experience; for some it was their first marathon and for others it was their thirtieth. The average age was forty-five. They were examined six to eight weeks prior to the marathon, immediately after the marathon and then three months later. The findings suggest cardiac stress similar to those that might be seen with a mild heart attack. There was inflammation and about 50 percent of the heart was involved. The less-fit runners had higher levels of stress. Regardless, by three months all signs of marathon-induced trauma were no longer present. But wait—there's more.

A study out of Britain examined the cardiac status of very athletic older individuals.[6] These people were competitive athletes their entire lives and continued to train rigorously even into their golden years. A comparison group was a similarly aged cohort, healthy in general but more of the weekend-warrior sort, as well as a younger group of athletes. The groups then underwent cardiac magnetic resonance imaging (cardiac MRI) to look for fibrotic deposition within the heart muscle. This is a type of scarring not unlike what happens after a heart attack. The results were a surprise. The younger athletic group had no significant scarring; neither did the older weekend-warrior types. But in the elder overachiever group, about 50 percent had scarring. Even more surprising, the degree of scarring seemed to correlate with the degree of training intensity and duration. A study looking at a similar phenomenon that occurred to intensely exercised rats found that the fibrotic changes resolved with a discontinuation of exercise.[7]

Exercise has a tremendous amount of benefit and is extremely important in achieving and maintaining both health and wellness. Exercise can even potentially blunt some of our vices. Americans, along with members of other industrialized nations, consume too much salt. According to some experts, the average American takes in about 3,375 mg of sodium each day.[8] The current recommended daily allowance (RDA) is about 2,400 mg, with some recommendations calling for less than 1,500 mg per day. A study looking at folks on around 3,000 mg per day looked at the effect of exercise after they were put on a high-sodium diet of about 18,000 mg per day. They found that physical exercise blunted the effect of salt on blood pressure, and the study's coauthor, Dr. Jiang He, admitted it was a "little bit of a surprise. . . . But this is the first study to look at this particular association between physical activity and salt sensitivity and blood pressure. But after thinking it over it makes sense, because we already know that physical activity will reduce blood pressure."[9] The highest-activity group saw about a 38 percent reduction in the risk of their blood pressure being significantly impacted by the high-salt consumption.[10] Yet some of this data suggests that doing a Forrest Gump and just jumping off the couch and running and running and running is detrimental. What is the answer? It is common sense. Working too hard all the time, physical or otherwise, is bad. The Japanese even have a specific word for death from overwork of the vocational variety: *karoshi*. Not engaging in any physical activity ever is also bad. What this type of information signals is that, like all things in the natural world, there are boundaries and balances. Nature, as I like to say, is all about Balance. So definitely exercise and find that balance that makes you feel good, that makes you feel well. Extremism and fanaticism of any type is never a long-term positive, no matter how noble or fundamental we believe the cause to be at the time.

Even things we think are bad for us can be found to have a positive purpose, depending on their magnitude. Interestingly, a recent animal study looked at oxidative stress on the heart. Conventional wisdom has held that oxidative stress causes a cardiac inflammatory response and thus is a bad thing. This type of reaction was the target of many studies looking to use high levels of antioxidants to reduce the effect or prevent oxidative reactions from occurring. The recent animal study showed that these lower-intensity oxidative reactions caused the heart muscle to respond by producing more blood vessels and this response to the inflammation helped make the heart less susceptible to permanent damage from major stressors down the road. Thus these reactions served to condition the heart to be more resilient and less likely to develop permanent heart muscle weakness. This may explain why, at the end of the day, the many studies looking for a benefit of taking high levels of antioxidants has not really panned out.[11]

There are also many more subtle traps beyond the obvious indulgence and overconsumption of mass quantities. For example, a tremendous number of shows and segments demonstrate how to cook restaurant meals. The meals, techniques and ingredients are presented just as if one had ordered the meal in the restaurant with all attention given to taste and pleasure. What is neglected is the barely perceptible caveat that restaurant eating is a treat, not a lifestyle. A restaurant is a business. Restaurant meals are designed to provide a product and experience that the consumer enjoys and wishes to purchase again. Restaurant meals are not designed to promote long-term health, nor are they concerned with anything other than the customers' immediate satisfaction. They are a product of pleasure for the moment. That is not to say we cannot prepare meals with an eye toward healthfulness *and* demand a gustatory encounter worthy of a great dining experience. But the constant deluge of restaurant meals makes for gourmands, not gourmets.

While the pursuit of pleasure can drive us to one extreme, avoidance of suffering can compel us to the other. Human beings are emotional creatures. Such emotions as guilt, pride, vanity, or desire can be used constructively and as motivation in the proper setting. Improperly used, they can become obsessive driving forces. The craving to appear a certain way can lead to anorexia or bulimia. A particular stance or opinion can cause us to alter our food choices irrespective of taste or nutrition. At the extreme it can become asceticism.

Asceticism forms the other boundary to hedonism. Commercials and advertisements nestled within the media programming of excess decry that the only path of true salvation lies in deprivation. Often coming from those persons professing association with the medical and health community and rallying under the banner of health, dispossession and denial are the battle cries for their so-called healthful living formula. Do not eat this even though it tastes good and you know you want it. Eat only fresh, raw vegetables and fruits—and small twigs and pebbles for fiber and bulk while you're at it. According to their pseudomedical gospel the only way to achieve health is by walking through the cleansing flames of nutrition perdition, where the only thing that is flame broiled is you. But this, too, is an extreme in every regard and as ill-advised as the former.

A fellow practitioner related an amazing story to me about one of her patients. He was an elderly gentleman who developed head and neck cancer. To treat this he had surgery, chemotherapy and radiation treatment. He survived but lost all ability to taste. He remarked several years later that although he had survived and he was very grateful for all that had been done, he still suffered. "You have no idea," he said, fighting back the tears welling in his eyes, and then he paused. He took a deep breath and continued with measured words: "You know, I just wish I had died. You don't know what it is like to live without tasting anything. I would give anything to be able to taste again."

There is nothing wrong with eating raw fruits and vegetables. Raw fruits and vegetables are tasty. There is no doubt that, as omnivores, fruits and vegetables are a large part of any balanced, healthful and delicious mainstay diet. However, we evolved, at least according to some anthropologists and paleontologists, a superior intellect specifically because we moved beyond consuming *only* raw vegetables and fruits. We began to evolve because we consumed meat and cooked foods. The extra protein supplied by meat and fish allowed for the development of increased cranial capacity. That increase was also dependent on the cooking process, which allowed us over evolutionary time to decrease the size and energy expended on the very large gut required to chew, digest and extract nutrients from a raw plant-based diet. According to Harvard professor Richard Wrangham,[12] that energy could then be diverted to cranial processes, and thus we grew bigger brains with more potential. We became human.

But now we seem to be humans caught between being at one extreme or the other. As a foodie/chef and as a healthcare professional/interventional cardiologist, I see the vast majority of folks puzzled. In speaking with people who view me from a culinary perspective, they discuss their love of flavors, textures, tastes and the entire eating experience. From those approaching me as a physician seeking answers to their concerns from a health perspective, they discuss their desire to feel good and be healthy. They may relate how an illness has caused a change in their diet or the diet of someone close to them. They may relate that certain foods hold certain emotional ties for them. They may reflect that their rushed and out-of-balance diet is just a microcosm of their lives. Many of these are the same people on different days at different events. They are all of them confused. We have become a torpid mass that wanders to one extreme, bounces to the other extreme, and goes back again. We resemble the little square blip from the game of "Pong," back and forth eternally between the paddles. Occasionally we collapse on the ground face down and "out of bounds." There must be a way to use these extremes like channel markers, avoid the potential wreckage and sail on through. There is, and that way is the Way of the Middle Path.

the middle path

THE BUDDHA was born in the sixth century BCE. When he was young, before he was the Buddha or Supreme Enlightened One, he was Prince Siddhartha Gautama. During his early years and by some accounts until he was about twenty-nine years old, the prince lived a life of excess, luxury and pleasure. Much like the New Testament, the teachings, stories and accounts were initially transmitted through oral tradition. It was not until several hundred years after the death of the Buddha that much of the material was written down. Nonetheless, the accounts agree that the prince was raised in a small kingdom in what is today Nepal. He lived in multiple palaces depending upon the season and was shielded by his father from religious teachings and exposure to suffering and the human condition. He was married when he was young and had a son. When he was about twenty-nine years of age, he left the palace to walk among his subjects. Despite the best efforts of his father to hide the frailties of the human condition, he reportedly saw an old infirm man. He then learned that we all would grow old and die. He continued his journeys outside the palace and came across disease and death. Because of his exposure to these conditions, he embarked upon the pursuit of enlightenment. He renounced a path of excess. He became a mendicant, for he felt there was no wisdom to be found in complete hedonism.

For a while he lived the life of an ascetic seeking illumination through deprivation. He eventually joined four other extreme seekers. Over six years his regimen became more stringent until he was consuming but a grain of rice a day. He became so frail through his austere practice that one day he collapsed and nearly died. He then had a glass of milk and some rice porridge and renounced the ascetic path. His four fellow journeymen abandoned him, regarding him as an undisciplined quitter. The prince, now about thirty-five years of age, had learned that there was no salvation to be found through deprivation. The answers he sought were not to be found in sensual deprivation or the rationing of the food he was allowed to eat. So the young prince, having learned what excess was by consuming too much and what deprivation was by consuming too little, set out to sit under the Bodhi tree. There he sat for forty-nine days and discovered Enlightenment and the Middle Path.

Today we find the food and health world caught at these same extremes. There at each extreme like moths around a flame, we flounder because we are ignorant. Our ignorance comes in two forms: an ignorance of not knowing and an ignorance of false knowing. The former is due to a gap or deficit of the requisite knowledge. It is remedied by acquiring that missing piece and acting upon it. The latter is based upon false assumption—believing that to be true, which is in actuality false. We must understand the nature of our own true food/health reality.

Food, at its simplest, is fuel. We require energy to live and we intake that energy as food. Anyone who has had to feed a baby knows what I was taught in medical school; a baby intuitively knows what it needs to eat. If it needs the nutrients in carrots, it will eat the contents of that jar of baby food containing the carrots. When it no longer needs what is in that jar but needs what is in the pea jar, it starts spitting out carrots. You try the pea jar and down the hatch it goes. When food was scarce in ancient times, adults learned to listen to their inner baby as well. For example, for many years it was unclear how the Inuit people survived in such a healthy way. The extreme environment severely limited their access to vegetables and fruits. For a time some necessary nutrients like vitamin C were thought to be found only in plant sources. The Inuit diet contained meat, blubber and lots of offal. Some of the organ meats were consumed raw. It was recently discovered that the vitamins and nutrients that in a Western diet are obtained from plant sources can be obtained from the raw meat. Heavy cooking destroys the vitamins and nutrients.[1] When we listen to our bodies free of addiction, we know what we need to eat.

But knowing what we need to eat and getting what we want to eat are two very different propositions. As we grow we mature and experience the full gamut of emotions that comprise the human experience. Food is no longer just fuel. It is part of a meal, part of the eating experience. And like any experience, it becomes inexorably attached to emotion. It is an activity in which we no longer engage for strictly nutritional purposes. Coming home after a rough day and pouring a glass of single-malt whisky from Scotland is soothing. The taste of the smoky peat takes me back to the Highlands and I can almost feel the salt spray. I begin to relax. The whisky is good. But that very same glass of whisky sipped in the Highlands on a rocky crag with the wind coming off the loch and the spray of the ocean reaching up to cool off a rare but potent Scottish sun is ethereal. Think of some meal you recall as outstanding; what you recall is the dining experience. The food was great because the experience was great. Bad food can ruin a dining experience and a bad experience can ruin great food. It is an additive equation.

That's one reason I think so much of these current TV shows where the "judges" try to critique the food is an entertainment wasteland. First, there is usually some gimmick or restriction to "test" the competitors, so you're not really seeing someone's culinary potential. Second, because dining is an experience, ultimately it's a subjective call, like art. If someone doesn't like you, they probably won't like your food. Serve that judge the same meal he just snubbed but tell him it was prepared by his favorite chef and it becomes an unbelievable masterpiece. I recall one show where a judge slammed a contestant for using raw onion, which he found unpleasantly strong. He remarked that he never ate any raw onion because he found that flavor too strong and offensive. He never told the contestant about his private onion issue. He has a weird aversion from some past-life onion trauma and then reams a contestant for something the majority of the dining public routinely enjoys? Really? That's how you pick the best chef? So yes, you can comment on the technical execution of a dish, but ultimately eating is experiential; the diner cannot be separated from what he or she is dining upon.

We can see this emotional connection in the name we give certain types of foods; "comfort foods," "treats," and even (most appropriately) "junk" foods. We hear about people feeling depressed and eating one or even several pints of Ben and Jerry's ice cream. Emotion affects our mental state. Our mental state affects our physical well-being. Anyone who has taken care of patients for any significant amount of time has seen people come in with an illness they should bounce back from, strictly medically and physiologically speaking. Yet they seem to have given up on life and are ready (sometimes even telling us they are going) to die and no matter what we do, they pass on. It is well documented that after many years of marriage, if one spouse dies, an inordinate number of the remaining spouses pass within a year. The excess mortality rate varies according to the method and seems highest in the first six months of bereavement. Yet it can last up to about three years and make no mistake, the phenomenon it is real.[2] Multiple studies have demonstrated the effect of depression impacting the immune system or mental stress precipitating bouts of angina. There is even a condition called takotsubo syndrome or broken heart syndrome. It affects mostly women middle aged or older. After experiencing a severe life stress they present with all the symptoms and findings of a huge heart attack, including the ECG changes normally associated with a blockage in a major heart artery. When we rush them to the cardiac catheterization laboratory, their heart arteries are all normal. When we look at their heart function, it looks for all the world like they had a blockage in that suspected artery and the huge corresponding area of heart muscle doesn't work. The name *takotsubo* comes from the abnormal shape the heart assumes with this damage, which resembles the pot fishermen in Japan (where this phenomena was first described) use to capture octopus. Treated with medicine and rest, almost all of the sufferers have their hearts return to normal in several weeks. So normal, in fact, that you cannot tell there was ever anything wrong. Left untreated, they can die.

Science, and particularly the science of medicine, most people do not understand, is an ongoing enterprise. Modern medicine has reached incredible heights in its ability to diagnose and treat. I am very proud to be part of the community that dispenses our current and for the most part, very effective remedies. Yet we have by no means reached the pinnacle of our knowledge or armamentarium. Not so long ago, we believed bleeding folks with leeches was a really good therapy for a host of ills. And before that we were sure that your tummy ache was the result of some tap-dancing gnomes in your stomach. Then we got our "real" science groove on and moved light-years beyond that ignorance. Except that today I use a derivative of leech spit to treat heart attacks and coronary artery blockages. Some things come full circle, and as Gandalf noted, "not even the very wise can see all ends."[3]

Our medical science is built upon the scientific principle. That principle is predicated on testing some hypothesis and observing the results. In medicine we generally accept that the data proves (or disproves) a hypothesis if the significant p value is ≤ 0.05. This implies that, if the rest of the statistics were done correctly, the likelihood that the results observed were due strictly to chance alone is 5 percent or less. In between these dots of knowledge in medicine, we must interpolate theories and treatments. And as in any branch of science, as we learn new things that for the moment we assume are correct, we discard old, disproven theory or assumption. People assume in medicine that we have all the answers because they want us to have all the answers, but we don't. It is a very fluid, moving enterprise. It is still a healing art. Consequently, trying to ascertain the effects of eating and health can be a bit like trying to understand chaos theory: "The flapping of a single butterfly's wing today produces a tiny change in the state of the atmosphere. Over a period of time, what the atmosphere actually does diverges from what it would have done. So, in a month's time, a tornado that would have devastated the Indonesian coast doesn't happen. Or maybe one that wasn't going to happen does."[4]

I remember when I was growing up eating real butter. I love butter; maybe not as much as Paula Deen, but I love butter in my own way. Then margarine was the rage. All the health-food gurus and government institutions told us not to eat butter. It caused coronary disease and death. Margarine was the new elixir from the fountain of youth. Margarines then were made by creating trans-fatty acids (TFAs), a class of compounds rarely seen in nature. While they are an unsaturated fat, they are not good. They are, in fact, highly atherogenic. They move from the bloodstream into the walls of the arteries like Katrina into New Orleans. I wonder how much of the coronary artery disease I treat today was the result of some misguided government directive; more on the Law of Unintended Consequences later. A patient shared a story with me that drives the point home. In the heat of the Florida summer, he put a tub of the margarine outside. He came back several hours later, expecting it to be full of bugs and other critters. Amazingly, other than partially melting, it was unperturbed. Nothing ventured into the margarine because neither bugs nor critters could recognize it as a naturally occurring food source.

I also remember learning in medical school other things that would later be disproven. We were taught that fiber was not necessary. Because it was not absorbed and thus provided no nutritional value, it was regarded as without any import. It was viewed as the food equivalent of an appendix. Only after this advice was debunked was the need for fiber recognized. We attended lectures where alcohol was demonized, no benefit in any way, shape or form. That fact struck me as strange at the time given that alcohol provides an energy source just below fat and ahead of protein and carbohydrates on the efficiency scale at 7 kcal/gm. Given the fact that the human body consumes alcohol as the preferred energy source when available provided another moment for reflection. Today there is overwhelming data that moderate alcohol consumption reduces the risk of cardiovascular events and has a plethora of other positive effects on health. The data also suggest that moderate drinkers are not only healthier but outlive teetotalers. Just remember: Once upon a time we physicians told you it was in good health to fire up a Lucky Strike.

So what are we to conclude from this constant barrage of contradictory information? Of the "eat this today, you shouldn't eat that tomorrow" ramblings? I conclude that trying to isolate single variables of causality in such a complex system as what we eat and who we are and who gets (or doesn't get) which disease is an exercise in chaos theory. It allows us to predict only when some of the variables are extreme in nature and, by being so extreme in value, dominate the equation.

I think that, in this setting, the more applicable data are observational in nature. Cultures that eat diets rich in seafood (excepting those who regularly frequent Long Dong's Seafood Hut) don't get heart disease—I don't care how much cholesterol you find in a shrimp. Populations that do not deeply partake of the Western fast food/junk food diet are healthier. Civilizations that consume fresh, unadulterated product are healthier. Societies that address how you eat as well as what you eat are healthier.

To walk the Middle Path, we must understand the ultimate nature of what drives us to consume certain items. We must be able to differentiate taste, where *we* decide what to devour, from addiction, where the *food* is the master.

taste versus addiction

IF HEDONISM is a rut you can get caught in, then addiction is the land from where few travelers return. Addiction can be defined as the "state of being enslaved to a habit or practice or to something that is psychologically or physically habit-forming, as narcotics, to such an extent that its cessation causes severe trauma."[1] Personal trauma, like any emergency, is a condition that can be said to exist in the mind of a person. It is the possibility that he or she mentally conceives that can constitute an emergency or personal trauma. For many people, not getting that morning muffin stuffed with some industrial meat-like product or an afternoon nugget of assorted chicken parts causes severe mental duress. Yet, you can't live without eating. That makes dealing with the potentially addictive components of eating difficult because they are omnipresent; salt, sugar, and fat are everywhere. The potential for addiction to these substances is also biologically hardwired into us, at one time serving to reinforce survival habits. Those very behaviors that helped the human species survive the last 50,000 years have been turned against us by some very clever and manipulative forces within the food industry that prey on our intrinsic vulnerabilities.

Salt has been around a long time. Our fascination with salt goes back even further than our ability to write about it. Evidence of humans seeking out salt predates recorded history. Early prehistoric man seemed to settle preferentially in areas where salt could be obtained. Because animals in the wild would actively seek these same locales, this is a logical place to set up shop and hunt. It is the earliest form of home delivery. Throughout history salt served not only as a source of vital minerals but also aided in the preservation of foodstuffs. Until fairly recently, salt formed the basis of entire economies. It was associated with the rise and fall of empires from Africa and Asia to Europe and America. It was considered so valuable that Roman soldiers were often paid in salt. The Latin *salarium* is the origin of our word *salary*, the root for both being the Latin word *salarius*, meaning "of salt." Hence the laudatory expression "worth his weight in salt."

Yet, what is this compound we call "salt"? In chemical terms a salt is any ionic compound produced by replacing a hydrogen ion of an acid with another positive ion. What we refer to as salt is actually sodium chloride. It is a compound composed of a positively charged sodium ion (Na^+) and a negatively charged chloride ion (Cl^-). The hydrogen ion of hydrochloric acid (HCl) is replaced by a sodium ion. The neutral $NaCl$ (+1 and -1 equals 0) when exposed to water splits into its respective components, Na^+ and Cl^-, each of which are surrounded by water molecules. Putting salt in water gives us the saltwater we are all accustomed to tasting when the ocean wave pushes some up our noses and down our throats. In fact, the salinity of our very blood matches the salinity of the ocean about the time our very distant ancestors wriggled out of the slime and onto the beaches. Over the millions of years since, the oceans have gotten saltier, which is why today the salt content of the ocean is higher than that of your blood and plasma. As such, when you drink saltwater, you actually are ingesting salt in excess of your internal salt–liquid balance and thus act to dehydrate yourself.

Both the sodium (Na^+) and chloride (Cl^-) ions are necessary for the human body to function. They are known as essential minerals. Both sodium and chloride are necessary for a number of important functions throughout the body. In fact, there are far too many to go into detail here; suffice it to say, without them we could not live. Animals need these vital minerals as well, which is why they seek out salt sources. For marine creatures, the salt they need is all around them. For carnivores, it is found in the flesh they devour. For herbivores it is in the ground, plants, and other natural sources, like salt licks. Thus we are physiologically wired through our animal brains to seek out sources of salt and consume it.

Although the sodium ion functions in many different capacities throughout the body, the regulation of how much sodium we retain is generally performed by the kidneys. The kidneys work closely with the cardiovascular and respiratory systems. The regulators of body fluid volume are related to sodium metabolism. When we speak of the need to avoid or decrease the use of salt, what we are really speaking of is reducing the sodium intake. If you look closely, you will see that most "salt substitutes" contain a substitute for sodium (usually potassium), so there is an X-chloride compound there. You still take in the same chloride content, but that's OK. It's the sodium that is the dickens. It is sodium's relationship to the body's volume status that helps relate sodium intake to blood pressure. An indirect measure (and not necessarily a great measure at that) of that volume is your blood pressure. In simple terms, increases in sodium increase your body fluid volume; that increases your blood pressure and thus reducing sodium would reduce your blood pressure. This would act to help people with high blood pressure, or hypertension. In fact, there is good medical evidence that lowering sodium intake does in fact lower blood pressure in both people with and without hypertension. Exercise seems to potentially protect from hypertension as a consequence of high salt intake.[2]

Unfortunately, not all of those with hypertension demonstrate sodium-sensitive hypertension. This means that only a fraction of those with high blood pressure will see it lower significantly with a reduction in sodium intake. In terms of sodium being a contributor to increased cardiovascular risks and mortality, there is not a clearly defined risk to specific populations (some studies show risk while others do not). The current thought is that sodium has an effect on the cardiovascular system that goes beyond simply looking at blood pressure and sodium's potential detrimental effects.

This is important as the per-capita use of salt in the United States has increased by approximately 55 percent from the mid-1980s to the late 1990s. In a parallel process, studies have shown that levels of potassium, magnesium, and calcium are lower than desired. This likely reflects the increased consumption of processed foods over their unprocessed natural counterparts. The daily recommended intake of salt is less than 2,300 mg (recently lowered from 3,000 mg), or only about 1 teaspoon. Some recommendations are to lower this to less than 1,500 mg.

Research has looked at the sources of sodium in the U.S. diet. Roughly 77 percent of sodium intake is from *processed and prepared foods*. Only about 5 percent comes from what is added to construct a tasty, well-seasoned meal during preparation. In addition, if your meal is well seasoned as it is prepared, it should not require any additional tabletop salt application. This reduces another 6 percent (6 percent of the total salt intake is added at the table during eating). The remaining 12 percent is found to occur naturally.[3] The take-home message here: 83 percent of all sodium intake can be accounted for by adding salt at the table and consuming prepared and processed food.

The key is to cook more fresh food and reduce the consumption of processed foods, which includes high-sodium prepared condiments, many salad dressings, prepared meats/meals, and things like energy drinks and sodas. Oh, did I mention not eating processed and prepared crap? A stealth offender among the prepared and processed garbage is mass-produced bread. A slice of bread, which not only ranks high on the sodium list (95–210 mg) for content, also contains about 15 g (about 3 tsp) of sugar. Increases in consumption of foodstuffs heavy in refined white sugar, among other items, have been correlated with increases in metabolic syndrome, obesity, and diabetes. However, there are few studies that look at the benefits of reducing refined sugar intake; this type of study lends more evidence to a cause-and-effect relationship than simply a correlative one. A study published in *Circulation* looked at the effect of reducing the consumption of sugar-filled soft drinks on blood pressure in persons with hypertension.[4] The study looked at 810 men and women aged twenty-five to seventy with hypertension. They underwent a lifestyle modification by decreasing their sugar-filled soft drinks by one drink (12 oz.) per day over eighteen months. The study found that after additional adjustment for weight change over the same period, a reduction in the sugar-sweetened beverages was still significantly associated with reductions in blood pressure readings. Consumption amounts of caffeinated or diet beverages did not have any effect. Another study published in the *Journal of the American Society of Nephrology* done at the University of Colorado at Denver investigated "whether increased fructose intake from added sugars associates with an increased risk for higher BP levels in U.S. adults without a history of hypertension."[5] The study looked at some data for over 4,500 U.S. adults previously collected for a study called the NHANES (National Health and Nutrition Examination Survey) for the period of 2003 to 2006. What they found was that "those who ate and drank more fructose from added sugars (as opposed to healthy sources like fresh fruit) had higher blood pressure than those who didn't."[6] This type of study is again a correlative study, not one of cause and effect, but Dr. M. Chonchol, the senior author, reports that the data is consistent with other studies. The exact mechanism for the possible cause remains unknown, but hypotheses include involvement of the nervous system, gastrointestinal system, and vascular system, and the production of uric acid. A consumption of greater than 74 g per day resulted in a 77 percent higher risk for a blood pressure greater than or equal to 160/100 mmHg.[7] These findings suggest that sugars may contribute to the observed association between hypertension and the consumption of sugar-sweetened beverages. In general, it seems prudent to avoid consuming mass quantities of anything containing refined, white, powdery substances.

But can we really? Sugar served an important evolutionary purpose. Imagine you are wandering the plains of the African savannah. You espy some fruit ripening on the tree. Being the lazy sort, you munch on the easy-to-retrieve, low-hanging fruit. You enjoy a delicious snack. To your dismay, Smiley, the resident sabertooth of the plains, has decided that fruit-stuffed *Homo erectus* is exactly what the kitty ordered for dinner. But the fruit you just ate gives you quick energy; up the tree and off to safety you go. Eating things with naturally occurring sugars readily and easily utilized by the body is a good survival practice. Hardwiring a behavior such as seeking sugar requires tapping into the pleasure center. Among the five senses, only taste has an all-season, all-access pass into our pleasure dome.[8] Remember: We naturally seek happiness, so when the little red pleasure light goes off in our brain and we feel good, we are inclined to repeat whatever experience brings us that pleasurable feeling. Sugar taps into the same circuitry involved in the brain's pleasure response to opioid narcotics like morphine and heroin. And it need not be sugar; artificial sweeteners stimulate those same sweet spots in the brain.[9]

While the white refined variety of sugar taps into our sugar-sensitive pleasure palace, it does not behave metabolically like the simple sugars (glucose and smaller amounts of fructose) found in fruits. Highly refined white sugar is not glucose. It is sucrose (also known as saccharose) and contains both glucose and fructose. While providing a rapid rise in blood glucose levels, metabolism of sucrose is more complicated than that of isolated glucose.

Excess sugar is transformed by the body into fat for storage and later use. From an energy perspective, fat is the biological equivalent of jet fuel. It provides more energy (9 kcal/gm) than any other available food. Thinking like a Stone Age hunter-gatherer unsure when your next meal might be (and the fact you may be something else's meal if not vigilant), consuming fat would be a good survival strategy. In addition, you would want to be able to pack in as much quantity as quickly as possible. Once you made a kill or came across some edible protein and fat, it is only a short amount of time before Smiley and friends show up for their cut. You can see the same event play out today after a leopard makes a kill; shortly thereafter come the hyenas and lions. Life on the savannah has not changed drastically in 100,000 years; only the names have changed. Thus, the built-in delay of twenty to thirty minutes from the time you start to eat until your brain signals satiety served another valuable evolutionary function, allowing you to gorge like the lions at the feast and pack away as much meat and fat in as short a time as possible. Unfortunately, we are packing in more fat than ever. Over the last several decades, consumption of fats has increased more than 60 percent, from more than fifty pounds to more than eighty-five pounds.[10]

Harvard psychologist Deirdre Barrett sums up our evolutionary-derived modern-day vulnerabilities. She describes how from a physiological perspective we are almost identical to our Stone Age ancestors. She observes how we are built to be omnivorous hunter-gatherers and how we are programmed to seek out sugar, fat, and salt because, at the time we were learning to become upright, these things aided our survival as a species.[11] Our bodies have evolved at a much slower pace than our society. At one time these mechanisms helped us survive. Now they are like an exposed security breach in Microsoft Windows, and we are being infected and hacked.

There are forces in the food industry that take advantage of these evolutionary backdoors. Just watch some TV and notice the volume of food-related commercials. See how many billboards by the side of the road have to do with food. We are constantly being cued and conditioned. Although our bodies are equipped with a homeostatic mechanism, this system is being overwhelmed by the manipulation of our evolutionary reward system.[12] This manipulation of our inherent survival mechanisms and senses serves to stimulate our desire for foods with salt, sugar, and fat.

In fact, it is the combinations of salt, sugar and fat that are so very addicting. One fast food chain glazed some chicken in extra butter to enhance optimal sweetness and achieve a "halo effect," making the food not just palatable but also addictive.[13] There are optimal levels of salt, sugar, and fat in certain foods, which is in some part determined by the food and expectation. We want salty potato chips, not a salty donut. So the optimum salt, sugar, and fat level is different for a potato crisp than it is for a donut. There are likewise optimal levels for the combination of salt, sugar, and fat for each type of food product.

As David Kessler notes in his book *The End of Overeating*, which examines this aspect of the food industry, the insiders responsible for hooking us turn to the "three points of the compass. Sugar, fat and salt make a food compelling. . . . They make it indulgent. They make it high in hedonistic value, which gives us pleasure."[14] Food for mass consumption is layered with salt, sugar, and fat that are layered with more salt, sugar, and fat and so on. The layers are constructed to provide maximal pleasure not only in the form of flavors but also in the form of textures as well. That pleasurable "mouth-feel" or "savoriness" is often referred to as the fifth taste, or umami. The physiological exploitation aims to involve all our senses, to seduce us with looks, sights, textures, sounds, and smells, as well as taste.

At a very basic level, the desire for salt, sugar, and fat will encourage animals to perform work to receive the triad of salt, sugar, and fat even if the animals are not hungry. The name for this hedonistic hardwiring is orosensory self-stimulation,[15] which, although it sounds like something done in certain parts of Amsterdam, is just an extraordinarily compelling impulse. In addition, the location of where these foods are available can become as potent a cue for the animals as the food itself.[16] We are vulnerable in the same way.

The combination of salt, sugar, and fat is potentially a gastronomic axis of evil. The effect of the combination of these three items is to literally hit that same direct-connect sweet spot of the pleasure response in the brain. The stimulation of the pleasure center links not only the location but also the entire eating experience with reinforcing emotional content. Here the biochemical manipulation becomes supercharged by associated emotional content. The endorphins (the natural opioid-like substances produced by our bodies) released when our pleasure center is tickled act just like exogenous opiates. They reduce feelings of stress, pain, and suffering. And the more supercharged the food, the greater the attention paid to it and the more vigorously we will pursue it.[17] The experience of eating is colored by emotion. After a fashion we can be manipulated not just by the actual process of eating the food but also by the very anticipation of the experience. We respond like Pavlov's dogs. Had a pleasurable dining encounter at Hoo Hoos? The commercial you just saw gets you salivating at the prospect of a return visit, and it's not just the Hoo Hoos.

In fact, when the experience is packaged in the right way, seasoned with novelty and administered as an intermittent reward, it resists habituation. Habituation is what can cause people to cheat on their spouse. They become less aroused to the same occurrence in the same routine. Their brain secretes less dopamine in response to the same stimulus that had them searching for the magic blue pill not so long ago. It is the same reason most diets fail because food choices are restricted and we quickly habituate to them. That, and most diet food sucks. But if the axis is packaged correctly, it behaves more like crack (which resists habituation) than coffee.

This should not be confused with the development of habits. Habits are routines of behavior that are repeated regularly and tend to occur subconsciously without one being conscious about them.[18] Consequently, the reason you are inundated by messages to buy certain foods or eat at certain places is to make that action a habit. Because with repeated exposure the experience will not habituate, if performing that action can be turned into a habit, you will likely continue that action again and again. Once a habit or pattern is formed, it is difficult to disengage and very resistant to change. It is the reason you stop for that muffin in the morning before you even realize you've driven there.

So how do we change? How do we break this vicious feedback loop? Patients, after receiving a stent or some other cardiovascular intervention, often comment to me when we discuss diet approaches about having to "acquire" a taste for healthy food. These folks are often the victims of the aforementioned food-industry, Pavlovian exploitation. What they really mean to say is that they have had to reacquire their sense of taste. Their sense of taste has become distorted. Through abuse it has become replaced by a desire for ever-increasing layers of salt, sugar, and fat. They have transmuted from sipping wine with the approach of a sommelier to guzzling antifreeze like a homeless wino. Commentary on "American" food or style of preparation from other cultures around the world echoes this sentiment. We disregard technique, spice, flavors, and textures in favor of ever-increasing layers of salt, sugar, and fat. We must recapture the palate of our innocence. We must learn to experience taste anew.

We need real food—real, good-tasting food. We need to get beyond this pathetic mass-produced, highly processed, self-addicting gruel we are being programmed to consume. We need to be the master of our own taste domain. Like the amazing Spiderman says, with great taste, comes great responsibility. OK, he didn't really say that, but he would have if Peter Parker was a chef and not a photographer. And if he were a chef, he'd be a Grassroots Gourmet.

diet or die

a word on obesity and weight loss

"Let food be thy medicine and thy medicine be thy food."

—HIPPOCRATES (460–337 B.C.)

MY **WARNINGS** often go unheeded. Go figure! Sometimes I feel like Rodney Dangerfield: No matter what I say, "I don't get no respect." As an interventional cardiologist, this often comes with the territory, as does trying to convince my patients they can enjoy the foods they love—just not as often as they might like. They—and let's face it, most of us, physicians included—just don't want to accept that we can't have that endless diet of cheese-slathered monster burger, five-egg omelet, and terrine of foie gras that is paraded before us 24/7 in the media.

Case in point: Though I had warned one of my patients about the dangers of his high-salt, too-much-saturated-fat diet, lack of physical activity, and heavy smoking, it didn't change his habits. The result: I had to put a number of coronary stents in his heart after he suffered a heart attack. Fortunately, we had intervened early, and he had suffered essentially minimal heart muscle damage. But the message was crystal clear: At forty years old, he had to change the way he lived. My whole team had worked hard to educate him. He was receptive to our strong recommendations to stop smoking, become less sedentary, and modify his eating habits to include more food that came out of the ground and less out of a takeout container. I really thought he would make these changes, at least in part. He was dedicated to getting healthy for his young children and had his wife's complete support. But three months later, I knew he hadn't changed anything. No weight loss, no change in cholesterol. But still he protested that he was exercising and had quit smoking. He said he only ate the vegetables his wife fixed, with some occasional fish on the side. Clearly, something was amiss.

Being a cardiologist is sometimes akin to being in an episode of *CSI*. When it comes to patients saying they have changed their dietary and exercise habits, nothing is as it seems. Actually, it's sometimes more like an episode of *Lie to Me*. So while my patient was getting a routine electrocardiogram, I cornered his wife. I needed to find the truth of what was going on: a conspiracy (I would break them down until I got to the truth about what they really ate) or maybe clandestine nighttime indiscretions at the local burger joint.

"He quit smoking, he works hard, and he exercises," his wife protested. "And I mostly fix him vegetables. Why is nothing working? We'll do whatever we need to, but I don't know what else to do." Not quite understanding myself how this could be, I asked how she prepared the vegetables. "Well, I'll make something like bacon or fried catfish for me and the kids. Then I cook something like green beans and maybe some tomatoes if we have them for his dinner. If there's not enough of it left in the pan, then I spoon in some that I keep by the stove. Then I serve that with some white rolls or cornbread. Maybe some fish now and again, too."

"What is it you spoon out?" I asked, already knowing the answer. "What do you keep by the stove to cook the vegetables in?"

"Why, lard and bacon drippings. The vegetables aren't any good without it, and he won't eat them any other way." This was the South, after all.

Mystery solved. And now the coup de grâce: "With deep-fried catfish?"

"Of course," she replied.

I carefully explained why cooking in bacon grease and lard was counter to everything we were trying to achieve, how we needed to change what they had been doing. "We've done everything you asked, doctor. But I can't make him eat like that. It's just not right, and he's not going to do it. It just doesn't taste good that way."

It just doesn't taste good that way.

This is really the dilemma everyone faces. You want to engage in a healthier culinary lifestyle, but you want to be able to enjoy things that taste good. All the things that seem to taste good seem to be the same ones on the governmental "no-touch" list. You may be a patient and need a change in diet because of a disease or condition you have developed. You may be at risk for developing a disease or condition and were told to or want to initiate some preventive practices. You may be the relative or spouse of someone who fits the above descriptions. You may be a foodie who loves to dine on gourmet food but realizes you can't have a chef's tasting menu every night. That death-row meal exists precisely because, in that setting, tomorrow is irrelevant. On the surface it seems as if we are stuck with two mutually exclusive options: Eat what you want and die, or eat what you should and live a life of gustatory monasticism. It is this apparent contradiction that sends us into endless mental mastication. It seems an unsolvable paradox, a timeless koan. But it is not, really. We have been hooked into craving salt, sugar, and fat and equating that with good taste. We have become complacent and allowed an industry to process, cook, and prepare our meals for us. Our nutritional needs are met (or not) by what we consume. Food is both the fuel that keeps us running and supplies the raw materials of our internal infrastructure. Most people do not realize the reality of our internal turnover. Our bodies are constantly replacing the very pieces, even atoms, of that which constitutes us. For example, an average person will produce about 200 billion red blood cells (RBCs) each day. There is complete turnover of that inventory about every 120 days. The skin is replaced in one to three months and bone broken down and replaced about every ninety days. The materials for that constant construction come from recycling some of the parts and from utilizing raw materials that we ingest to construct new parts. If the bulk of what we consume is sugar, salt, and fat, is it any surprise we've become fat, hypertensive diabetics? And contrary to popular myth, these people are not generally jolly.

I think the medical response, of which I am a part, on the whole has not really done a good job. I think a large part of that is a reflection of the current medical system. The system is constructed to address acute illness in a diagnose-treat-discharge fashion. The payment of medical services is based primarily on quantities of documentable procedures. There is not a lot of money put forth to prevent something that someone might get sometime down the road somewhere. Thus, less effort is put forth in the area of prevention. Although there are breezes of change, this is the unfortunate reality for the foreseeable future. The resultant response from the medical community has resembled an issuing of the Ten Medical Commandments: We are your Lords of Health;

1. You shall have no other health-care practitioners before us (especially chiropractors and New-Agey folks).
2. You shall not make for yourself an idle; in other words, exercise—no excuses, and we don't care if you need a knee replacement.
3. You shall not make wrongful use of your prescriptions, or at least you shall remember the names when you show up because we don't all have electronic medical records yet.

4. Remember the appointment day and keep it holy and totally free because sometimes we run really behind.
5. Honor your copay.
6. You shall not deep fry.
7. You shall not commit unapproved snackery.
8. You shall not smoke.
9. You shall not bear false witness if you smoke because I can see the nicotine stains on your fingers and smell the cigarettes.
10. You shall not covet Little Debbie, nor shall you not covet anything that looks like Little Debbie.

These strict guidelines are backed up by studies, data, graphs, charts, slides, and expert consensus recommendations from the governmental and scientific houses of the holy. They make for a strong, logical argument. They don't make anything taste better. The problem seems to be that we're asking people to sprint a fifty-yard dash when the race is really a marathon. After fifty yards they slow down or stop. Then they get pissed on when they can't finish the last 45,710 yards.

A word here about diets for weight loss: As I have mentioned, if a person is overweight and needs to shed some pounds, then fine. If you need to undergo some restrictive regimen to get you to the weight you want or need, by all means pursue that goal. If you need one of those programs that sells you meals and all you can eat is what is on their order list to lose some pounds, again fine. I just don't think you need to eat that stuff forever. I call it *stuff* because I guess it's sustenance, but I would not classify it as food. I don't know anyone who has tried it and really finds it delicious and satisfying. I've tried that stuff, and I think it tastes really crappy. The microwave pizza meal caught on fire. What the hell do you construct a pizza out of so that it bursts into flame in the freaking microwave? It should be dough, sauce, and cheese. This resembled something more like evidence from an X-files case than something to eat. If you need to call Jenny, again that's fine, but just realize that doing so does not commit you to a lifetime relationship. The aforementioned aside, the longer-term problem is that they try to snare you into a lifetime program. It's like Hotel California. You can check in, but you can't check out.

This is not a weight-loss program. However, I do believe that, if you consume a typical American or Western diet and follow the principles outlined here, you will most certainly shed some pounds. Add a little bit of exercise, and you'll shed more. Especially if you've been consuming a lot of highly processed, pre-prepared foodstuffs, both your waistline and your well-being will benefit. This program is here for you when you want to get off the weight loss–weight gain funhouse crazy train. I believe that most diets fail not because people can't or won't follow them but because, when people achieve their desired weight loss, there is no sensible program to shift to that rewards their hard work and sacrifices and allows them to enjoy eating. They are thrown back into bouncing from the extreme they just encountered (deprivation) to the other side of the road (excess). That, I believe, is why according to some studies up to 95 percent of weight-loss diets fail over the long term, usually measured at about five years.[1] A weight loss program should be a short-term sprint to some goal, not a lifetime journey. As a physician, as an interventional cardiologist, I understand the health aspects of diet and the need for weight control. As a chef and a foodie, I want to enjoy my eats.

Health hazards of obesity have been recognized for centuries, appearing, for example, in writings attributed to Hippocrates.[2] In the simplest terms, weight gain is primarily due to overeating. At the end of the day, it is calories in the pie hole versus calories expended. People and children who eat more weigh more. While exercise is important for a number of reasons, physical activity alone does not predict weight gain. Correspondingly, many obese people actually burn more calories and have a higher basal metabolism than those who are not obese.[3] Despite the appeal of attempting to reduce the equation to simple calories in versus calories out, how we arrive at a certain weight and why we trend toward maintaining a higher weight is not as straightforward as it seems. Once gained, excess weight is difficult to manage. It is well accepted that long-term maintenance of successful weight loss achieved by behavioral and/or pharmacological means is generally relatively modest and difficult to maintain. This is true even though people are aware of data that clearly show the benefits of weight loss for control of cardiovascular risk factors.[4] Kessler promotes the settling point theory of weight, suggesting that the weight at which we "settle" is the balance point between both the motivation to seek food and the availability of food versus expenditure.[5] This discussion surrounding the issue of the expanding American waistline is a weighty one. One need only pick up a paper or magazine or turn on the news to see reports on obesity and the overweight condition. By the latest statistics, 67 percent of Americans are either overweight or obese. The condition is similarly present in many other industrialized countries around the globe.

But where exactly do these statistics derive? What measure finds two out of every three Americans outside the desired norm? We currently use the body mass index, or BMI. It is what is currently used to define normal, overweight, and obese individuals. This is a measure the government will be requiring all health-care providers to report on every electronic medical record (EMR or EHR) by 2014. The BMI is not new; in fact it dates back to 1832. At that time a celebrated Belgian mathematician, astronomer, statistician, and sociologist named Lambert Adolphe Jacques Quetelet came up with the Quetelet Index of Obesity. This index measured obesity by dividing a person's weight (in kilograms) by the square of his or her height (in meters). Quetelet worked with life insurance companies and wrote a book that detailed his research on height and weight for men at different ages. His original research focused on data collected on several hundred of his male countrymen. He found that weight varied in proportion to the square of height (people 10 percent taller than average tended to be about 20 percent heavier). In 1972, Professor Ancel Keys published a landmark study of more than 7,400 men in five countries. Keys examined which of the five various height-weight formulas examined correlated best with each subject's body-fat percentage as measured more directly. The result was that the best predictor was the Quetelet Index of Obesity. Keys renamed this measure the body mass index. The BMI became an international standard for obesity measurement in the 1980s. In 1998, the National Institutes of Health lowered the overweight threshold for BMI from 27.8 to 25 to match international guidelines.

As a measure of fat, the BMI is an indirect measure, although at some level an increasing BMI is always associated with increasing health risk, but the BMI at which this occurs varies across studies and populations.[6] The BMI is indirect because it measures the total body mass, both lean (like muscle) and fat. Thus someone who is extremely fit, like Sly Stallone in the *Rambo* movies, Arnold Schwarzenegger in the *Terminator* movies, or any number of professional athletes, can be "obese" by the BMI measure because they contain a lot of muscle. Because of this there is an ongoing debate about the accuracy of the BMI. The relationship between BMI in the overweight range and total mortality risk is controversial. There is evidence of an adverse relationship in some studies but not in others.

Is the BMI an inaccurate or outmoded measure? How well does just BMI correlate with risk? Are there more accurate measures we should use? Should we be looking at fat distribution and body polymorphisms? Further complexity is added by the fact that the association of an overweight state with mortality may vary according to such variables as sex, ethnicity, age, and body fat distribution.[7]

Even direct measures of fat, like skinfold thickness and hydrostatic testing, often do not address the distribution of body fat, which makes a big difference when it comes to health risks. Visceral fat distribution, or fat around the waist (also known as visceral adipose tissue, or VAT), has been more closely correlated with health risks than BMI. A study published in 2010 in an issue of *Archives of Internal Medicine* examined over 100,000 men and women over the age of fifty and followed them for ten years.[8] The study demonstrated that the waist circumference was a predictor of death, regardless of the BMI. For men the risk increased with a circumference greater than 120 cm (compared to less than 90 cm), and for women that number was greater than 110 cm (versus less than 75 cm). Other factors beyond just consumption can affect abdominal fat deposition. Hormones, stress, and certain medications are known to increase abdominal fat deposits. One of the earliest signs of dysfunction of the circulatory system is the impaired ability of blood vessels to dilate. A study from the *Journal of the American College of Cardiology* noted that people who gained "even a little weight around their middle hinder the function of cells that line their blood vessels, increasing the risk for high blood pressure and other problems."[9] Centers for Disease Control and Prevention director Dr. Thomas Frieden has said, "Over the past several decades, obesity has increased faster than anyone could have imagined it would," and should the trend persist, "more people will get sick and die from the complications of obesity, such as heart disease, stroke, diabetes and cancer."[10]

While we refine our measures, the variables involved in the calories in–calories out equation are simply not quite as straightforward as the hawkers of quick-fix, miracle–weight-loss programs would have you believe. Such things as a lack of sleep, from whatever cause, may contribute more to obesity than what and how much we eat. The hypothesis is that there are several key hormones involved. The sleep cycle appears to impact weight via the hormonal system. Among the important compounds, the hormones leptin and ghrelin appear to play prominent roles. Both these hormones affect appetite; ghrelin, which is produced in the gastrointestinal tract, appears to stimulate appetite. Leptin is produced by fat cells and seems to signal satiety in the brain. When you don't get enough proper sleep, leptin levels fall, and ghrelin levels rise. In a study looking at people who were sleep deprived, their desire for high-density, carbohydrate-rich food increased by 45 percent. Interestingly, despite eating more, they felt less full.[11] However, even this relationship is not as simple as it seems. Individual responses to these hormones are quite variable. These variable responses to hormone levels may represent some degree of intrinsic or acquired resistance. Other factors, such as environment, dietary habits, exercise patterns, personal stress levels, and particularly our genetics, may all influence the production of leptin and ghrelin, as well as our response to them.

I find this particularly fascinating from an anecdotal point of view. I see some very obese patients with a fat distribution one would expect from simple overconsumption; they are fat everywhere. Very often they do not have significant cardiovascular problems. They often have joint problems, are short of breath with limited endurance, but otherwise remarkably well except for those at the very extremes of obesity. Then there are patients whom I see who are slightly overweight or borderline obese. Their fat distribution mimics what we see with steroid-induced weight gain. That is, they have a central type of obesity. Their bellies are fat with the dangerous visceral type of fat accumulation around the middle, but there is not an equal distribution of fat in the extremities. They often have diabetes and cardiovascular problems. Therefore, although the quantity and quality of what we consume matters tremendously, we see other important variables in the obesity equation, such as:

- What is added, or not, to what you eat
- How much you eat over how much time
- How the food is prepared
- How (over-) processed the food is
- Amount of exercise or physical activity
- Quantity of sleep
- Quality of sleep
- Hormones
- Medications
- Stress
- Genetics

Even our prenatal environment has also been potentially implicated. A study in *Lancet* suggests that women who gain excessive weight (more than fifty pounds) during pregnancy are more likely to have high–birth-weight babies. High–birth-weight babies are more likely to develop obesity during later life. More than 1 million babies from more than 500,000 women from Boston and New York City were followed. Babies over 8.5 pounds were considered heavy. Women who gained more than fifty pounds had twice as high a risk of developing heavy–birth-weight babies.[12]

Because physical inactivity and excess weight have been independently associated with mortality in several studies, there are additional advantages to overweight and obese persons adopting an active lifestyle as well as healthy eating habits. So in order to avoid Dunlop's disease (where your belly Dunlop over your pants), both healthful eating and physical activity have roles. Managing weight and reducing cardiovascular risk should be encouraged in all. In the long term, because weight gain is progressive and weight loss is difficult to maintain, it is vitally important to start early.

I am all for a more-healthful population, but simply focusing the discussion on BMI in this range or that range and looking only at total mortality may miss broader implications.[13] We must strive for individual wellness, not government-mandated numbers. Wellness (which includes good physical health) should be each individual's goal. It must be individually nurtured, not uniformly impressed. Wellness requires choice and participation by election. To try to achieve some "ideal" without any respect for the individual situation, while perhaps expedient, is ultimately poorly conceived. When I was an attending physician at the teaching hospitals and universities, I always taught to treat the patient, not some lab result. I cannot tell you the number of times interns, residents, and fellows went off to initiate some procedure based solely on some arbitrary lab value. When we stepped back, treated the patient, and repeated the measurement, we often found the first lab value was in error.

When we look with that slightly broader perspective, we see things like our external environment and our own emotional state come into play. Factors like where you live affect how you live (and die). For example, the American Heart Association reviewed data regarding heart disease and air pollution in 2010. They reached the conclusion that there appears to be a correlation regarding worsening air quality and the rate of heart attacks. They also mentioned correlative evidence to link poor air quality with "heart failure, stroke, irregular heartbeats, cardiac arrest and vascular diseases."[14] Perhaps most worrisome was a "'small yet consistent' link between short-term exposure to high pollution levels and death."[15]

Emotions can also affect our physical well-being in untoward and unexpected ways. A study out of New Zealand suggested that those having a stressful, troubled childhood may be more prone to health problems as adults, including heart health. One of the researchers suggested that adolescents may be "more vulnerable to cardiovascular risks if they are exposed to various stressors because of their hormonal changes and their sensitivity to peer rejection, acceptance and how they interpret others' attitudes towards themselves."[16]

Thus we must consider these additional factors when we engage in our pursuit of happiness. We must expand our goal to achieve wellness as opposed to simply attaining an arbitrary weight. We must understand that a weight-loss program, if needed, is a stop on the way—not the whole journey. We must understand that, although calories consumed are very important, weight and weight-associated health risks are a very complex equation. We must understand that, in striving for wellness, the equation is exponentially more complex than simply attaining a mandated weight on some chart. And attitude counts. So have a plan, and as I was told in my martial arts training, "Keep going." The measure is not in if you fall down, because you will, but how you get back up. Once you have achieved weight loss, you should be able to construct a sustainable program that doesn't require special meals, gimmicks, or anything that is emptying your wallet on a regular basis; that's what ex-spouses and taxes are for. The question becomes, Can you have a regimen that supplies you with what you need to maintain a healthy existence and also supply you with what you need to be happy existing? The answer is yes. You don't have to diet or die. What you have to do first is become a Grassroots Gourmet.

the grassroots gourmet

THE GRASSROOTS GOURMET is a modern construct derived from my experience as a physician (interventional cardiologist), chef (and foodie), and martial artist. Although contemporary in conception, it is more of a "rediscovery" than a twenty-first-century invention. It has been built upon ancient roots, roots that run deeply in philosophy, gastronomic application, and medicine. It is a premise with medical origins that reaches back to at least the time of Hippocrates. Hippocrates of Cos (circa 460–370 B.C.) lived during the classical period of ancient Athens and is known as the father of Western medicine. He is credited with originating a systematic approach to clinical medicine and perhaps most famously for the Hippocratic oath. Most people recall this as the famous "first do no harm" recitation, but actually that is not even in the original oath. The original text reads, "I will prescribe regimens for the good of my patients according to my ability and my judgment and never do harm to anyone."[1] The classic version includes this twist on that famous phrase "I will apply dietic measures for the benefit of the sick according to my ability and judgment; I will keep them from harm and injustice."[2] Perhaps this is an integration or a reference to another quote of Hippocrates reflecting a forgotten tenant in the practice of modern medicine: "Let food be thy medicine and medicine be thy food."[3] In today's modern version of the Hippocratic oath, this important principle has been reduced the generic allusion, "I will prevent disease whenever I can, for prevention is preferable to cure."[4] Yet even that is something modern medicine does not actually do very well at all beyond inoculation and vaccination. The tendency of modern Western medicine is to isolate and fix the critical issue of the moment, often at the expense of a more integrative approach.

As an interventional cardiologist who has practiced in environs ranging from a faculty position at teaching universities to solo private practice, I have seen this isolate-and-fix approach pervade all levels of our current health-care–delivery system. As a provider of care within the U.S. health-care system, I am proud of our service to patients in the United States and what we have accomplished to date. I believe it is one of the finest, if not the finest, health-care systems in the world. In the course of my studies while completing my health-care–focused executive M.B.A. degree, we extensively studied health-care systems from around the industrialized world. Here is the result of that analysis in a nutshell. There is no perfect system; each has benefits and drawbacks. Our current system's ability to focus deeply, isolate, and address critical needs is second to none. Our system is effective in this type of operation because that is the way it has been constructed and the way it has evolved. It is a system of triage, built upon reacting to a crisis and dealing with a critical or life-threatening situation and remedying that particular situation. Think of battlefield medicine, and you get the idea. If you break a leg, we are good at fixing it. If you are having a heart attack, I can open that artery and place a stent. We are not as good at treating chronic conditions and preventing certain types of illness. The effects, consequences, and repercussions of events that occur slowly over longer periods of time, including the end products of our consumption, are less well understood and less well addressed. The number of variables interacting in the chronic disease process increases over time. The intensity of the variables themselves fluctuates. Thus this result is not surprising. The very technology that has enabled us to make these huge strides in successfully treating acute situations has also acted to remove us from our more holistic healing roots. In focusing deeply but narrowly, we lose the broader but shallower viewpoint.

Having studied martial arts for more than thirty years, I have long been acquainted with the concept of such a duality. The notion of these broader perspectives is often found within more traditional Eastern approaches. Where the Western approach can give you the genus, species, and health of the individual tree, the Eastern approach tells you of the state of the forest. Indeed, there are places in the Orient even today where your health is treated not necessarily by a pill, poultice, or potion but by a delicious meal crafted by highly trained chefs based on a food prescription written by a doctor of oriental medicine. Thus do the origins of healing, whether Eastern or Western, from the Yellow Emperor to Hippocrates, seem to spring from the common campfire of what it is we consume. For whether by Eastern or Western approach, as Jean Anthelme Brillat-Savarin said, "Tell me what you eat, and I will tell you what you are."[5] But that is only half the story.

As a chef I know that the food has to taste good. If it does not taste good, if it consumed without pleasure and only for perceived health benefit, then it is not what I call food. That is my definition of medicine. An ascetic approach to eating does not lead us to culinary nirvana. There is no salvation through deprivation. It is a Faustian ruse. Achieving culinary nirvana without having to buy in or sell out is the goal of the Grassroots Gourmet. It is the place he or she strives to reach, for it is there that you achieve epicurean enlightenment; it is there you get to have your cake and eat it, too—just not all at once.

The Grassroots Gourmet seeks this enlightenment in the sacred space of the kitchen. Being a Grassroots Gourmet means eating well by eating real food that is good for your body. But most importantly, it means eating food that tastes good because that is what nourishes your soul. You don't need anyone telling you what you need to eat. Acquiring the ability to taste is also simply the process of rediscovery, of reclaiming that which had been lost due to the abuse/addiction at the hands of those doling out fast food, junk food, and adulterated food as I previously mentioned. I recall a conversation in which someone who had suffered detrimental health effects from an excessive "junk food" diet discussed their current eating habits. They told me that, if they were confronted now with what they used to consume on a regular basis, it would make them nauseated. A similar phenomenon occurs quite frequently among those cigarette smokers we can actually get to quit. After successfully breaking the addiction, they often cannot stand to be anywhere near cigarette smoke. They did not "learn" or "acquire" the pleasure of air free from smoke and toxins; they remembered how pleasant it is to actually breathe. Therefore, what they do not like is not breathing. A fundamental tenet of medicine is that in most circumstances oxygen is a good thing, literally a breath of fresh air.

The act of eating is also a transformative process. It occurs in part as a result of the associations that are formed between the food, the act of consumption, and social and emotional experiences that surround the event. As we mature the memories of prior experiences scent the present. Our individual food preferences become shaped by our exposure to what we eat, where we eat it, and with whom we dine. We form our own individual perceptions and palates. While we all have our own appreciation of what exactly tastes good to us as individuals, much like we each have our own appreciation for music and art, we must avoid addiction. What is often peddled to us as fast food is truly junk food, and it has that moniker for a reason. A weakness for fat, sugar, and salt is hardwired into our craniums and has been for at least the last 50,000 years. Preying upon our primeval lust for fat, sugar, and salt, the junk food peddlers overwhelm our taste buds until they are so comfortably numbed we just crave our daily fix. It is the culinary equivalent of a crack addiction and robs us of our sense of taste; life becomes nothing more than obtaining that daily McMortem and pasty shake. That temptation is always at every meal, with every bite. Like a yo-yo we seem to bounce between extremes; so often we never seem to find the balance.

Nature is about balance; the "Tathagatha [Buddha] avoids the two extremes, and talks about the Middle Path."[6] The method to achieve the harmony between the yin of taste and pleasure and the yang of sustenance and healthful is the threefold path. It is the path of the Grassroots Gourmet. It is the Threefold Path of the "Bes":

1. Be aware and avoid the call of the junk food/fast food siren.
2. Be fresh—but no adultery.
3. Be on time and in proportion.

It's so simple, but that doesn't mean it's easy. In fact it can be quite difficult at times. Perhaps some of our most difficult food decisions come about during or after an illness. Perhaps it is not even we but those close to us who are affected. Or perhaps you just want yourself and your loved ones to feel good not only about what you eat but also while and after you eat. Regardless the reason, we follow this path realizing that it is but a guidepost, not a definitive text nor a final commandment emblazoned in stone. We realize that all our current knowledge, tenets, beliefs, science, and recommendations must not contradict itself or our own direct evidence.

Or our own reason.

Or our own taste.

In the next few chapters, I take you through what it means to be a Grassroots Gourmet—how to have your cake and eat it, too, without sacrificing good health or great taste!

first

good escape make; avoiding the junk food siren and her weapons of mass consumption

"Tell me what you eat, and I shall tell you what you are."

—Jean Anthelme Brillat-Savarin

I WAS SPEAKING with another cardiologist recently over a cup of coffee about some medically related topics. Amid the smells of the lovely pastries wafting about the coffee shop, our conversation drifted. We began to discuss the current explosion of Dunlop's disease among our respective practice populations, indeed among the U.S. population in general. Now for those not in the medical field, Dunlop's disease is where the belly Dunlop over the pants. This has become a real health issue for a majority of Americans. While there may be some genetic component or some aspect attributable to our genes, clearly from an aesthetics point of view there is a real jean issue. Like a glance from the Gorgon sisters, prolonged viewing can be harmful to the viewer's health; however, it can be fatal to the viewee. Knowing that the masses are generally aware of the downsides of upsizing, why does Mr. Potatohead waddle away from the counter while trying to devour a cinnamon roll slightly larger than his entire cranium? Why do we behave like junkies?

One reason that we crave junk food is that, well, it is associated with pleasure. It can be part of a pleasurable experience, some of which is hardwired into the crevices of our brains as we have touched upon. David Kessler notes in his book *The End of Overeating* that sugar, salt, and fat make us crave more sugar, salt, and fat.[1] That may seem obvious, but think on it for a minute. The basic role of food is to provide our bodies with fuel to run efficiently and to provide the building blocks for us to maintain our own personal infrastructures. Because we are hardwired to seek out sugar, salt, and fat, these taste combinations are identified as pleasurable to reinforce the seeking behavior. If it is associated with happiness or pleasure, we will seek it out. In terms of pure day-to-day nutritional survival, good taste is really a bonus. It's because of this land of plenty that we have the opportunity to be persnickety about what we put into our pie holes. There are biological precedents for our current yearnings. As hunter-gatherers what sort of things helped us survive, as both individuals and as a species? In terms of fuel, it is the instinctual preference for fats. On a per-gram basis, fats supply more energy (at 9 kcal/gram) than carbohydrates or proteins (both at 4 kcal/gram). Only ethanol comes close to fats in terms of a preferred energy source (at 7 kcal/gram), but more on that later. Another survival advantage is the ability to convert extra calories into fat. This allows an individual to survive periods where food is less abundant. It is hypothesized that the ability of our ancestors to diverge from primarily vegetarian fare to a diet higher in protein (fish and meat), along with cooking our food, was a stimulus for the human species to improve our cranial prowess.

Salt is an essential nutrient. Animals instinctually seek out and consume salt. Any deer hunter will tell you about the success of salt licks in acquiring venison. It is an animal-brain-hardwired component. In addition to providing essential nutrients, the availability of salt allowed for the preservation of foods, such as meats and fish.

As for sweets, they've been hardwired into our brains for about 2 million years. The desire for things like ripe fruit and honey provided immediately usable forms of energy from carbohydrates.[2] The neural pathways in the brain involved in sweet attractions are the same as those involved in drug addiction. Kessler writes how the combination of sugar, salt, and fat affect not only our bodily composition but also our very brain centers as well. So things like sweets, fats, and salt do have a hardwired basis for our attraction to them. Morgan Spurlock noted in his *Supersize Me* movie that after a while he began to actually crave the fatty, salty fast food products he was eating when he hadn't craved them before. You ever wonder why the people eating at those fast food joints look like they always eat there? It's because they do. Salt, sugar, and fat are addicting.

Some food responses can trigger opioid production in the brain. Opioids are the class of compounds to which heroin and morphine belong. So our dietary habits are affected not only by a true nutritional need but also by a potentially captivating component that can be associated with sugar, salt, and fat. It should not be surprising that these responses are programmed. They may have not only helped the human species survive but also evolve. However, as with anything we are instinctually attracted to, in the right circumstances and with a little push, sometimes just a gentle breeze with a sweet, salty tinge, attraction can transform into addiction. And we are not led gently into that good bite; we are double dipped and deep fried. I have heard of and/or read about nearly every crazy diet fad, program, and "miracle pill" that is out there. The plethora of diets and programs and quick-cure pills represent a clear panic reaction, like the man who drowns in three inches of water.

One of the more interesting and valid ideas as to the cause of our concern is that way too much of what we consume is over-processed junk. When we look at these items, we find that most of what is offered consists of empty calories. A great example is a soda or "energy drink." These are often artificially flavored, sweetened with refined sugar or high fructose corn syrup (HFCS) and contain coloring agents as well. Some of these items are available in colors that do not seem to be found anywhere in the natural biosphere. Unlike the water they contain, which all alone can quench thirst, they also contain calories. These are calories with no nutritional value. When you drink these, you get calories but really nothing else. A breakfast muffin likely contains refined flour, artificial butter flavor, oil, sweeteners, and other artificial flavors. Your topping is a processed-cheese, food-like substance; powdered egg substitute; and processed, reformed meat-like patty. Not a whole lot of nutrition there. In the processing of food, many compounds are removed or destroyed. Many of these products are then fortified or enriched, which means some things like vitamins and minerals may be added back.

There are intangibles that nature put there that are altered and/or removed, and thus the Law of Unintended Consequences may apply. Along with Murphy's Law, I believe the other universal truism is the Law of Unintended Consequences. The universe is always in a cause-and-effect mode. The glass falls off the table and breaks. Cause then effect: The glass never jumps from the floor and reassembles itself on the table. The universe never operates in an effect-then-cause fashion. Whenever you alter something, no matter how slight, it has some consequence. Some consequences do not translate into any meaningful effects; homeostasis is maintained. Some cause major perturbations. But make no mistake, there is *some* effect. With our keen science, we do our best to foresee what those effects will be and appropriately address them. That is where the Law of Unintended Consequences comes in; there are things that occur to a system that anyone neither can foresee nor ever intended to happen.

For example, at one time fiber and its various forms, such as bran, were thought unimportant from a dietary perspective because they are not processed for nutrition and pass through the gastrointestinal tract. Now we recognize they are necessary for gastrointestinal health, nature's little colon sweepers. When I was in school, we were taught that the DNA sequences between genes, known as introns (intervening sequences), were unnecessary leftovers from evolution, an evolutionary genetic appendix. Now it turns out they are crucial to correctly process and express genes. Nature is nothing if not necessary and frugal. If our diet consists primarily of processed foods, we are missing out on nature's intangibles. The currently used industrial processes often result in food products that contain little fiber, few active enzymes or any enzymes at all, and reduced or missing nutrients. What they do contain is artificial flavorings, colorings, and preservatives. In the 1940s there was research done by a Dr. Pottenger. He studied nine hundred cats over several generations and divided them into five groups. The first two groups he fed raw food. They remained healthy. The remaining groups were fed processed foods. The cats that were only fed processed food developed degenerative health conditions like arthritis, allergies, diabetes, and so on. There are a number of caveats about this study, including reproducibility, the role of taurine in the feline diet, and other issues. The point is not that cooking and some processing is inherently evil but that it creates a situation of unintended consequences by potentially removing things we are unaware of or consider unimportant and turn out to be crucial. Cats are not people, but the general takeaway principal applies. In consuming a diet consisting primarily of the readily available junk food stuff, you get extra addictive goodies and may be missing out on some potentially necessary items. These are things we need. Hardwired into our brains is the knowledge and desire to seek out and consume what we need. Your body is still telling you it needs fuel.

Your body is trying to tell you what it *needs*, and as adult humans we have the incredible capacity to replace what we need with what we *desire*. And what we desire is made readily available. We are inundated with a message to consume these readily available substances. This is constantly pounded into us every day from every venue. Notice the amount of food ads, food shows, and cooking pieces on television, billboards, radio ads as you drive, and the volume of enticements in all the various forms of media we are exposed to daily. And there within the gamut of fruit hanging from this tree of knowledge lies the snake. It is misinformation; it is the shadow realm of the Information Age. It entices us with what we desire under the cloak of what we need. If it is "homemade style," that must mean it's good for us. Kessler describes how sugar, salt, and fat, this nonnutritious axis of evil, is made easily and cheaply available and how it is used to addict us. Like any good junkie, we listen to what we are being told we need/desire by those pushing the product. So we consume more of the items exported from the nonnutritious axis of evil: the sugar, salt, and fat. In short, it's culinary crack.

But wait, there's more. It is precisely because we do not have to eat only for sustenance alone that we're in the shape we are in. That's because food or meals or mealtime has other components beyond the mere nutritional components, percent saturated fat, and other things people pretend to read about before stashing their favorite treat in the bottom of the grocery cart. How we feel when we eat the food affects us as well. The link to what we eat is accompanied by secretions of not only opioids but also dopamine, which is associated with emotion and memory, and other neural transmitters. This starts to blur the distinction between craving and needing, of choice and addiction, of conscious thought and desire and instinctive reflex. I believe this is a crucial factor.

I have some observational data. I know it is not as good as the double-blind, randomized, placebo-controlled trials, but there are some things about the human animal that just don't fit into neat boxes or double-blind, randomized, placebo-controlled trials. Quitting tobacco, I believe, has some of the same challenges that people face in trying to change their dietary lifestyle. Some people enjoy the act and sensation of smoking. Smoking must be pleasurable for them. The fact that tobacco contains some addictive components like nicotine is a given. This is like the salt, sugar, and fat found in addictive fast food. If those smokers trying to quit are given chemicals to block the addictive nicotine or are weaned off their chemical dependency over several weeks, we should, in theory, get everyone to successfully quit smoking. That would be so if their pleasure was just derived from a chemical process. Yet, clearly that's not the case. People keep smoking. What I think keeps some of these folks puffing away is some emotional component. Whether stress relief, social reinforcement, or whatever, there is some emotional attachment. I think the same can be said of food cravings. The difference is that you don't have to smoke to live. You do have to eat.

Eating is a requirement for life, yet the biochemical processes associated with it and the emotional trappings surrounding the endeavor make it a heady brew indeed. Add to this mix the fact that our modern cornucopia has truly provided too much of a good thing. Like Internet porn or cheap little blue pills, the modern food industry has provided us with too much opportunity for what we desire. It's no longer eating a few bronto burgers to make it through the winter with your cavemates. It's the "new and improved" antibiotic and preservative-laden Barry Bonds steroid dog on a bun amped up for your pleasure and served up by Honest John and Gideon. Next thing you know, just like Pinocchio, you're working *for* Stromboli, except, for this rescue, Jiminy Cricket is going to need more than wishing upon a star. He's going to need Seal Team 6.

Like any good supplier, the food industry makes access easy by the sheer number of venues where the goodies can be acquired. It manipulates this craving by tempting people to consume more and more. It is not just that the food is "junk" food in composition;

it is also easy to acquire, readily available, and competitively priced. We are being told what we desire by those pushing the product, and the product is in our face everywhere 24/7. Add to the equation that people are being driven to consume not just by addiction and desire but also because they are trying to fulfill a real physiological need. That physiological need manifests as hunger, which ends up being misinterpreted and filled with more "junk" food. You end up craving more from the addiction, and your body is telling you to eat more, trying to get you to down the right stuff. So in the midst of mass consumption, people are starving.

Many of the items consumed are made from things like refined and processed flour or fortified milk, which have some minerals and vitamins added back. Therefore, the effects are not those of vitamin deprivation, like scurvy or pellagra, that one may see in a specific form of dietary insufficiency. As mentioned, these things are loaded with calories, so there is not a wasting phenomenon as would be seen in overall caloric insufficiency. In fact, because of the caloric intake and the dual drive to consume driven by a dependence upon the nonnutritious axis of evil and a misinterpreted physiological need, we end up with excess calories. Trends like this are seen in reports that show while sodium intake is rising, levels of potassium, phosphorus, and other essential vitamins and minerals are declining. This is felt to be secondary to the ever-increasing consumption of these highly refined and processed foods.[3] We end up "starving" in the midst of excess. We are seeing what one would expect: increasing obesity and problems like diabetes, heart disease, chronic fatigue, fibromyalgia and many others.

An article in the *New York Times Magazine* highlights where this road ends.[4] In the article it ends in places like Huntington, West Virginia. An Associated Press article based on a 2006 Centers for Disease Control report proclaimed that the five-county Huntington metropolitan area was the country's fattest and unhealthiest. The *New York Times Magazine* article chronicles the travails of Jamie Oliver, celebrity chef from across the pond, as he travels to Huntington. Now I have never met nor even eaten at any of Jamie's establishments, however I have enjoyed his televisions shows and found his recipes easy to use and tasty. He seems genuinely committed to his cause regarding promoting healthier eating habits—particularly among the younger crowd.

With great endeavor and mixed success for previous tries at intervention in his native Great Britain, the article gives an account as Jamie brings his efforts (and of course a new TV show) to Huntington. He aims to redirect the locals' eating habits from neighborhood favorites like fifteen-pound hamburgers (yes, fifteen pounds of meat, bun, and toppings) and fifteen-inch, one-pound, eleven-toppings hotdogs to more healthful fare. No doubt little butt bombs like this are responsible for the extremely high incidence and prevalence of obesity, diabetes, and heart disease found in that region. As reported, Jamie seeks to initiate change through nutritional education and instruction in cooking from scratch. I will say unequivocally I agree with the principal aim here: Change the current self-destructive dietary habits in favor of far more healthful ones.

As a physician, an interventional cardiologist, I can add that trying to change the habits or behaviors of individuals can sometimes be next to impossible. If people have not experienced any physical harm from their ongoing condition (e.g., they haven't had heart attacks or strokes), the vast majority does not change. It is like telling someone fire is hot and burns therefore do not touch it; until that person feels the heat and/or gets a burn, he or she really does not understand. The people of Huntington, and America in general, may be overweight and have high blood pressure and diabetes, but they still want to eat what they perceive as tasting good. As we have seen, what we perceive as tasting good may simply be cravings from the sugar, salt, and fat addiction. Jamie's plan was to supply nutritional education and impart some basic culinary skills. His program was "about scratch cooking, which to him means avoiding processed and fast food, learning pride of ownership, encouraging sparks of creativity and finding a reason to gather family and friends in one place. If you can make pancakes or an omelet, a pot of chili or spaghetti sauce and know how to perk up some vegetables, you can spend less and eat a more healthful meal that's delicious."[5]

Nutritional education and cooking from scratch are only part of the successful equation. After initiating this program in institutions like schools as well as teaching people in their homes, there was only mixed success. The article notes that "only half the schools are functioning properly; the other half are still experiencing difficulty training cafeteria staff and enforcing new guidelines. And follow-up reports show that while students now understand the benefits of eating healthfully, many still opt out of their school-lunch plans, reverting to fast food instead."[6]

Deprivation and doomsday preaching alone do not work. They do not work because the basic human desire is to pursue happiness and flee suffering. Anyone raised on the addictive refined fast food can come to crave that greasy, salty, sugary fix. It's the same for the long-term smoker who wants a smoke because it tastes good. People will pursue these activities until they wind up in the deep repose afforded by a diabetic coma or receive smoking's little free gift called cancer. Given these proclivities, food that satisfies these unwholesome desires makes us feel good in that undeniably American, instantly gratified way. Particularly with current tough economic conditions, a rational person does not inflict upon himself or herself additional misery, even if it is for some down-the-road, as-yet-unrealized benefit. It is simply a very hard sell.

When I first started training in the martial art of Bujinkan Budo Taijutsu, I wanted to learn how to punch, kick, and throw effectively. I wanted to know not just how to fight but how to really kick ass. But in the world of real life-and-death combat, there are no rules, no winners and losers—just survivors and the dead. Opponents do not have to necessarily be more skillful than you, sometimes just luckier. During my early training in my current style of martial arts, one of the senior Japanese instructors would help us newbies out. While we struggled to learn the basics of the proper forms, he would walk around and critique us. He would demonstrate the proper form that we were supposed to emulate. One evening, while displaying a particular pose, he positioned his rearward foot at an odd 45-degree backward-facing angle. Someone asked him why his foot was set that way. With broken English he replied, "In any potential conflict, rule number 1: good escape make." I wish someone had told me that before my first marriage. If the situation allows, always escape if you can. Do whatever you need to do to always survive. Do not let your ego get you killed.

Consequently, we must first learn to avoid being manipulated by the call of the junk food siren. It truly is a siren song; we have been seduced into an addiction masquerading as taste and convenience. We are being seduced into what to eat, and we are being driven to eat when we're not even hungry. It is like some subliminal message tucked into the white noise that sits incessantly in the background of our everyday lives. The lure of the junk food/fast food siren is all around us and ever present. She is a two-headed, bewitching enchantress who addicts and poisons. We are under attack. We must good escape make. The junk food out there is not junk. Junk is stuff you throw away. Junk doesn't hurt anybody. These things are weapons of mass consumption.

And these weapons of mass consumption are everywhere visible. A good escape starts with awareness. The saying goes that the best swordsman is the one who never need draw his blade. By being aware and recognizing a potential problem before it is a predicament that requires extrication, it can be successfully reconciled. It can be eliminated before it ever has the chance to manifest into a difficult quandary. If we are not aware of potential dangers, then we spend our lives putting out fires. The medical equivalent is to simply continue to treat symptoms without ever identifying the cause of the illness: expensive, futile, unsatisfying for all, and inevitably fatal. Awareness requires knowledge, of our own weaknesses and vulnerabilities and those of our potential dilemmas, for there are those on the dark side of the food industry who are only too ready to prey upon our personal shortcomings with their weapons of mass consumption.

For example, processed foods are not just processed for preservation. Look at a typical piece of fast food chicken. I include a lot of the chain restaurants when we speak of processed, fast food/junk food. It is something you might order when eating out, thinking you will get a healthy piece of delicious, wholesome chicken. It is highly likely that the chicken has been chopped, processed, and reformed before being frozen and shipped. During the reforming process, the chicken has preservatives added, as well as flavor enhancers like yeast extract. Yeast extract contains glutamate, which acts to ramp up weaker flavors. Think taste steroids, and you get the picture. Moisteners, protein extracts, and enzymes are added to soften the food. Softening the food is important. Chewing takes work and can add to the unpleasantness of a meal. But from the dark side's perspective, chewing means you eat less because you spend more time chewing. It takes twenty or so minutes after you start eating for you to start to signal to your brain you're full. They need you to consume as much as possible in that time period, which is why they don't want you to have to chew, just shovel as much down your gullet as possible. Water, hydrolyzed protein, salt, and chemical augmentation produce a sensuous, soft, melt-in-your-mouth mouthful. All the while the chicken is subjected to high levels of salt, sugar, and fat manipulation. It becomes, as they say, "ultra-palatable."[7]

It is not just meat products that are made with scientific calculation and precision. Things like cakes, cookies, and breads are all constructed to perform similar tasks. A sweet homemade cinnamon roll made with fresh ingredients and love is a welcome treat. I have made them for many folks on special occasions. They are about the size of a small bun, and rarely does someone eat more than one. I have watched people blindly consume the fast food/junk food version in malls and airports in amounts that require an insulin chaser and then go back for more. That's how these things are constructed, to hook you in with all your senses. It is why the breads, cookies, and cakes are made with refined flours. By removing the bran and refining and processing the flours, the end product is airy and soft and has an ethereal in-your-mouth texture—and no nutritional value. That's why the buns at the fast food burger joints contain HFCS and oils. Not enough for you to taste the sweetness or fat flavor but just enough to provide a subliminal and devious backdrop. The smell, the look, the feel, and the taste of every single molecule of that salt, sugar, and fat is packaged so it becomes focused on slamming the pleasure spot in your brain again and again and again. They are deceptively pleasurable gastronomic improvised explosive devices (IEDs).

These gastro-IEDs also include chemical munitions. Processing includes many additives and chemically modified additions. Flavor additives are in almost all the processed foods in one form or another. These machinations are used to mimic through emulsified compounds everything from nuts, fruits, and sweets for drinks and desserts to artificial smoked, grilled, and roasted flavors for vegetables and meats. There is even an artificial butter flavor for that homey butter-baked-in taste for breads.[8] Beyond the flavors there are artificial colorings. There are also artificial textures, things added to give a snap or a crunch and improve the artificial experience. In the same way, any potential unpleasant or piquant flavors or textures can be processed out. It can be homogenized for the masses.

Because we develop a Pavlovian response to these temptations, the desire can be initiated by the suggestion of the enticement: the packaging, the commercial, the billboard. When you enter the establishment, the smells caress you. By the time you've been seated you're wiping the drool off your chin with the napkin.

Modern eating is a multisensory experience in the short attention span theater. For many fast food/junk food venues, it has become "eatertainment."[9] Remember that the goal of the places offering meals to you is to make money. It is big business, with about $0.49 of every food dollar being spent dining out, that amounts to more than $580 billion per year in the United States alone.[10] They do not exist for your health. The way that they make money is by selling the people what the people want. Unfortunately as we've seen, what the people want has become what they're addicted to—salt, sugar, and fat. Profit margins are enhanced by artificial flavorings and chemical additives that lower costs and extend shelf life. Foods come parcooked so they can be assembled (usually by dropping into a fryer) in a kitchen by a staff that does not have any culinary skill or training. Vegetables are prechopped, and any prepping of fresh food is eliminated. These act to reduce labor costs. You are not being sold nutrition, satisfaction, or even really food. You are being sold edible emotion.[11] The difference between fresh, wholesome food made with real ingredients and love and the siren's offering is the difference between sex with a prostitute and lovemaking with your soul mate.

The food is manipulated to appeal to our weakness by layering on the salt, sugar, and fat in as many permutations as possible. Then the whole thing is redressed, and we gladly let in this Trojan horse. And like any good general, the food industry manipulates this craving to tempt people to consume more and more. The soldiers inside the horse open the gates, and lo and behold, access is made easy by the sheer number of venues where the goodies can be acquired. It is not just junk food—it is easy-to-acquire, readily available, competitively priced addiction. It is everywhere and always available.

Once aware, how do we avoid the siren song? I remember a martial arts training session when my *soke* (grandmaster) was asked an entertaining but bloody stupid question. Someone in the audience who had obviously already taken some head shots asked, "Well, how do you win a bar fight?" *Soke* looked right at him and without missing a beat said, "Don't go to a bar." It may seem absurdly obvious, but that is the short answer. But you have to eat, and sometimes you have to stop at a bar. I remember doing a radio show, and one of the hosts was a mom. She asked, "Well, if you had to stop at a fast food place with the kids, would you get the chicken so and so? Would that be a good choice?" A pause, Zen calm, and then, "Why no, I just wouldn't stop at any of these places. If you have to stop, maybe find someplace, some mom-and-pop place, any place where they use real food. If you have nowhere else to go, if your survival and sanity depends on it, then stop. Eat whatever you like and make a special time of it. Get everything on the hotdog. Just make it infrequent; all things in moderation, even moderation." She loved me.

I have been in many pressure situations, lives-on-the-line pressure situations during code-blue heart attacks. I've had thirty six-inch razor blades buzz by my head, with very angry men holding them. But one of the moments that chilled me to the core came when I was reading David Kessler's book *The End of Overeating*. He was doing an interview with a top executive in the fast food industry. When the executive was asked what the goals of the food industry are, he replied, "*The* goal is to get you hooked."[12]

Therefore the next step in taking control is learning (or relearning) what not to eat. If you avoid the bait, you can't get hooked. It is as simple in theory as not walking into the bar. But any recovering alcoholic will tell you that, while it is simple, it isn't easy. You may need to adjust this based upon your lifestyle. For example, if you travel on a family vacation once or twice a year and that is the only time you're munching on fast food or feasting on foie gras, then you're probably OK—all things in moderation and clearly no addictive patterns. If you are a truck driver and on the road all the time and that is where you get 90 percent of your meals, you've got to make some dining choices because those dining choices are your lifestyle choices. And like the great sages of Metallica have sung, "My lifestyle determines my deathstyle."

There are a lot of references, programs, and data out there to provide a good starting point. Find one that works for you if simple avoidance seems impossible. But do understand it is about more than just calories and a nutritional scorecard. You can opt for the salad at one of these places and it can taste terrible and may not even be that good for you. It is not because salad in general is bad but because *this* particular salad is not good. The tomatoes are underripe, and the lettuce, carrots, and cucumbers were cut two days ago and are in need of veggie Viagra. So it tastes terrible, and you have a terrible-tasting meal. But wait, there's more. Because the veggies were precut days ago, they contain about as much nutritional value as the cardboard they now resemble. The prepackaged dressing list of ingredients reads like an organic chemistry text written in Farsi. It is loaded with empty calories, additives, salt, sugar, and fat. So the salad is also terrible at the nutritional/caloric level—a terrible dining experience on multiple levels. We need to avoid or at the very least limit our junk food exposure. This requires some planning. If you know you will be traveling and will be eating out, make that your "culinary holiday." Enjoy eating what you want wherever you want guilt free. Yet when you return home realize that it is back to acquiring more healthful meals. To participate in a program of constant deprivation is like working with no vacation or time off. After a while there is a point of diminishing returns. I remember one of the worst workdays ever. All the rumors and myths you hear and read about the horrors of internship and residency are true—it is extremely abusive. I did a twelve-hour shift in the emergency department that ended at 8 a.m. At 8 a.m. I reported to my new ward rotation and was on call that day and evening and worked the entire day after that before I had a break. It was forty-plus hours straight. When I finally got to bed and I next awoke, I had slept more than twenty-four hours. I have never experienced anything like that before or since. Since then there have been all these studies and data reporting that the lack of sleep is bad for you: impaired judgment, decreased responsiveness, and detrimental physical effects (like weight gain). Now they limit the number of hours interns and residents can work in a week; some break time is mandatory. That's probably a good idea we should all apply.

The same principles can be applied to escaping the junk food trap. Here's a way to get a handle on the situation:

1. Make a food diary by writing down everything as you currently eat now. Do this for at least one and up to several weeks. No cheating (it's for you anyway), and write down everything in your current regimen, including portion sizes (approximate if you need to).
2. Analyze what percentage of your meals and/or snacks come from dining out, fast food, prepared meals, or a snack bag.
3. With your calendar, see where/when you are most vulnerable, that is, consume the most junk or when you find it difficult not to indulge (at friend's dinner party or business dinner).
4. Set a goal to limit your exposure to no more than 10 percent.

For example, let's say in one week, the diary looked like the one shown in table 8.1. This is not the end-all list but meant to be some preliminary data gathering from which we can start a long-term program. We can see that we were eating six meals (including snacks) a day. First we tag the takeaway meals and preprocessed junk food snacks. Now we see what appears in table 8.2.

We have forty-two meals per week (six meals a day times seven days a week). Of those forty-two meals, 36 percent (fifteen out of forty-two) are either fast food takeaway or preprocessed junk. That is over a third of what is being consumed, although a little snack here and there may not seem like it. We notice that Tuesday and Wednesday we are busy at work and eat office goodies. We also order out all during the week while we are at work. So we plan our menu for the next week knowing we are going to have some hot-dogs, fries, and beer on Sunday as we watch the football games after Sunday brunch. We also have a business dinner Thursday. We want to reduce our intake to around 10 percent. To allow for that, we are vigilant about what we do during lunch at the workplace during the week. It's like knowing you're going on vacation for a long weekend, so mentally you buckle down and finish the work before you leave so you can take the time off and enjoy it. It's the same principle here. If you do not want to do the planning, there are groups like Weight Watchers that offer programs that do this; you just have to pay for it. So our template for the next week might look like table 8.3.

TABLE 8.1. Sample Food Diary

	Mon.	Tues.	Wed.	Thur.	Fri.	Sat.	Sun.
Breakfast	coffee	coffee	coffee	coffee	coffee	coffee	coffee
Snack	1 apple, 1 banana	2 takeaway chicken biscuits	2 glazed donuts	none	none	1 orange	none
Lunch	2 slices of pepperoni pizza, soda; delivered	1 order of takeaway nachos with chicken	1 takeaway steak sub, fries, and soda	1 takeaway pork BBQ sandwich, 1 order of hushpuppies, sweetened iced tea	large Greek salad, water	fast food sub, 12 inches	2 eggs, 2 slices of toast, 4 slices of bacon, bloody Mary
Snack	1 candy bar	1 vending machine snack	½ bag of raisins	none	none	⅓ bag of chips	none
Dinner	homemade salad, chicken breast, baked potato, 1 glass of wine	homemade chili, 1 cup, with cheese topping, 1 beer	fast food double cheeseburger, large fries, large soda	homemade pot roast with carrots, potatoes, water	homemade spaghetti with marinara sauce, 2 pieces of garlic toast, 1 glass of wine	home-cooked steak, 1 ear of corn with butter, 1 piece of garlic toast	2 hotdogs, fries, 1 beer
Snack	none	none	none	popcorn with butter	½ bag of chips, 2 beers	½ bag of chips	½ pint of ice cream

The key is really in achieving a balance. That also applies to the constitution of a meal. To taste good a meal needs balance: not too much salt or sugar or spice. Out-of-balance food tastes awful. Yet without any of these elements it is not any good, just bland cardboard pulp. Likewise the way we eat and enjoy must reflect the very balance we find desirable in our food. For the long haul, you need a reasonable pace. That's not to say you can't exit for a double bacon cheeseburger with fries now and again. We're human, and we like those things every so often. And really, I can't say as an interventional cardiologist that if you smoke a cigarette or cigar three or four times a year and have a Kobe steak with foie gras for dessert on a rare occasion it's really going to negatively affect your overall health. We are descended from opportunistic scavengers. We have canines. We grew our

TABLE 8.2. Sample Food Diary with Tags

	Mon.	Tues.	Wed.	Thur.	Fri.	Sat.	Sun.
Breakfast	coffee	coffee	coffee	coffee	coffee	coffee	coffee
Snack	1 apple, 1 banana	**2 takeaway chicken biscuits**	**2 glazed donuts**	none	none	1 orange	none
Lunch	**2 slices of pepperoni pizza, soda; delivered**	**1 order of takeaway nachos with chicken**	**1 takeaway steak sub, fries, and soda**	**1 takeaway pork BBQ sandwich, 1 order of hushpuppies, sweetened iced tea**	large Greek salad, water	**fast food sub, 12 inches**	2 eggs, 2 slices of toast, 4 slices of bacon, bloody Mary
Snack	**1 candy bar**	**1 vending machine snack**	½ bag of raisins	none	none	**⅓ bag of chips**	none
Dinner	homemade salad, chicken breast, baked potato, 1 glass of wine	homemade chili, 1 cup, with cheese topping, 1 beer	**fast food double cheese-burger, large fries, large soda**	homemade pot roast with carrots, potatoes, water	homemade spaghetti with marinara sauce, 2 pieces of garlic toast, 1 glass of wine	home-cooked steak, 1 ear of corn with butter, 1 piece of garlic toast	2 hotdogs, fries, 1 beer
Snack	none	none	none	**popcorn with butter**	**½ bag of chips, 2 beers**	**½ bag of chips**	**½ pint of ice cream**

brains by eating meats and proteins. Fats sustained us through tough times. A sugar high from the honey pot gave us the speed to outrun Smiley the sabertooth. Salt preserved us. We can handle it in small doses. The converse is not true; if you grab a snorkel and dine at the trough 95 percent of the time, a salad now and again will not cure what ails you. I'm not sure there's a high colonic that could do that.

The solution has to come from both ends. We need to approach this with a stethoscope in one hand and a chef's knife in the other. There is medical and nutritional education and guidance. There is the preparation of delicious fresh food. There is a chef's sensibility to utilize fat, salt, and sugar as a surgeon wields a scalpel, providing for us

TABLE 8.3. Sample Planned Food Diary

	Mon.	Tues.	Wed.	Thur.	Fri.	Sat.	Sun.
Breakfast	coffee	coffee	coffee	coffee	coffee	coffee	coffee
Snack	fruit or none	fruit or none	fruit or none	fruit or none	fruit or none	fruit or none	fruit or none
Lunch	home packed	home packed	home packed	home packed	home packed	homemade sub	**2 eggs, 2 slices of toast, 4 slices of bacon, bloody Mary**
Snack	fruit or none	fruit or none	fruit or none	fruit or none	fruit or none	fruit or none	none
Dinner	homemade salad, chicken breast, baked potato, 1 glass of wine	homemade chili, 1 cup, with cheese topping, 1 beer	fast food double cheeseburger, large fries, large soda	**business dinner**	homemade spaghetti with marinara sauce, 2 pieces of garlic toast, 1 glass of wine	home-cooked steak, 1 ear of corn with butter, 1 piece of garlic toast	**2 hotdogs, fries, 1 beer**
Snack	none	none	none	**business dinner**	none	none	none

consumption in moderation, not unlike the approach to responsibly utilizing alcohol. A constant barrage of sugar, salt, and fat not only is physiologically detrimental, but it also dulls your palate. It is like smoking a cigar, licking the ashtray, and then trying to discern the finer points of a French Bordeaux Chateau Petrus. So to avoid the siren call, we must perform the equivalent of Odyssey's lashing to the mast and plugging the crew's ears with wax. We avoid and limit with foreknowledge. First, we made sure we had a good escape route. We become aware of the junk food siren, and now we can avoid her song. We begin to reclaim our palates and our lives. Once you reclaim your palate, then you get to taste anew. It is gastronomic rebirth. And the first step toward culinary nirvana.

get fresh, but no adultery

"Nothing great in the world has ever been accomplished without passion."

—CHRISTIAN FRIEDRICH HEBBEL (1813–1863)

WE HAVE made our escape from overindulging in fast food and junk food by becoming aware of the siren's presence and avoiding her call. Yet in doing so, we have created a void, a void previously filled with tempting nibbles and bits. The next phase is to fill that void with the results of some fresh Grassroots Gourmet–style cooking. This is not a diet of deprivation. We are not talking about gastronomic masochism here. The process is the sensible use of proper, fresh, nonrefined, and nonprocessed ingredients cooked with good technique and consumed in rational servings.

Being a Grassroots Gourmet is all about using fresh, wholesome ingredients. It is about being a "localvore" by local sourcing where and when you can. It is about the judicious use of salt, sugars, and fat to create wonderfully appealing and tasty, restaurant-worthy dishes. You do not need to be a trained chef; a few simple techniques go a long way. It is important, however, to differentiate between cooking with a long-term view and for a lifetime of tasty great eats versus cooking for a single service as in a restaurant.

Remember that the goal of places offering meals, whether in a sit-down restaurant, fast food drive-through, or preprepared frozen to take home in the grocery store, is to make money. They do not exist for your health. The way that they make money is by selling the people what they want. Unfortunately, as we've seen, what the people want most has become what they're addicted to—sugar, salt, and fat. When they panic and find themselves at the other extreme of the spectrum, they are offered "diet meals," which are often overprocessed, tasteless rubbish.

The home cook has, I believe, the hardest job of all and often receives the least amount of respect for performing the tasks at hand. The fact is many home cooks perform at a level more worthy of the title "home gourmet." To achieve that level, all that is needed are some basic planning, techniques, and education along with a healthy dose of passion and enthusiasm. This is like anything else; if you are not willing to put a little effort into the undertaking, you will not succeed. There are no magic pills.

Let's look a little more closely at those who strive anonymously in the daily kitchen grind. What must the home gourmet do compared to the restaurant professional chef?

- While both have to work within budgets, the home gourmet cannot simply pass along any increased costs in the form of increased prices to his or her customers; he or she and family are the customers.
- Going out to a restaurant is often somewhat celebratory in nature. The vast majority of customers do not dine at the same restaurant every night. Unlike the home gourmet, the diners are not relying on the restaurant chef to provide for their long-term nutritional and health needs.
- The folks at home (and the home gourmet) want the food to be as tasty as when they dine out.
- The home gourmet often does not have access to the resources of a professional kitchen.
- The home gourmet may be under a different but equally demanding set of time constraints compared to the restaurant chef.
- The home gourmet often has to do it all without additional sous chefs: shop, prep, cook, plate, serve, and clean.
- The skill set of the home gourmet is often self-taught and trial and error.

Ultimately the environment is one in which meals and dining are prepared to have the presentation and taste appeal of a good restaurant meal with an eye toward the repercussions on the diner's nutrition and health. While professional restaurant chefs can offer some "healthy options" on their menu, the home chef is often limited to a relatively fixed daily menu in terms of the number of offerings. In some ways this seems an even more daunting albeit different challenge from a culinary perspective than the daily challenge facing a professional restaurant chef. As a consequence of these unique challenges, a Grassroots Gourmet approach to cooking presents an opportunity to successfully address these issues within the given framework. Here are the general concepts, principles, and basic skills needed. It only requires practice and passion to elevate you from mere cook to Grassroots Gourmet.

The concepts are few and simple; in fact the most effective martial arts techniques are often the simplest. When we operate in the hospital, we do it in the simplest manner that is effective. Simple lends itself to successful repetition. As I was told in my first year in medical school, "repetition is the mother of all learning." These operational concepts allow you to stay focused and execute successfully on a consistent basis. The concepts in Grassroots Gourmet cooking involves keeping it fresh, maintaining quality, retraining the taste buds, keeping it simple, and watching content. The more I cook, eat, study, and learn, the more I am convinced that the seventh commandment, "Thou shall not commit adultery," refers to your food.

FRESHNESS

Fresh food has great flavors. In the simplest, chef-foodie speak, I say this because fresh food just tastes better. It has a vitality that is missing in preserved preparations. Truly fresh fish should smell like the ocean. If it smells fishy, it is actually on the spoiled side. While eating sushi and sashimi in Japan, I was told that the fish must be very fresh. Now there are obvious health concerns about eating raw seafood in a timely manner. However, an additional concept relative to timing consumption was that, after the fish is killed, it immediately starts to lose its vital essence, its chi, and by consuming it as close to the bada-bing moment as possible, we capture some of that fundamental essence for ourselves. It is their belief that it is this quintessential component that provides the real life-sustaining nature of food. It is not unlike the belief of many native peoples across the globe that by consuming parts of a kill (often raw or minimally altered) immediately after it occurs, a bit of the essence of that animal is transferred to the person. The same reasoning holds for many fruits and vegetables. Nothing you can buy compares to a freshly picked, right-out-of-the-garden, vine-ripened tomato. For many types of food, the decline in vibrancy and taste correlates with a loss in its nutritional value. Fresh bread is not only far superior in taste to packaged, but also the smell strikes a guttural response. It is such a powerful smell that having that scent present when would-be buyers come through your home can aid in the sale. Once you have had fresh pasta and a fresh sauce, any other option becomes a bland substitute. Nature has put an expiration date on everything and with good reason. Therefore, we should strive whenever possible to work with the freshest, most minimally processed ingredients. When Michelin stars are awarded, the prospective chefs know that the inspectors will evaluate the freshness of their produce and product as well as their final creations.

QUALITY

Hand in hand with freshness walks quality. Everyone is always looking for a bargain, and sometimes we find one. Yet more often than not, the old adage that you get what you pay for applies. Something may be fresh, but that does not mean it is always of quality. The tomatoes at the farmer's market may be freshly picked, but they can still be bruised with insect bites and thus of poor quality. A steak may have been purposely dry or wet aged and thus not technically fresh but may be of excellent quality—and the aging process just adds value in this setting. A great example is the sweet pea. I often only use frozen sweet peas. The reason is that, once the peas are picked, they immediately start to convert sugars to starch and quickly lose their sweetness. The flash freezing done as they exit the field stops this process. Thus, unless the peas are field fresh and unshelled, frozen peas can constitute a higher-quality ingredient than never-frozen peas that have been sitting on the grocery shelf for several days. Quality also applies to how the product has been prepared or, in the case of meats, how it has been raised. I am not a believer in mass-produced, industrial, factory-farmed birds that grow up crammed into gobbler ghettos. I realize most people are far removed from their food sources, just purchasing the end result, ready for the stove or oven, direct from the supermarket. However, if you're traveling down the road, particularly the highways in Virginia, the Carolinas, or Georgia, you may encounter the smell. It's not a bad smell; it's *the* bad smell. Imagine for a moment a combination of bloated roadside carcass, nasty baby diaper, and dog farts. That begins to describe the stench, a result of the excrement and waste where these birds are raised. I have visited some of these commercial mills, and the conditions are crammed. Forget the genetics for more breast meat and so on; all creatures are in some way products of their environment. Mordor was clearly not the breadbasket of Middle Earth. If you want a tasty, delicious, nutritious bird that hasn't been pumped up with chemicals, you may want to try something like a free-range, vegetarian-fed bird. I realize it costs more than an industrial bird, but it is worth experiencing because prepared correctly there is no comparison in taste and texture. Next time you go out to shop, start shopping for quality over quantity. Learn as much as you are able about where your food comes from, and show it a little respect. Remember: what we shove in our pie holes is what we are destined to become.

RETRAINING THE TASTE BUDS

Particularly when we first start, our palates are often quite unsophisticated. A large part of the cause can be due to ingesting the overprocessed junk food offerings. They will, in effect, make our taste buds comfortably numb. We seek salt, sweet, and fat, registering those tastes and basically ignoring everything else. A key component to successfully avoid being lured into junk food overindulgence and addiction is the development of your palate. A sophisticated palate will start to shun the junk. It will seek a balance that uses sweet, salty, and fat to create textures, tastes, and flavors and are not ends unto themselves. In speaking with many folks with whom I have helped send down this path, I notice a pleasantly consistent commentary. Several weeks to several months after cutting out junk and working on developing their palates, folks often will have some fast food or junk food encounter. At a gathering or on the road, a situation arises when that's all there is to eat, so they do. Almost universally there is an amazing response. They ate something they used to crave, and it did not taste good. Often they put that burger or sandwich down and speak about how it just tastes awful to them now. I think it is not unlike someone who finally quits cigarettes and lights one up only to wonder what they hell they were ever thinking putting this crap in their mouths and lungs. This occurs because they have learned (or relearned) how to taste. Everyone can do it. You will develop your own likes and dislikes. That is OK. It is a lot like appreciating art or wine. In the end it is about what you prefer. Understanding the need for both fresh and quality items is necessary to retrain the taste buds. When you have that fresh piece of quality produce, taste it. You have to learn what the individual components are supposed to taste like. Taste the fresh green bean you bought at the farmer's market that was picked that morning from the field. Now taste a green bean from a can. Now taste a previously frozen green bean. Now taste one of those freshly picked green beans a week later. You should always be tasting and working. When I taste wine, I put forth a conscious effort to examine and experience the components. I do the same with food. This is part of the work, but it is also the fun. You must constantly taste, identify, recall, and experience. This is one way we train our taste buds to recognize the subtle flavors of fresh, quality components so we can present them most favorably upon the plate.

A great example of learning how to train the buds for me occurred during a trip to Canada for a weekend to participate in a martial arts seminar. It was a fantastic weekend full of great training with new and old friends. Traditionally, everyone gets together following the big training session for a feast of food and drink to relax, unwind, and nurse a few bruises. Often, the hosts choose a Japanese venue. I suppose as the martial art we study has its roots in Japan, this is a logical extension of the activities of the day. But in Canada we got a treat. We went to a local area bistro. I got to speak with the chef, and he convinced me to try the local Alberta beef steak.

The Alberta beef in Canada is unique. They can track every piece of meat from start to finish. There is a "raised right" campaign in place to ensure the proper and ethical treatment of the animals. All this produced a lean and fantastically flavorful steak. I learned about the new cut and the unique flavor of this Alberta cut of beef. You should know what you taste, so inquire and pair the knowledge with the sensation.

Sourcing fresh may and often does conflict with convenience. An everyday example can be found in the produce sections of most grocery stores where you can find pre-chopped veggies. There are few prep jobs more loathsome than chopping vegetables. However, as soon as the vegetables are chopped, they start to lose some of their nutritional value as well as some of their flavor. That loss includes the phytochemicals. *Phytochemicals* is an all-encompassing term that refers to the chemical properties found in plants. It includes sterols, flavonoids, sulfur-containing compounds, minerals, antioxidants, and many other compounds whose modes of action are still poorly understood. It also includes even more compounds that are little known and poorly characterized.[1] The potential loss of unknown players in the complex equations of how "what we eat is what we become" starts horrific visions of chaos theory, butterflies in China, and thunderstorms in New York.

Now unless you are part of a commune, it may be near impossible to get everything fresh, but when and where you can get it fresh and wholesome, you need to make that effort. Buying the vegetables fresh and whole and chopping them yourself is a good start. Sourcing reliably fresh product is an important part of the acquisition process. Once again, tomatoes are a great example. Tomatoes just picked from the garden or from a farmer's roadside stand have a smell and taste that makes grocery store tomatoes less appealing. The reason is that although the tomatoes in the megachains look bright red, ripe, and juicy, they have not ripened naturally on the vine. They are often picked green and forced to ripen by exposure to ethylene gas. The sugars thus do not get to be produced as they would if the fruit ripened on the vine. I just don't want my produce to have been forced into any unnatural acts.

SIMPLICITY

To highlight fresh and quality products, we want to keep the preparation methods simple. Any sauces and additional elements to the meal should complement the natural flavors. Heavy, cloying sauces are what you need when you have tasteless, overprocessed food or you're trying to hide the fact that the ingredients are inferior. If you keep it fresh, you need to keep it simple in preparation and allow the food to express itself. As in the martial arts and the cardiac catheterization laboratory, just K.I.S.S.—Keep It Simple, Stupid. Combining flavors and techniques from previously disparate regions or ethnicities is fine.

It is often referred to as fusion cuisine and defined as "combining usually widely differing ethnic or regional ingredients, styles, or techniques."[2] In fact, our Grassroots Gourmet cooking is a form of nouvelle cuisine that incorporates fusion. Nouvelle cuisine is a lighter cuisine based on natural flavors, shortened or simplified cooking times and techniques, and utilizing innovative combinations such as those found in fusion cuisine. Therefore let me declare my love for all food things fusion. Yet anything lovely can be twisted into a nightmare. As an example let's look at sushi: "cold, boiled rice moistened with rice vinegar, usually shaped into bite-sized pieces and topped with raw seafood (nigiri-zushi) or formed into a long seaweed-wrapped roll, often around strips of vegetable or raw fish, and sliced into bite-sized pieces (maki-zushi)."[3] Now I realize sushi in reality refers to the rice used, but in the American vernacular it has come to mean sushi rice topped with raw fish and other things. A recent experience demonstrated a loss of simple, tasty preparation in the name of trying to appear cool and trendy with "fusion cuisine." The chef forgot K.I.S.S. and wound up more like WHAM. Now in the name of fusion cuisine, I can abide smoked salmon with a shmear of cream cheese and onion (the "jewshi roll") or the so-called cowboy roll with some cooked steak inside, although I avoid the brokeback mountain roll even if it claims "You won't be able to quit this roll." I can also tolerate the "crabby roll" that contains no real crab, which is why I suppose it is "crabby." What I cannot abide is subjecting the sushi to a technique that so fundamentally alters its core it resembles sushi in no way, shape, or form. Fusion demands skillful combining and melding. Destroying the essence of ingredients leads to travesty cuisine, not fusion. When sushi is combined with bacon and deep fried, it is no longer sushi. It is a southern fish fry, plain and simple. Sushi is sushi, and deep-fried fish is deep-fried fish. Sushi and a fish fry are both delicious, but they should never be cross-pollinated. Keep it simple and focused.

CONTENT

As you prepare the recipes from later chapters, you'll notice a consistent theme. Lots of vegetables and fruits are used that either stand on their own or subtly complement a focused entrée: a chicken breast, a fresh fillet, or a reasonable amount of fresh meat. In having the privilege to have dined at various places around the globe and noticing healthy native cultures, this concept of fresh, quality content seems to be a unifying principle. For example, here are some commonalities of content that are highlighted in the report from the American Heart Association referencing the Lyon diet heart study and the Mediterranean diet:

- high in fruits, vegetables, bread and other cereals, potatoes, beans, nuts, and seeds
- includes olive oil as an important source of monounsaturated fat

- dairy products, fish, and poultry consumed in low to moderate amounts; little red meat
- eggs consumed zero to four times weekly
- wine consumed in low to moderate amounts[4]

I would add that those corresponding principles seem to apply to healthy Asian diets as well. A recent study looked at a number of previous trials from across the globe comprising over 500,000 participants.[5] It was found that a Mediterranean diet was associated with:

- decreased waist circumference
- higher HDL (good) cholesterol
- lower triglyceride levels
- better blood pressure control
- better glucose (blood sugar) metabolism

All of these positive findings are associated with a reduced risk in the likelihood of having a cardiovascular event. Another study looked at the Mediterranean diet in nondiabetics with high cardiovascular risk.[6] The Mediterranean diet, as described in this study, utilized:

- olive oil for cooking and dressing
- increased consumption of fruit, vegetables, legumes, and fish
- reduction in total meat consumption, recommending white meat instead of red or processed meat
- preparation of homemade sauce with tomato, garlic, onion, and spices with olive oil to dress vegetables, pasta, rice, and other dishes
- avoidance of butter, cream, fast food, sweets, pastries, and sugar-sweetened beverages
- in alcohol drinkers, moderate consumption of red wine

There are a couple of important points to highlight here. There is liberal use of olive oil, which is a natural fat. Yes, it is a fat. Fats are not only good, but also they are essential. You just shouldn't abuse them. The fruits, vegetables, legumes, and fish are of the very fresh and minimally processed variety. The meat, likewise, should be minimally processed. The sauces to dress the dishes are of the homemade type. Avoidance of prepared fast foods and products using highly refined components like flour and white sugar is key to the diet.

When this high-risk population consumed this diet for four years versus a low-fat diet, the incidence of new-onset diabetes was reduced by about 50 percent. As Dr. Jordi Salas-Salvadó, a principal investigator, notes, "The diabetes risk reduction occurred in the absence of significant changes in body weight or physical activity, so the reduction can be attributed only to the diet, not to weight loss."[7] Stephanie A Dunbar of the American Diabetes Association comments that "previously, a randomized controlled trial, the Diabetes Prevention Program, showed that it was more the weight loss that helped to prevent diabetes, but in this study they are showing that by changing the foods you eat, you can reduce your risk without weight loss."[8] Notice that this study in which folks consumed fat and alcohol was more beneficial than a low-fat diet.

Interestingly, the study PREDIMED (Prevención con Dieta Mediterránea) also had a substudy that randomized folks to a Mediterranean diet with extra virgin olive oil, a Mediterranean diet with nuts, or a low-fat diet as the control group. Diets were without limits, and no advice on physical activity was given. The main outcome was incidence of diabetes as diagnosed by the 2009 American Diabetes Association criteria. The study is still ongoing, but the preliminary data from a Spanish site shows that after a median followup of four years, incidence of diabetes was 10.1 percent, 11.0 percent, and 17.9 percent in the Mediterranean-diet-with-olive-oil group, the Mediterranean-diet-with-nuts group, and the control group, respectively.[9] This equates to a 52 percent reduction in diabetes due to the diet, not weight loss or physical activity.

In a classic book by Dr. Weston A. Price, *Nutrition and Physical Degeneration*, he examined the health of groups of people around the globe. He also looked at their diets. He did this in the early part of the twentieth century before the rampant globalization and homogenization of today was widespread. At that time there were still many pockets of people relatively isolated and consuming the local foods as they had done in their respective regions for centuries or longer. What he found was that good health did not necessarily correlate with a specific type of diet or food. In great contradistinction to the super foods and miracle diets hawked everywhere in the United States today, he found that health correlated to consuming the fresh, local, wholesome foods and avoiding what he called the "displacing foods of modern commerce"—sugar, refined grains, canned foods, pasteurized milk, and devitalized fats.[10] For instance, in a remote Swiss village, the diet consisted of unpasteurized dairy products such as milk, cheese, butter, and cream as well as breads with whole grains like rye. Proteins were occasional meats and soups made with homemade stock. Another locally sourced diet was found in a remote Scottish village where the diet was seafood and hearty whole grains like oats. In all cases the native populations consuming the local fresh whole foods were extremely healthy—until embarking on the more "civilized" Western diet.

Even today, in remote villages where the Inuit people live a traditional lifestyle, they continue to consume a traditional diet high in fat and meat with little vegetables as their ancestors did centuries ago. Their overall health tends to be better than someone consuming the typical Western or U.S. diet. In some villages in northern Quebec, where adults get about half their calories from native foods, the myocardial death rate is about half of that for Americans. That food, according to Patricia Cochran, an Inupiat from northwestern Alaska, is

> seal and walrus, marine mammals that live in cold water and have lots of fat. We used seal oil for our cooking and as a dipping sauce for food. We had moose, caribou, and reindeer. We hunted ducks, geese, and little land birds like quail, called ptarmigan. We caught crab and lots of fish—salmon, whitefish, tomcod, pike, and char. Our fish were cooked, dried, smoked, or frozen. We ate frozen raw whitefish, sliced thin. The elders liked stinkfish, fish buried in seal bags or cans in the tundra and left to ferment. And fermented seal flipper, they liked that too.[11]

The greens and roots were what they harvested during short summers along with native berries, like blueberries, crowberries, and salmonberries. Despite a diet heavy on meat and fat—hardly the raw fruit, nut, vegetable, twig, and small pebble regimen hawked by today's taste Nazis—the population is extremely healthy, with low rates of cardiovascular disease. The interesting conclusion reached by Dr. Harold Draper is that "there are no essential foods—only essential nutrients. And humans can get those nutrients from diverse and eye-opening sources."[12]

In turning our gaze inward, in the typical Western diet, we derive much of our vitamin A from plant sources and vitamin D from fortified foods like milk and exposure to sunlight. Yet vitamin A and vitamin D are also readily found in the oils of coldwater fishes and sea mammals, especially in the livers.[13] Vitamin C, which humans cannot synthesize, is often obtained in the Western diet from fruits (especially citrus) and fresh vegetables. However, in doses needed to avoid diseases like scurvy, which is to say about 10 mg per day, those amounts can be obtained by meat—especially organ meat—when it is not overcooked.

Similar adaptations utilizing different foodstuffs can be found in the diet of the Maasai tribes of Africa. Their diet is based on meat, milk, and blood. The equally healthy diet of the Quechua peoples of the high Andes region conversely consists primarily of potatoes and quinoa grain. The Kuna Indians, who live off the coast of Panama, consume enormous amounts of cocoa daily—sometimes even with salt. Their daily sodium intake exceeds that of the average American. Yet they have lower-than-average blood pressure and no age-dependent decrease in their kidney function. Their cardiovascular mortality is roughly just 10 percent of other Central American peoples (9.2 versus 83.4 per 100,000 people).[14] Okinawans have one of the longest life expectancies on the planet, yet they consume lots of fresh pork and seafood and do a lot of that cooking in lard.[15]

As a physician, I do my best to heal my patients. I address symptoms and perform procedures when necessary. As an interventional cardiologist, that at times involves treating heart attacks and placing stents or other devices to open up blocked heart arteries, restore blood flow, and reverse years of damage. I try to help restore their health so they may enjoy the rest of their lives. Yet after the procedures are done and the prescriptions written, after a time, all I can give is advice and guidance. It is ultimately up to the patient. As a chef and a fellow foodie, I realize very few people are interested in salvation through deprivation. If the food on the menu doesn't taste good, no one will stick with it long term. Counseling often involves trying to establish a balance about what to eat. It also involves building a palate to appreciate flavors beyond the typical fast food culinary speedball of foods high in salt, certain types of fat, and refined sugar. Knowledge is power, and knowing this, everyone can achieve the realization that your food is your best medicine—or your worst poison.

In my study of martial arts, the first thing I was taught and the first thing I teach is not how to punch, kick, or throw your opponent. The first thing I teach is how to avoid being hit, how to avoid taking damage. In medicine we don't just treat by throwing random therapies at a patient; we acquire information and make a diagnosis. By increasing our awareness and knowledge, we can avoid the call of the junk food/fast food siren. But we still have to eat. That's why such a strategy to procure unadulterated product is so important. It does no good to avoid that siren call only to stock our own pantries with the very refined, overprocessed, prepackaged, and prepared foods we strove to shun outside our doors.

Why is it important to avoid adulterated food? Because once again it invokes the Law of Unintended Consequences. For example, the Grassroots Gourmet approach to eating healthful is not by necessarily skimping on the steak but by choosing the right kind of steak and a reasonable portion. We avoid what is offered from the Sizzlin' Salmonella Corral because it is a highly processed, adulterated, reformed meat-like creation. We procure not a just a fresh steak from the grocery store but a free-range, grass-fed product. Beef from free-range, grass-fed cattle is low in saturated fats and rich in omega-3 fatty acids and other goodies. When beef cattle are allowed to do what beef cattle do, which is walk around fields of grass and eat, what you get resembles more in composition a salmon filet than a standard megamart piece of beef. It is because of its composition that things like salmon are considered "smart and healthy" choices. Interestingly, when you subject salmon to the same treatment as beef cattle, things change. When the salmon are penned, fattened, and given antibiotics to prevent disease because they are unnaturally overcrowded, they become higher in undesirable saturated fats, lower in things like omega-3 fatty acids, and tend to lose flavor.[16]

Recently the data has been coming in to support this hypothesis about choosing less-adulterated products and including them in a tasty, enjoyable, and healthy diet. A meta-analysis from the Harvard School of Public Health was published in 2010.[17] It suggests that the cardiovascular risk associated with red meats comes primarily from the highly processed and chemically treated varieties such as bacon, sausage, hotdogs, and other processed lunch and deli meats. The nonprocessed meats examined were beef, lamb, and pork (not poultry). They examined the regular, standard, megamart options, so the difference had they examined our suggested grass-fed red meat choices might have been even more dramatic. Nonetheless, the results were impressive.

While both the highly processed and standard red meat choices contain fat, cholesterol, and saturated fat, the highly processed choices are much higher in salt, preservatives, and additives. The analysis combined data from twenty different studies involving more than 1.2 million people worldwide. The findings revealed that daily consumption of about two ounces of processed meat was associated with a 42 percent increased risk of heart disease and a 19 percent increased risk of diabetes. Conversely, a four-ounce daily serving of red meat from beef, hamburger, pork, lamb, or game did not increase the risk of heart disease, nor did it significantly increase the risk of diabetes. The rates of smoking, exercise, and other risk factors were similar between the two groups.

The study concluded people, especially those already at risk of heart problems or with high blood pressure, should consider reducing the consumption of bacon, processed ham, hotdogs, and other packaged meats that have a high salt and nitrate content. The heavily processed choices had four times the amount of sodium and 50 percent more nitrates than their unprocessed counterparts. I would add to that the processed versions also contain high levels of additional compounds and preservatives. This combination is what may have led to an unintended consequence in the effort to keep food preserved. The levels of saturated fat and cholesterol are roughly equivalent between the highly processed and unprocessed meats.

Renata Micha, a research fellow in the Harvard School of Public Health's epidemiology department and a lead author of the study, explains that there are "factors that have made all red meats potential culprits in raising the risk of cardiovascular disease. . . . But when you try to separate processed from unprocessed meats, you get an entirely different picture."[18] Victoria Taylor, senior heart health dietician at the British Heart Foundation, echoes our Grassroots Gourmet viewpoint: "If you like red meat, this can still be included as part of a balanced heart-healthy diet. . . . Aim to cook from scratch."[19] Lumping all meats together is like talking about cars in general. A Yugo and a Ferrari are both cars but very different animals. A previous meta-analysis released in March 2010 involving twenty-one different studies found that intake of saturated fat wasn't linked to a statistically significant increased risk of heart disease, stroke, or cardiovascular disease.[20]

The importance of context and whether whole foods or isolates are studied is gradually becoming understood. A recent study from the Netherlands prospectively looked at the value of omega-3 fatty acids in patients who recently had a heart attack.[21] Most of the previous recommendations showing benefit had come from smaller studies and a large meta-analysis suggesting a 20 percent to 36 percent risk reduction for animal-derived omega-3 fatty acids. Omega-3 fatty acids can be obtained from animal sources (principally marine) where they are found in the form of n-3 fatty acids, eicosapentaenoic acid (EPA), and docosahexaenoic acid (DHA). Plant sources are primarily found as n-3 fatty acid alpha-linolenic acid (ALA), and their benefit has been of borderline significance.

The study looked at more than 4,500 men and women aged sixty to eighty over a four-year period. They were given placebo margarine, an EPA-DHA–enriched margarine, an ALA-enriched margarine, or an EPA-DHA– and ALA-enriched margarine. There was no benefit to adding the omega-3 fatty acids to margarine, although there was a trend toward benefit in women receiving ALA-enriched margarine. In looking specifically at a diabetic subgroup, there appeared some benefit, especially with the EPA-DHA–enriched margarine. The authors concluded that the lack of benefit may be due to the composition of the study group, new treatments, and medicines that reduce the benefit of omega-3 fatty acids and thus make it difficult, statistically, to show a protective effect, or there simply was no benefit. I submit that an additional possibility is that, by taking the omega-3 fatty acids "out of context," additional and necessary compounds that work with these molecules were not present.

Similarly, many studies have shown health benefits for populations consuming moderate amounts of wine, yet studies with large doses of isolated antioxidants have, for the most part, not demonstrated the same level of benefit. Despite that, the conclusion consistently reached is that it is the effect of these antioxidants that are responsible for the benefit. To grow an oak tree, you need acorns. But a thousand acorns scattered in the Sahara or Antarctica will not yield any oak trees. Dumping omega-3 fatty acids in an entirely artificial construct may not yield any positive effects.

These studies do not establish a cause-and-effect relationship; it is correlative. They do, however, validate the universal truism held within the Law of Unintended Consequences. In our Grassroots Gourmet philosophy, we choose the path of least perturbation. Eat for health by realizing that what you put in your body should make you feel good afterward as well as good while you eat it. Fresh and unadulterated may not be easy, but it's pretty damn simple.

The basic techniques are likewise straightforward. They involve securing some fundamental skills and acquiring some basic knowledge so that, when it comes to ingredients, you know what you are getting as well as how to acquire it. It involves reading labels and understanding grading. Figure 9.1 is an example of blackened redfish from our blackened redfish tacos recipe. Realize that with any of these nutrition labels, there is a 20 percent variation because of the natural variation between samples. First, look at the serving size. Here, it is half of a fillet, about 100 g. The whole fish has two fillets and thus four servings. If you were to eat a whole fillet, then you would have to double all the values. Next, look at the total calories and calories from fat. The general guide to calories is

<table>
<tr><td colspan="2">Nutrition Facts</td></tr>
<tr><td colspan="2">Serving Size 1/2 fillets (99g)
Servings Per Container 4</td></tr>
<tr><td colspan="2">Amount Per Serving</td></tr>
<tr><td>Calories 120</td><td>Calories from Fat 45</td></tr>
<tr><td></td><td align="right">% Daily Value*</td></tr>
<tr><td>Total Fat 5g</td><td align="right">8%</td></tr>
<tr><td>Saturated Fat 1g</td><td align="right">6%</td></tr>
<tr><td>Trans Fat 0g</td><td></td></tr>
<tr><td>Cholesterol 65mg</td><td align="right">21%</td></tr>
<tr><td>Sodium 75mg</td><td align="right">3%</td></tr>
<tr><td>Total Carbohydrate 0g</td><td align="right">0%</td></tr>
<tr><td>Dietary Fiber 0g</td><td align="right">0%</td></tr>
<tr><td>Sugars 0g</td><td></td></tr>
<tr><td colspan="2">Protein 17g</td></tr>
<tr><td>Vitamin A 4%</td><td>•   Vitamin C 2%</td></tr>
<tr><td>Calcium 6%</td><td>•   Iron 4%</td></tr>
</table>

* Percent Daily Values are based on a 2,000 calorie diet. Your daily values may be higher or lower depending on your calorie needs.

	Calories	2,000	2,500
Total Fat	Less than	65g	80g
Sat Fat	Less than	20g	25g
Cholesterol	Less than	300mg	300mg
Sodium	Less than	2,400mg	2,400mg
Total Carbohydrate		300g	375g
Dietary Fiber		25g	30g

Calories per gram:
Fat 9 • Carbohydrate 4 • Protein 4

- 40 calories is low
- 100 calories is moderate
- 400 calories or more is high[22]

Next, look at the nutrient listing for two things. The first is the items to limit, such as sugar, salt, and fat. The second is for items to maximize, such as vitamins, fiber, minerals, and so on. Finally, note if there are any footnotes and things such as percent of daily value. Here they are shown for both a diet of 2,000-calorie- and a 2,500-calorie-per-day diet. The values per gram are also shown, so if the fillets are large, say 400 g, which is twice the size of what is listed, you can adjust accordingly. You should also be familiar with a number of terms:

- ingredient substitute: the replacement of one ingredient with another presumably similar, although not identical, ingredient
- ingredient alternative: the replacement of one ingredient with another of differing flavor, texture, or appearance
- X free: containing no or physiologically insignificant amounts of fat, saturated fat, trans fat, cholesterol, sodium, sugars, or calories, depending on the "X" labeled
- X low, little, few, or low source of: can be consumed frequently without exceeding dietary recommended guidelines for fat, saturated fat, cholesterol, sodium, or calories, depending on the "X" labeled
- low fat: less than 3 g of fat per serving
- low saturated fat: 1 g or less of saturated fat per serving; not more than 15 percent of calories from saturated fat

- low sodium: 140 mg or less per serving
- very low sodium: 35 mg or less per serving
- low cholesterol: 20 mg or less per serving
- low calorie: 40 calories or less per serving
- X reduced, less, or fewer: the nutritionally altered product contains at least 25 percent fewer calories than the reference
- light or lite: the nutritionally altered product contains at least 50 percent fewer calories than the reference
- high: 20 percent or more of the daily value of the desired nutrient per serving
- more: at least 10 percent or more of the daily value for protein, vitamins, minerals, dietary fiber, or potassium than the reference product
- good source: contains 10 to 19 percent of the daily value per serving for the specific nutrient or dietary fiber
- lean: meat, poultry, game, fish, or shellfish that contains less than 10 g of fat, less than 4 g of saturated fat, and less than 95 mg of cholesterol per serving (100 g)
- extra lean: meat, poultry, game, fish, or shellfish that contains less than 5 g of fat, less than 2 g of saturated fat, and less than 95 mg of cholesterol per serving (100 g)

Along with understanding the labeling process, it is important to understand the classification, inspection, and grading processes. As an example we will use turkey. The process is basically the same, with the labeling and some other changes based on whether it is beef, pork, poultry, or fish. There are a lot of different terms being thrown around out there. Know the lingo so you don't get a jive turkey. Table 9.1 lists the U.S. Department of Agriculture (USDA) classes of turkey and what they mean.

All these birds, indeed all poultry consumed for public consumption in the United States, are inspected. This is the round stamp on the packaging. It indicates that the products are processed under sanitary conditions fit for human consumption. It is not a measure of quality. The grading process for poultry is voluntary, so what you buy may or may not be graded. If it is graded, this is the shield-like emblem on the packaging marked A, B, or C. An A bird simply indicates it is free from deformities; has thick flesh; and is free of pinfeathers, cuts, tears, or broken bones as well as free from discoloration. It has no bearing on tenderness or flavor. The following are explanations of some other terms.

One of the first things to understand is exactly what is meant by *certified organic*. The ability to label a product "organic" or "100 percent organic" is regulated by the USDA. To meet this requirement, the food must be grown and manufactured without using any hormones, synthetic fertilizers, pesticides, and so on. To be "100 percent organic," single-ingredient foods are produced by organic methods, and foodstuffs made from more than one ingredient must be made completely from ingredients that meet the

TABLE 9.1. U.S. Department of Agriculture Classes of Turkey

Class	Description	Age	Weight (lbs.)
Fryer/Roaster	Immature bird of either sex	Younger than 16 weeks	4–9
Young	Tender bird with smooth skin	Younger than 8 months	8–22
Yearling	Mature bird with somewhat coarse skin	Older than 8 months but younger than 15 months	10–30
Mature	Older bird with coarse skin and tougher flesh	Older than 15 months	10–30

organic definition. If it is grown in soil, the soil cannot have been treated with synthetics for at least three years prior to harvest. To meet the requirements to display the "organic" label on the packaging, the product must contain at least 95 percent organic product by weight. For a processed product to be labeled "made with organic ingredients," it must contain at least 70 percent organic ingredients. Less than 70 percent, and the product may list those ingredients on the information panel but cannot use "organic" anywhere else on the packaging.[23] The USDA defines organic food as follows:

> Organic food is produced by farmers who emphasize the use of renewable resources and the conservation of soil and water to enhance environmental quality for future generations. Organic meat, poultry, eggs, and dairy products come from animals that are given no antibiotics or growth hormones. Organic food is produced without using most conventional pesticides, fertilizers made with synthetic ingredients or sewage sludge, bioengineering, or ionizing radiation. Before a product can be labeled organic, a government-approved certifier inspects the farm where the food is grown to make sure the farmer is following all the rules necessary to meet USDA organic standards. Companies that handle or process organic food before it gets to your local supermarket or restaurant must be certified, too.[24]

There are many organizations that use the terms *organic* or *natural*. Many smaller farmers and producers may adhere to organizational or USDA standards but not go through the expense and rigmarole associated with acquiring the USDA seal. Also, realize that the terms *natural, all-natural, free-range, antibiotic-free,* and so on are not regulated, and while they may be truthful, they do not necessarily have the same implications as an organic label.

Therefore, you will have to carefully read the labels. There does seem to be a bit of irony in the fact that we now have to identify and pay more for food that was produced in the fashion that most agriculture has used since farming began. However, if we are going to pay more for organic products, then we need to understand where the potential benefits lie.

Organic foods therefore are not necessarily any more nutritious than their nonorganic counterparts. There really is not any definitive data on the subject, but you should not pay more for organic food expecting it to be more nutritious. Some of what determines the product's nutritional value, especially with produce, is its freshness. So whether you buy organic or not, it is important that you shop for fresh goods. This often means looking locally and taking advantage of what is available seasonally. This type of fresh, local sourcing is often referred to as being a "localvore," and it is a practice I diligently follow and heartily recommend.

Organic foods in theory might be safer because of the limitation in terms of artificially and synthetically manufactured additives, including the routine addition of antibiotic and hormone therapy. In my opinion this lessens the effect of the Law of Unintended Consequences. Although the amount of additives may be small in each particular item, we do not have a grasp upon cumulative and long-term consequences. Although conventional produce does not exceed governmental safety thresholds, organic produce does contain significantly less pesticide residue. By definition organic products are severely restricted in the use of additives, including enhancers, extenders, preservatives, and the like. This is one of the main reasons I prefer to use organic products where and when possible. I find organic particularly useful when I use thin-skinned produce and produce where you may consume the skin, like apples and tomatoes. There may be less benefit to a thickly skinned product like grapefruit, unless you use the skin for zesting. I also like the fact that the farming practices are more in line with an approach that emphasizes a natural balance.

Does that result in tastier food? That is up to the individual. Whether a tomato is organic or not, what makes it taste spectacular is that it was allowed to ripen on the vine and was just picked from the garden. For me some items, meats in particular, taste distinctly better and are more flavorful. Again, part of that is because I look to local and fresh first, and that in and of itself is a great flavor enhancer. So while the choice to pay more and use organic product is a personal and economic one, it always makes sense to be fresh and avoid adulteration the localvore way.

There are also many other organizations that "certify organic," but they cannot display the USDA organic seal. Generally this means that

- the land on which organic food or fibers (e.g., cotton) are grown must be free of chemical additives/pesticides for three years prior to being certified

- farmers and processors must keep detailed records of methods and materials used in the production process, particularly those that replenish soil fertility
- all methods and materials are inspected annually by a third-party certifying agency (under the jurisdiction of the USDA)
- as previously indicated, products must be free of chemical additives, such as pesticides, chemical fertilizers, hormones, and antibiotics

Naturally grown indicates that the producer may prefer not to pursue an organic certification but does follow organic principles in growing produce.

Certified Naturally Grown (CNG) is a grassroots certification program created specifically for farmers who sell locally and directly to their customers. CNG's certification standards are based on the National Organic Program but with some variation.

Grass-fed/pastured animals are raised on pasture as opposed to being kept in confinement and fed primarily grains.

Heritage breed is a breed of turkey as opposed to the broad-breasted white. The broad-breasted white is what 99 percent of Americans consume on Thanksgiving. It is a quick-fattening, genetically bred bird specifically for the industrial-scale setting.[25] This bird likely would, if not slaughtered, be unlikely to survive to a mature stage; they often get so heavy that their legs collapse and they are incapable of flying, foraging, or mating. They are bred specifically for consumption. The heritage breeds were derived from the wild turkey and bred for flavor. They can forage, fly, strut, and mate (and, gosh, that's got to make for a happier bird)—in essence a "real turkey" that hasn't been supersized for another tasteless meal. Tables 9.2 and 9.3 list some additional classes for poultry.

Like poultry, grading for beef, lamb, veal, and pork is voluntary. For beef and lamb, the grading can be on the basis of quality, quantity (yield), or both. The yield for beef and lamb is a shield-like stamp that has "yield grade" and a number of 1 to 5 on it. The number 1 is the greatest yield and 5 the smallest. The yield refers to the usable amount of meat (as opposed to fat and bone) on the carcass.

The quality grades of beef consist of prime, choice, select, standard, commercial, utility, cutter, and canner. Prime beef is of limited quantity and is well marbled with a thick covering of firm fat. Choice is well marbled but with less fat than prime. The standard and select grades are less flavorful and tender than choice or prime. They are sometimes referred to as "no roll." Lower-grade beef is usually reserved for processed or ground meat products. Additional beef descriptors include "boxed," "certified Angus," and "Kobe" beef. Boxed beef generally refers to vacuum-sealed primal and subprimal cuts. Certified Angus was created in 1978. It is high-quality beef produced from descendants of Scottish Angus cattle. It is usually found as prime or high choice. Kobe beef is beef produced in Kobe, Japan, from the Wagyu cattle breed. The meat is extremely flavorful and tender

TABLE 9.2. U.S. Department of Agriculture Classes of Chicken

Class	Description	Age	Weight (lbs.)
Game hen	Young or immature progeny of Cornish chickens or of a Cornish chicken and a white rock chicken	5–6 weeks	2
Fryer/Broiler	Young with soft, smooth skin, relatively lean	13 weeks	Less than or equal to 3.8
Roaster	Young with tender meat	3–5 months	3.8–5
Capon	Surgically castrated male, tender meat	Younger than 8 months	6–10
Hen/Stewing	Mature female, flavorful but less tender	Older than 10 months	2.8–8

TABLE 9.3. U.S. Department of Agriculture Classes of Duck

Class	Description	Age	Weight (lbs.)
Fryer/Broiler	Young and tender	Younger than or up to 8 weeks	3.8–4
Roaster	Young with tender meat	Older than 8 weeks and younger than or up to 16 weeks	4–6
Mature	Old, somewhat tough	Younger than or up to 6 months	4–6

with characteristic marbling. The breed raised outside of Japan may be referred to as Wagyu- or Kobe-style, but the methods used to rear the cattle may not be identical as those used in Kobe.

Veal can be graded according to quality into prime, choice, good, standard, or utility. The meanings are the same as those applied to beef, with the good grading being somewhat analogous to select. Specific terminology regarding veal includes *formula fed* and *free range*. Formula-fed veal is fed only nutrient-rich formula. They are often kept in pens prohibiting their movement. Free-range veal refers to calves allowed to roam free and eat grass and other natural foods.

Lamb is graded as prime, choice, good, or utility with meanings the same as those for veal. An additional term usually associated with lamb but can be used with other meats is the term *frenched*. This simply refers to a trimming method whereby the eye meat is left intact while all other meat and connective tissue is removed from the rib bone of a rack or individual chops.

Pork is graded as acceptable or utility. Many pork producers use a private grading system, which in some instances is more stringent than the USDA in terms of requirements. Only acceptable is sold for consumer purchase. Utility is used in processed products.

Unlike the mandatory inspection for meat and poultry, inspection of fish and shellfish is voluntary. Inspections are done for a fee by the U.S. Department of Commerce, not the USDA. There are three types of inspection. Type 1 covers plant, product, and processing from raw to finished product. It assures a safe and properly labeled product produced under inspection at an official institution. If the products are inspected under a type 1 inspection, they receive a circular "Packed under Federal Inspection" (PUFI) stamp. Type 2 covers warehouse or storage facility locations. These usually ascertain compliance with condition, weight, labeling, and packaging. Type 3 deals only with sanitation. Seafood that has received a PUFI is eligible for grading. The grades are A, B, and C. A is the best quality, free from defects, and with good flavor and little odor. B is good quality. C is fairly good quality. Grades B and C are mostly canned or processed. Additional terms with regard to seafood include:

- fresh: is not nor ever has been frozen
- chilled: the item was held between 30 and 34 degrees Fahrenheit
- flash frozen: quickly frozen within hours of being harvested
- fresh frozen: frozen but not as quickly as flash frozen
- glazed: frozen dipped in water
- fancy: usually means previously frozen

It is clear to see that, with many confusing terms and product options, sourcing fresh, quality items can actually be a bit challenging. While there definitely seems to be a movement toward increasing access to local quality ingredients, we still seem to rely on mass production and distribution. Although the local supermarket may be convenient and a good place for staple items, really great quality items can be had with only a bit more effort. Sometimes it is a bit more money, but often there is no difference in price, or there may even be savings.

Sourcing great fruits and vegetables can be as simple as going to a local farmers' market or locating a roadside stand. Wherever you go, ask questions. Establish a relationship if you like the product, and support your local farmer. The Internet can be a great source of everything from exceptional common fare to hard-to-find items. The most amazing blood oranges I have ever had I ordered through a local harvest website from an all-organic family farm. Although the supermarket carries them, these were cheaper and unbelievable. It's like flying first class; once you experience that, you can't go back.

Most of the fish and shellfish in the large supermarket chains are imported or previously frozen. I always find a great local fishmonger and establish a personal relationship with him or her. If you have ever had food poisoning from shellfish, you will go to great lengths to ever avoid that again. Establish a relationship with your local butcher. He or she can explain "new" cuts—like the "California" cut of Alberta beef I had in Canada. The "California" comes from the same part as the traditional New York strip, just cut differently. More importantly, they can get you hormone-free, grass-fed beef with knowledge about the how, when, and where of production. I also have some other sources that supply similar meat when I need it. It may cost a little more, but I think it is worth it for the taste and quality. I'd rather have something a little less often and have a quality experience than a whole lot of mediocre.

Grow what you can, even if it's just some fresh herbs in the windowsill. Try to source product locally for freshness and quality when you can. If we look at the locally produced or more artisanal methods of production, if they deliver on their promise of superior product, we should consider spending the bit extra. Supporting these endeavors helps us in the long run. And there are ways to be economical about it as well. For example, I prefer a free-range, vegetarian-fed chicken. The meat actually has flavor. My butcher gets these for me, and they cost more than a ghetto bird raised in one of those atrocious, stinky avian tenements. If you don't have access to a butcher, with the Internet you can access quality producers who can overnight these items. I get a whole bird, butcher it myself, and in the end spend as much as, if not less than, buying some breasts, thighs, and so on as separate parts. I use the bird, beak to tail, and nothing goes to waste. Any leftover carcass is used for stocks and such. Chickens are easy to butcher, and with a little practice, it takes no more than ten minutes, if that.

While you do not have to be a culinary graduate to master Grassroots Gourmet cooking, some basic knowledge, methods, and techniques are extremely helpful. It's like being an EMT or paramedic. While you don't have to go to medical school, if you're going to be transporting in the ambulance, you should know at least some CPR.

As for techniques, basic knife skills are always a good starting point. If you are going to invest in only one thing in your kitchen, arm yourself with a really good chef's knife— not an infomercial crap special but a real, honest-to-goodness chef's knife. A word of experience here: I have gotten many cuts in the kitchen. Universally, the worst ones have been from using a cheap, dull blade. A dull blade causes you to exert more pressure to try to cut. The cheap knives often have a poor center of balance as well. The combination results in wounds. A sharp chef's knife is much safer, but make no mistake, it requires respect. I have a Global chef's knife I finally bought after years of procrastination. I look back now and don't know how I survived without it. Splurge; when you can count to ten on all your fingers years from now, you'll be glad you did.

How to hold the knife appears to be a no-brainer, but you would be surprised how many people have no clue as to how to do this properly. There are a few simple grips. Just pick one you are comfortable with using. I use what is probably the most common grip; I grasp the handle with my fingers and grip the spine (back end) of the blade between my thumb and index finger. Another grip is to use all fingers to grip the handle with your thumb against the flat portion on the front of the blade. Do not grip the blade as you would a sword or bat because it becomes difficult to exert fine, directional control of the blade. Even with a grip that allows fine, directional control, you want to protect the fingers on your nongripping hand. When you cut something, keep your fingers on the nonknife hand curled back. This prevents you from cutting the tips off your fingers. Finally, when you are chopping, slicing, and dicing, you want to either keep the tip of the blade fixed as a fulcrum or keep the heel fixed and using a rocking motion cut at the tip. As you use either the tip or heel as the fulcrum, there is a gentle rocking motion forward and back with each cut.

The best way to acquire knife skills, like anything else, is to practice. You do not need to know every single kind of cut in the chef's arsenal, but it is good to be familiar with some of the more common cuts and terms. You need to be able to read a basic recipe and understand what it is asking you to do. For example, you should know the difference between slicing, chopping, mincing, and dicing, as they are all forms of cutting something.

Slicing means to cut something into thin pieces. A common form of slicing is something called a chiffonade. A chiffonade is often used to slice things like basil. Take the leaves, reach back into your high-school memory (or more recent memory, depending on where you live), and roll it like you're going to smoke it. Holding the rolled herb, slice across it. The other common slicing method is to butterfly. This often used to prepare shrimp or other meats. Here you take the item to cut, say a boneless pork chop, and place the palm of your noncutting hand on top. Arch your fingers upward while applying a gentle downward pressure to fix the item in position. Hold the knife parallel to the cutting surface and cut the item almost in half. Now if you pull the chop open, you should have two identically shaped halves of equal thickness attached together by a thin band of uncut meat. It should resemble a butterfly.

Chopping simply means to cut into small pieces. The exact size and uniformity are not important. Mincing just means to finely chop, in other words, cut into very small pieces. Dicing means to cut into cubes. This is when uniformity of size and shape is important. Having things about the same size is important not only for aesthetics but also for even cooking. Things of different sizes cook at different rates given the same heat, so when we use a particular cooking technique, to properly cook all of the pieces of our particular item, they need to be uniform. The way to do this is simple. You first slice an item into a particular length and thickness. The most common are julienne, which is roughly ⅛ inch × ⅛ inch × 2 inches long (3 mm × 3 mm × 5 cm long), and batonnet, which is roughly ¼ inch × ¼ inch × by 2 inches long (6 mm × 6 mm × 5 cm long). These slices are then laid together and a final cut is performed to form cubes. If the cut is ⅛ inch (making a ⅛ inch × ⅛ inch × ⅛ inch cube) it is called brunoise. If the cut is ¼ inch to make a ¼ inch × ¼ inch × ¼ inch cube, it is called a small dice. You can also dice larger if you need.

To properly cook the food we have prepared, we need to recognize a few different methods. Basically, there are two ways to cook, a dry method or a wet method. The easy way to remember is that wet uses water or water in steam form. Everything else is dry. Deep frying is considered a dry method because it uses fat, like oil, to cook. Common dry methods include broiling, grilling, roasting, baking, sautéing, pan frying, and deep frying. Broiling and grilling are opposites of the same method. Broiling employs an overhead heat source. Grilling employs an equally hot heat source but from the bottom. Roasting and baking are essentially the same thing. Both apply to cooking by surrounding the item with dry, heated air in a closed environment. The term *baking* is generally used for fish, fruits, starches, breads, and pastries. *Roasting* generally applies to meats or poultry, although it seems in vogue to serve roasted vegetables. Sautéing is a dry heat method that uses high heat applied to a sauté pan with a small amount of fat added. Pan frying is the same thing with just more fat added. It is somewhere between sautéing and deep frying. Deep frying really needs no explanation if you live in the United States or the United Kingdom.

Common wet methods include poaching, simmering, boiling, and steaming. Poaching uses water at between 160 and 180 degrees Fahrenheit to cook food. Just for the record, you poach at 160 to 180 degrees, simmer at 185 to 205 degrees, and boil at 212 degrees Fahrenheit. So add a thermometer to your Christmas wish list if you ever want to get this right. If you are steaming items, place them in a basket or something that places them above the water that is boiling and turning to steam, otherwise you're boiling as well.

Two common combination methods include braising and stewing. Braising generally involves sautéing an item first to develop some flavor and color by browning. A liquid or sauce is then added about one-third to halfway up the sides and the item finished with a low, slow cook. Stewing is basically the same process. The difference is that the items browned are usually smaller pieces and they are then completely covered in liquid.

Whatever method is called for, a commonly ignored factor is carryover cooking. The tendency is to cook on the stovetop, grill, or oven until 100 percent done. The item is then removed. The problem here is what is known as carryover cooking. The cooked item still contains the residual heat once it is removed from the heat source. It will continue to cook for a bit even when removed, especially if you just remove the pan from the heat and leave the items in it. This results in food that is consistently overcooked; fish is a classic example. The trick, through practice, is to realize that the items need to actually be removed from the heat a tick shy of being done. When you are looking for a certain temperature, remove the item 5 to 10 degrees prior to reaching that desired temperature. The carryover will finish the cooking, and it will be perfect. Now we are ready to properly enjoy our repast.

on time and in proportion

> "We have more ability than will power, and it is often an excuse to ourselves that we imagine that things are impossible."
>
> —François de la Rochefoucauld

IT'S HARD to change. I think everyone can agree on that. Certainly all my patients over the years have let me know that in no uncertain terms. Despite warning, cajoling, begging, and demanding, people often refuse to change behaviors that they intellectually know are detrimental in the long run. Even when confronted by death in a very personal way—like you were actually dead—people resist changes. I took care of a woman so addicted to cigarettes she could not stop. The first time I met her was in the emergency room at 1 a.m. She presented in cardiogenic shock, which is medical-ese for damn near dead (DND). Her systolic blood pressure was around 80 mmHg (the normal is around 120 mmHg), she was having all kinds of abnormal heart rhythms, and she was barely conscious. Her right coronary artery was 100 percent blocked. We opened the artery up quickly and restored normal blood flow. We also put a stent, a type of metal tube to help the artery stay open, in her right coronary artery, and she recovered completely after a few days. Despite being so close to the light that she received a tan, the lady still would not quit smoking cigarettes. Over the next three weeks, she came into the hospital DND three times. Every time it was within hours of lighting up a coffin nail. If "Reaper, Grim" shows up on your e-Harmony perfect compatibility match based on your lifestyle choices, it's you who needs to make a change. The individual has got to want it for themselves. Someway, somehow you have got to find that self-motivation. If you do not initiate some type of transformation, then by the process of elimination you're adhering to the status quo. That status quo is a commitment to self-eradication. You're as committed to the "die early and leave a good-looking corpse" philosophy as the pig is to breakfast. When you have eggs and bacon for breakfast, the chicken—well, she's involved; the pig—now he's committed.

I've seen this stuff up close and personal. I consider it a real bit of good fortune to be involved in people's lives in such an intimate way. As an interventional cardiologist, I look for and treat diseased arteries, and I've gotten to see the pathology from a number of perspectives. I have seen the entire gamut of the disease process. I've seen miracles and unspeakably difficult tragedy. There have been times I've thanked God, and there have been times I wondered if God even existed. I have seen people given reprieves, young people escape big heart attacks with no residual damage. I've seen people beyond repair, hearts with massive damage and no options, surgical, medical, or otherwise. I have seen mothers die weeks after childbirth from peripartum cardiomyopathy. Intellectually and practically, I treat people with cardiovascular disease. I know the data, the numbers, and the facts. I understand the science. I do my best to communicate that information to my patients in a way they can understand. I give them the best advice I can and try to guide their decisions with respect for both their needs and their wants. I evaluate them as thoroughly as possible. I try to fix the deficiencies, pathologies, and anomalies to the best of my ability, but ultimately it comes down to the patient. It comes down to the individual. It is their choice, as Yoda noted, to either do or do not—there is no try.

As best I could, I always chose to be present at as many martial arts seminars as was feasible to continue to enhance my progress. I remember attending a martial arts function in my early twenties. I think it was a *tai kai*, which can roughly be translated from the Japanese as "big party." The *tai kais* then were the occasion where the *soke*, or grandmaster, would come over from Japan and teach outside of Japan for a couple of days. He always seemed to make a stop on the tour somewhere in the United States, and I would always try to attend, if logistically possible. It was a big event. There would be a hotel ballroom or equivalent venue for three to four hundred students who would show up from around the world to learn and train. I specifically remember him talking about mastering the Art. He spoke about not even remotely considering mastering anything until you were at least forty years old. Although forty is a bit of an arbitrary number (Japanese always loses something in translation), it was, I believe, used figuratively to represent half a lifetime. That's a long time. He continued speaking, telling us we needed to "just keep going." As an impatient twenty-something, I was indignant. Of course I could master this and anything else for that matter; isn't that the mindset you're supposed to teach in martial arts? Conquer quickly without fear or remorse? It was as if he could read my mind or sense the indignation in the room. He remarked that we were like children who thought we knew the world but in truth had no worldliness about us. In short, as all good cooks know, we needed a little seasoning. Just as a great meal is built in flavor levels that must be properly seasoned at each stage, so must we be properly seasoned with each experience as we move forward in life. Only then will we have the depth of experience upon which to start to grasp the essence of the Art. Only by acquiring this understanding could we appreciate the Art as a living thing. He went on to comment that this understanding of vitality was necessary before we could even hope to grasp basic technique.

Almost thirty years later, I continue to try to grasp basic technique. During my studies I came across some writings attributed to Miyamoto Mushashi, arguably the greatest Japanese swordsman who ever lived. He fought more than sixty duels and never lost. Many were life-and-death matches, and he fought many using a wooden sword, even if his opponent used a real one. He also became an artisan whose writings, paintings, carvings, and castings remain priceless today. He had been asked about how he could paint and carve so well, how he could be such a talented artist, when all he had ever studied was the way of the warrior, *budo*. He answered, after long reflection, that it was because it was all the same, all derived from the same source. I see, as usual, that *soke* was right. I now appreciate that the feeling cannot be separated from the action. You cannot remove the mapmaker from the map. There is no technique without vitality. There is no way to express vitality without perfect technique. Like yin and yang, *in* and *yo*, heads and tails, they are different reflections of the same coin.

Like the big bang theory in which the universe at its origin was a singularity, the *in* and *yo* must converge. I spoke of cooking a perfect risotto with a chef at a local Italian restaurant not too long ago. It reminded me of my lessons from the martial arts. No matter how fast you wanted it done or the customer wanted to eat it, to be perfect it had to arrive in its own time, the perfect risotto time. Too long and it might finish a pasty mush; force it too quickly and it may be like a plate of crunchy gravel. There I realized that cooking, medicine, martial arts, really any endeavor in which we engage with our passion, comes from a single place, a single source. It comes from a singularity. We are supplied with strength, speed, and resilience when we are young because we need it to survive. At that point in our lives, we do not have the wisdom of which *soke* spoke, which now seems so long ago that recalling it is like listening for echoes. It is this youthful abundance of reserves that allows us to survive despite our errors in judgment and execution. We need the time to become seasoned and acquire and utilize superior wisdom. But this grace period is not the unlimited checkbook the real housewives on Bravo seem to have; this bill comes due. It often comes due with interest like some forgotten credit card purchase that shows up six months later. The ability to avoid those debts comes from gaining that life experience and life flexibility to make the necessary changes. That insight is only acquired by living and paying attention. It is achieved by focusing on the now and understanding that what we got by with at an earlier time does not allow us to assume that we have a free pass to continue to do the same. Just because you could eat and drink whatever you wanted without repercussion when you were twenty doesn't mean you can do it at forty.

I've studied the martial arts for more than thirty years. It has provided a very direct motivation to me for staying in reasonable shape and more importantly for me to listen to my body. My technique is not the same as it was when I was twenty. I am older, slower, and less flexible, among many other things. If my technique had not changed, adapted, and matured, I would have very little left. This is the difference between some sports and Arts. In some sports once the physical gifts start to fade, you're done. My martial skill is much better than it was all those years ago despite losing some of the physical aspects. This is the way of Art if you "keep going." An interesting thing about treating patients with heart disease is that it appears to be something older patients really respond well to compared to younger patients. Advising people about their health seems to rely on them having a bit of life experience, a bit of seasoning. It is, unlike most things in America, not really a young man's game. Perhaps it is just that the patients need to understand that the veil of invincibility we wear so well in our youth is a removable garment. A successful plan requires that you think about not only the immediate pleasure/consequences, but how will it make you feel for the long haul. It requires an understanding of expenditure. It requires that one appreciate, however subtly, that this one action creates a reaction. This is what lifestyle choices are about. What I have noticed is that when patients make choices regarding a diet, they often view them as isolated diet choices, not really lifestyle choices or even modifications.

These are important choices we make along the way. Some may call them compromises. I do not think you should compromise your principles, but there are decisions that allow you to enjoy the best of both things. In the martial arts, you must adapt and change. If you don't adapt, you will get your ass kicked, or worse, in the most public and humiliating way possible. And if it doesn't kill you, it will hurt—bad. And I'm not talking just about the pride aspect. I still carry my share of training scars from which I have learned. I also, like everyone else, carry my share of other battle scars. I have also battled my weight since I was a little pudger having to shop for pants in the Sears' "husky boy" section. Despite the pediatric trauma, I still like to eat. I like to eat food that tastes good. As a result I can appreciate the struggles on a personal note. But I think we have to realize that we can have the food that tastes good if we are willing to understand the relationship between quality and quantity.

Within the realm of my culinary experience, I find that the concepts of quantity and quality are like the martial concepts of *in* and *yo*, yin and yang. The best meals strike a balance. Let me explain some definitions here. When I speak of quality in this sense, I am not referring to the quality of the ingredients. As a Grassroots Gourmet, we always want to use the highest-quality individual components. When I speak of quality here, I speak of the composition of the entire meal. A quality meal has components of fat, salt, and sugar for all the reasons we have discussed. It has fiber, fresh veggies, and exquisite subtleties of flavor. It is a quality meal, perfectly balanced and delicious. To provide us the nutrition without causing waistline addition, it must be served in the proper portion. The quantity must act to help balance the quality. Without the balance of proper portions, we become grassroots gluttons.

People make choices like this for things every day. Whole advertising campaigns, markets, product developments, and economies utilize these principles. Here is an example: If you had one thousand dollars to spend on your TV purchase and you could buy either fifty black-and-white TVs or a new big-screen LED HDTV, which would you buy? Most folks would choose the HDTV because although the quantity is less, the long-term enjoyment from this TV beats having old black-and-white TVs everywhere, even if you could have a black-and-white TV in every room and positioned so that you could watch TV without moving. When it comes to eating strategies, it is as if people choose to try to have fifty LED HDTVs.

One of the key concepts in learning to prepare delicious food that you can continue to partake of on a regular basis is learning portion control. Avoiding the siren call of fast food and junk food is important. Learning how to prepare a delicious meal with fresh ingredients that delivers a satisfying essence while maintaining food fidelity is also important. So is retraining our taste buds to appreciate, crave, and savor those very subtle flavors. Yet it is all for naught if we cannot learn to limit ourselves appropriately. Portion size is one reason the U.S. population is suffering an obesity epidemic with more than one third of the United States classified as obese and a full two thirds as overweight or obese.[1]

I remember vividly my first trip to Japan. We were in Tokyo for a bit, and we stayed near the very first McDonalds to open in Japan. It was weeks old. The lines were out the door and down the street. I remember many women in traditional dress, kimono, obi, and geta, walking the streets. I recall a generally fit and handsome population. One thing that struck me was how glowing their skin was, men, women, boys, and girls. Now, I return quite often for continued martial arts training. If I look now with fresh eyes, I see fast food on every corner. I see an overweight, generally unhealthy population. I look at the adolescents, many overweight and with terrible acne. I see everything being supersized. In essence, I see America. America has done wonderful things that we should be proud of: exporting freedom, democracy, technology, innovation, and many other praiseworthy things. But like a plague rat on a ship, we also exported a hidden death. I found it ironic in looking at Japan, which has embraced all things American, that the kamikaze lifestyle is actually an American creation.

And size does matter—a lot. Forget everything that you've ever heard from men with small penises. Smilin' Bob ain't smiling because he just won two tickets to the Donnie and Marie reunion tour. He's smiling because he can club the competition, literally. So size matters, and bigger is generally better, except here. In this instance, smaller is better. Cut down the portions. Many people eat like they are competing for a role in *Man vs. Food*. Try to focus on the bigger picture, not a bigger picture of yourself. Think not only of how the meal will make you feel now but how you feel afterward. It's focusing on the now (I am enjoying this meal) with a bit of seasoned wisdom (but I am satiated with this small serving—I do not need more). In fact, more in this situation will end up being less because it will make you feel like a heap of dung later on. That is grassroots gluttony.

How do we achieve this? Serve an appetizer-size portion for the first or starter. Serve a slightly larger but reasonable size for the entrée. The human body is about 60 percent water. Consume lots daily. I recommend a glass (8 oz.) of water prior to the meal, or at least with the starter. Also keep a glass of water with the main as well, even if you are having a glass of wine or something else to drink. The daily recommended water consumption is 64 oz. Just remember the 8×8 rule: eight glasses of 8 oz. each. Daily caloric intake for the average woman is 2,200 kcals (what we refer to as a calorie is actually a kilocalorie, or 1,000 calories) and 2,900 kcals for the average man. The urge to eat and grab some calories before we really need to is an ancient, hardwired, survival mechanism. We are biologically programmed to eat before we really need to get looking for food. We want to eat before the body starts to break down its reserves of fat and protein. Because we were originally an omnivorous scavenger, protein was likely a luxury when we could get it. Fat was a survival lotto supplying the most available energy per gram at 9 kcal/g. So as previously mentioned, our metabolism and biological predilections are predisposed to a dining opportunity different from what exists today.

Healthy eating in the midst of plenty requires some planning, focus, and execution. It is like knowing how to enjoy some wine without having to wake up face down in front of the porcelain altar every time you pour a glass. Where appropriate I've included recommended serving sizes along with the nutritional information at the ends of recipes to provide some guidance. Caloric information is provided as well. Adding calories is not really a challenging higher-math problem. Use both as guides. You can have your cake and eat it, too. You just need to eat it one slice at a time and not all at one sitting.

Einstein showed there is no isolated space without time, nor time isolated from space. It is one unalterable reality known as space-time. The space within our bellies is filled by the proportions we ingest. In the culinary world, that reality is proportion-time, and it, too, is an unavoidably linked proposition. From an evolutionary perspective, it was once advantageous to seek the biggest portion possible; more is more desirable than less.[2] That holds true when you do not know when your next meal may be found. Lions and other wild carnivores can gorge themselves on a fresh kill because that is perhaps their last meal for a while. The built-in time delay between the onset of gorging and the satiety signal allows them to pack away reserves. We still have that Stone Age set of wiring.

We have seen how that actuality can be perverted against us by altering the food products so that you end up eating much more in a shorter amount of time. During the time you eat, the proportions you are served go way beyond what is needed to properly satiate your hunger. If a rat receives two pellets of food, it will eat them. If a person gets two scoops of ice cream, it will be consumed in its entirety. As Kessler notes, "Portion size matters."[3] The fact that *to supersize* is now an accepted verb really says it all.[4] But it's not just the portion; it's the timing as well.

I remember watching *Schoolhouse Rock* growing up. There was the bill named Bill, conjunction junction, and that place where Lolly got her adverbs quickly. That series ran concurrently with some spots about a guy named Timer. He was this yellow amoeboid-looking thing with a huge pointy nose and pencil-thin arms and legs. He wore a ridiculous-looking cowboy hat and bandana around his neck, and he was always hanging around, hankering for a hunk of cheese. There were times when he even wore a bowtie and top hat. Either way he looked like a cartoon member of the Village People. To this day I am not sure exactly what he was supposed to be, but symbolically I suppose he represented our biological sense of timing—timing in that it is now time to eat, now time to stop eating, now time to sleep, and so on. He promoted eating when you're hungry and offered some healthy choices for snacks and other tips to help prevent overeating. He was utilizing the concept of timing and proportion. This was more than thirty years ago. Today Timer's message is even more needed and relevant, but that message seems to have been silenced. We find today that Timer is missing in action. We are eating all the time, often when we are not that hungry. Even if we prepare healthy food in reasonable portions, it does us no good if we stuff our faces nonstop. People should eat, not graze. So I ask, "Who the hell killed Timer?"

I wonder if he was done in by that pocket watch that he carried around. We have become slaves to schedules and appointments. With the ever-increasing availability of information and access to each other, it has become a 24/7/365 nonstop rat race. The longer you work, the longer you work. There are really very few ending points for days anymore, as the task list is endless. Only five o'clock Margaritaville time and Jimmy Buffet bring any sanity and relief these days. If we are lucky, we have thirty minutes to eat lunch, whether we are hungry or not. We have a dinner meeting at 7 p.m., whether we feel hunger pangs or not. We wake up and are told to eat a hearty breakfast, whether we are hungry or not. I am not a breakfast guy. Generally, being an early bird, it's a pot o' joe for me until late morning. However, I was reading an article by the venerable Dr. Oz, and he spoke of the importance of breakfast. Now, whether you are a true believer or really pay no attention to the man behind the surgical mask, Dr. Oz does raise an interesting discussion point. He states his usual breakfast is "steel-cut oatmeal, usually mixed with raisins, walnuts, and flaxseed oil."[5] Now that may be a little too much granola for some, but I think his general concept is right, with one important caveat. As I mentioned before, when I get up early, I am not hungry. But once in a blue moon, I do get the munchies in the morning. I recommend listening to your body. That whisper of hunger is the ghost of Timer, and I try to channel him. In general, I eat when I am hungry, not at specific times during the day. Eating at a consistently fixed time can set up an expectation response. Eating becomes a habit that is a function of the time, not of an actual need to eat. At a certain time, you feel you are hungry because it is time to eat. You eat because it is 6 p.m. and you always eat at this time. You look at the clock and see it is 6 p.m., so now you say, "I need to be hungry. I need to eat." You dine on a schedule instead of eating when you are hungry. If you can, allow some flexibility around the dinner hour so it is served when everyone is hungry. If you simply can't adhere to this schedule, then allow some light snacking beforehand for those who need it but reduce their dinner portions. Many studies have shown that obese people actually eat less frequently than the average person. Although they eat less frequently, they consume substantially more than they need to at a single sitting. They may only eat one dessert, but it's the whole damned cake. That kind of behavior is what you want to avoid. That is why many weight loss and diet programs encourage multiple episodes of small snacking throughout the day.

So if you're like me and not a breakfast person when you get up, don't eat if you don't want to eat. Where I think Dr. Oz has a valid point is that when you do get hungry in the morning, this is the perfect time for a sensible snack or meal. I may not really want an apple or banana for dessert after dinner, but as a mid-morning stop on the Crazy Train, it makes perfect sense; even a quick bowl of healthy cereal or oats, granola, and so on, is not only tolerable but can be quite delicious this time of day. So whatever time of the morning is right for your "breakfast," eat it then. The term *breakfast* literally means to break the fast from sleeping the night before, thus whenever you eat the first meal after arising it is, by definition, breakfast.

If you indulge in a champagne Sunday brunch from time to time, that's OK, too. Unlike marriage, successful fidelity in nutrition is a function of frequency, not absolution. Statistics say that roughly between 60 percent of men and 40 percent of women have cheated on their spouses. The numbers who have cheated on their weight loss regimens and general diets, based on the 95 percent diet failure rate in some studies, must make this number pale by comparison. Fortunately for us it is okay to satisfy our extra-nutritional yearnings in an occasional Romanistic orgy of gustatory pleasure. The key is frequency. A "night out" a few times a year for holidays and celebrations (let's say 10 percent of the time, or roughly thirty-six days a year) will not, I think, negatively impact your overall health. A caveat, of course, is that you can't do all thirty-six in a row. Then you become an addict like Morgan Spurlock after he spent thirty McContinuous days being supersized. Allow yourself the rewards of the occasional guilty encounter. By keeping it sporadic, you can keep enjoying the thrill of the affair, which is often based in its very nature of infrequent and emotionally charged rendezvous.

There are simply times you want or need to heed the call of a food vacation. In his book, *How the Irish Saved Civilization*, Thomas Cahill describes how the original Catholic Church confession process was originally a very public two-strikes program. Before the Irish advent of private confession, "sin was thought to be a very public matter, a crime against the Church. . . . Penance was a once-in-a-lifetime sacrament: second theft, a second adultery and you were . . . irreversibly excommunicated."[6] He goes on to comment that the Irish made "all confession a completely private affair between penitent and priest . . . on the theory that, oh well, *everyone* pretty much sinned just about *all* the time."[7] This is an important realization because almost all of us will fall. It is important not to become guilt obsessed or quit the program. I have asked many fitness experts, trainers, and exercise physiologists about training or exercising when people go on vacation. Should people do it? The near universal response is no. The down time, the recharging time, is as important as the training time in the long run. There is an analogous martial arts "sickness" that one can get from overtraining. In addition to the physical maladies, one can lose perspective and suffer illness of mind and spirit. In the martial arts, we say, "Keep going." It's the getting up and continuing forward on the path that is important.

That's because if you use this time correctly, I believe it can help you eat more responsibly the rest of the year. The only certainties, they say, are death and taxes. We must eat to live, and living is a prerequisite to be involved in the former certainty. If we pay taxes, then we must also work, a prerequisite to the latter certainty. Having a guilt-free fun feast is like a dietary holiday. But you can't go on holiday endlessly. We often plan to enjoy our holidays by perhaps doing some extra work before you leave or a little catch-up when you return—we schedule. Perhaps we also put away a little savings beforehand for extra "fun" money while we vacation—we budget. You schedule and budget beforehand to afford a proper vacation. The key is you plan for the time off, budget responsibly, and accommodate. Multiple studies have shown that to be the best worker, one needs some vacation:

- Taking time off work, however short, is necessary in maintaining the stress levels of work and home life. Workers who are under extreme stress experience headaches, irritability, eyestrain, digestive disorders, and panic attacks, which all directly lead to less productivity.

- Employees who work ten to twelve hours per day are significantly less productive and efficient than employees who work six to six and a half hours a day, according to a long-term study done by the Organizational Psychology Program at Rutgers Graduate School of Applied and Professional Psychology.[8] The most effective executives (a high-stress and high-demand position) take mini-breaks throughout the day to give their brains a rest. This is not to say those who work less or take multiple breaks throughout the day are lazier than their counterparts but that the human brain and mind become tired and less efficient while focusing for an extended period of time. To be more efficient, workers should take time to stare out the window, take a walk, or even make a phone call to a friend.
- Taking time away from work does not just improve productivity; it also improves a person's health. People who take vacations are more positive and healthier, as many studies show.[9]

So if you know you are going on a food holiday, make the necessary plans for it just as you would plan for a holiday away from work. Plan it, enjoy it, and then back on the path. Learn to listen to your inner Timer. It turns out Timer is not dead, just strung out, but we can close our eyes and bring him back.

We're talking about some simple, time-related concepts. Take time to taste your food. Sounds simple enough, but watch a few people chow a supersized, double-stuffed, extra-bacon McMortem sometime, and you'll realize that to consume that volume in that time frame they actually must defy known physics. It is as if they create a miniature black hole within the space of their pie hole. They are literally sucking in the tasteless matter, and all available light, into that maw. There is no way they tasted anything; if they did, they wouldn't inhale that stuff in the first place. It is interesting to note that in some forms of meditative practice, they actually address this issue. They tell their practitioners to chew the food slowly, savoring and acknowledging the taste by chewing between eighteen and thirty-six times for each bite. Try it sometime; it's like a dietary caution lap. The practice of light snacking between meals also helps keep us from overeating. Finally, consider time between courses. It takes at least twenty to twenty-five minutes for your stomach to tell your brain you're full. The time you allow from a first course to the main course helps you to develop some feeling of satiety before the main course.

Timing goes hand in hand with portion size. Using timing correctly as you dine also allows you to use portion control. Portion control, I believe, is one of the most neglected contributors to dietary-related issues out there. We seem to want to supersize everything. To counteract that supersizing urge, serve that appetizer, or first, before your main meal of the day. It can be a salad, fruit, cheese, bread, soup, or more complex offerings like risotto. Conversely, if you don't offer a first, then serve a light dessert course consisting of a small dessert portion after a well-proportioned main course. I generally keep my protein servings to 4 to 6 oz. per person. I increase the sides, which are usually a starch and veggie of some kind as needed.

Remember: It will take about twenty minutes for your stomach to tell your head you're full. Slow down, enjoy the meal, and sip the wine. Enjoy the experience. Even if it's just a meal for one, take some time to reflect on your day. As soon as you start to feel full, then stop eating. I am not sure what the clean plate club, what me finishing all my food, had to do with starving kids in Africa when I was growing up. Somehow my mother was convinced this would end famine. It just made me fat.

We are often in a rush in our fast-paced, needed-to-be-there-twenty-minutes-ago world. On the run from appointment to appointment, we stuff our gullets like Kobayashi on the Fourth of July. We have become a nation of not only "supersize me" but also of "I want that 'supersize me' ten minutes ago." Thus what originated in our genes as a recipe for survival becomes in our contemporary world a recipe for disaster in our jeans.

Learn to be on time and in proportion; allow the time for the stomach to signal the brain it has started to eat; consume reasonable portions that will appropriately engage our satiety response. It allows Timer to do his job and hit the "off" switch as well as the "on" switch. He likes to be useful; it keeps him out of rehab.

chapter eleven

food porn

"The difference between pornography and erotica is lighting."

—Gloria Leonard

THE HUMAN animal is exactly that: an animal at heart. We may clothe ourselves in the thin cloak of civility, but we still indulge our animal instincts. NASCAR is reportedly one of the fastest-growing and largest spectator sports, but if you are not rooting for your driver to cross the finish line first, you're rooting for the others to wreck, and wreck big time. It's no more than a twenty-first-century circus maximus. The fans may tote beer instead of togas, but the emotional experience seems much unchanged. It is a primal catharsis through violent voyeurism. These basic instincts are visible even at the international governmental level, where it is pack dominance that rules the day. As a nation we may try diplomacy first, which I think is a good idea, but we probably do it first because talk is a lot cheaper than tanks and bullets and there are no body bags. Yet if at the end of the day we don't get our way and we're sure we can kick their ass, we do. Ultimately it does become a "might makes right" philosophy. After we beat the hell out of them and destroy their country, then we give them money so we don't feel guilty about it. If I do the same thing to that guy down the street, I get arrested and sued. The logic falls under what my mother used to tell me: "It's because I'm your mother, that's why I can." At all levels from international to individual, our animal instincts drive us.

We have discussed the evidence of how our biological hardwired animal instincts affect our desires, cravings, and food choices. When they dictate our behavior, we can wind up with junk food addiction. But you can't just cage the beast. Repression and deprivation don't work long term. Many diets don't work long term exactly because repression and deprivation are the cornerstones of their programs. They may work over the first few months, but then the majority of participants gain the weight back and revert to previous habits of consumption. Data suggests that up to 95 percent of those dieting to lose weight regain it within one to five years.[1] Diets are a like a focused sprint when in actuality you're running a marathon. It's a pace you can't sustain for the duration of the event. These diets also often require an abrupt change. There is a sudden onset that focuses on immediate deprivation for some future goal. The motivation for this goal is usually some form of fear/threat: You must do X and avoid Y, or you will die.

We hear this dietic diatribe issued forth like an edict from government hallows and the sacred halls of medical academia. The high priests of Medicine preach what you must avoid and where and what you must do, lest you endure a fall from grace and suffer eternal damnation in the emergency room, where like Sisyphus you are brought to an exam room only to be bumped to the back of the line to wait again because another emergency has just arrived. But this is fear mongering: fear of death, disease, disability, or disfigurement. Fear mongering of any type, while it may be initially motivating, is never a successful, long-term strategy. This is especially true when many people who need to make changes are older. To them the idea of total deprivation of many of the things they have enjoyed their entire life for the few days of a now-miserable existence (occurring years down the road, mind you) becomes a very short film at the Short Attention Span Theater. This is the kind of advice that transforms Grandma and Grandpa into total GOBs (grumpy old bastards). After life's grand journey of a thousand miles, you ask them to sprint the last fifty yards, and after they sprint those fifty yards, they're done—because they're dead. But wasn't that last fifty yards really good for them? They burst across the finish line a geriatric model of health. Depending on the situation, I may just choose to cross the finish line in my jazzy, with a cup holder for my margarita. Again, it comes down to an understanding of the need for balance. Life is truly about making a journey and enjoying it along the way. Lifestyle choices are about how you feel now and down the road *and* where you are on that road.

We must keep perspective depending on where we are. It's about the whole journey, not just focusing on one stop to visit the world's biggest double cheeseburger and evil clown at exit 666. It involves balance, both in the balancing of time (past reactions, present experiences, and future consequences) and the balancing of quality and quantity.

Sometimes we seem stuck in that "more is better" mantra. Here's some free medical advice: "Yes, gravy with that" or "Yes, please do super-duper-size me for only $0.39

more" is not always the correct answer. Trust me: I'm a doctor. And trust David Kessler, an M.D. and former FDA commissioner, who has several pertinent observations in his book *The End of Overeating: Taking Control of the Insatiable American Appetite*.[2] He remarks that we must change how people in the United States look at food. I couldn't agree more. George Santayana said that "habit is stronger than reason."[3] I would add that instinct is stronger than habit. Thus we must not only change the way we look at food but also engage in an honest dialogue with ourselves regarding what we need for daily sustenance and what we desire that results from the impulse of gustatory self-gratification. We must come to terms in a realistic way to balance the two.

We can acknowledge and control the impulses. That is what sets the human animal apart. You may want to smack your loudmouth neighbor in the face sometimes, but you don't. That's the veneer of civility. When we use our brains to manage the food impulses and we don't drink the entire gravy boat, it's that same principle. It is culinary civility. We acknowledge and manage those instincts every day. Those instincts include the desire for sex and candy. They include "food porn."

Pornography (not the food kind) is a big business. Estimates range anywhere from more than $2.5 billion to $14 billion per year in sales.[4] Dietary supplements are an industry of similar size, with annual sales estimated around $16 billion.[5] The fast food and food service industries had sales estimated at $560 billion in 2009.[6] The market for appealing to our baser instincts in sex and candy is huge.

What is food porn? What is the difference between indulging in food porn and a complete descent into junk food depravity and addiction? Isn't food porn exactly what we are trying to avoid; if not, what is it? This exercise would be easy if the human animal were black or white. We're not. We are various shades of grey. We are not pure. We're all mutts.

Because we are all so different, it is somewhat easier to define what *food porn* isn't as opposed to defining exactly what it is. In 1964, Associate Justice of the Supreme Court Potter Stewart defined *pornography* by famously remarking concerning the case of *Jacobellis v. Ohio*, "I shall not today attempt further to define the kinds of material . . . but I know it when I see it."[7] Food porn is not mindless craving and dull consumption of fast food and junk food. That's addiction as we described. The best example of what constitutes our individual food porn fetish is to borrow the chef's game from Tony Bourdain. Fans of his shows have often heard him recount the details of the "death row meal." Basically, if you were on death row and were to be executed in the morning, what would be your last meal? What would you have in that one meal? That gives you an idea of your particular food fixation; you can be an uptown foodie and devour foie gras and Sauternes or go cheap and slutty with a couple of corner chili dogs, all the way of course.

Regardless, we all have that obsession. There are 10 percent of people who will admit to self-masticatory pleasure, and the other 90 percent are liars. But now that we have confronted the salacious shadows of our own food depravity, how do we deal with these instincts? Unchecked, these demons could derail any successful endeavor to eat well and be well at the same time.

The beauty is that we have already done it. It is akin to taking a vacation. If you vacation all the time and never work, then you are unemployed or very rich. Multiple studies have shown that to be the best worker, one needs some vacation, as previously described.[8] If you work all the time without a vacation, it affects your productivity at the job place and can also affect your health.[9]

Again we return to the concept of Balance. Nature is about Balance, but Balance is not equality. A pound of bricks is equal (in mass) to a pound of feathers, but it takes a lot more feathers to make a pound. They are not equal in number. It takes a lot more interns to do the job of one good senior resident. You get the idea. We need to return to our original "schedule." We need to retrain our palates and enjoy delicious, fresh, Grassroots Gourmet cooking for 90 percent of our allotted meal time. We "work" at maintaining an enjoyable, nutritionally sound, and appropriately portioned cuisine. We allow ourselves a "culinary vacation" the other 10 percent of the time. We budget our money and our time to take a vacation. There is no reason we shouldn't do the same with our diet. Food fidelity does not require absolution, just that you're pretty good most of the time. You can have that burger or be tempted by that devil's food cake. Enjoy your indiscretion guilt free. But after you're done dining with the devil, you need a come to Jesus meal of great food and discover for yourself God, food, and the art of cooking.

great food, God, and the art of cooking

"Arsenic is edible. Only once."

—Anonymous

WHAT MAKES something delicious and something else disgusting? Preparing food is making Art. That's why it's called the culinary arts. Thus, like Art, the line between disgusting and delicious can be a thin one. In terms of art, there seems to be a lot more of things like crappy paintings, sculptures, and so on that try to pass for art than true art. I think crappy food is like that as well. It is not just being "different" that makes something bad or tasty. Just watch Andrew Zimmern's show sometime. He eats some really nasty bits he says are delicious, but the guy can't stomach a walnut. New or old, some things just don't appeal to some people. That is OK. And it is not just about price. There is stuff for sale in galleries for amounts I could never afford that look like a colonoscopy in HD. There are plates that I could likewise never afford from celebrity chefs that look and taste just like the aforementioned Art. Spending a lot may increase your chances but is no guarantee.

I had the opportunity to dine in what at that time was one of the top fifty restaurants in the world. It was an opus to the chef's massive ego. It was plate after plate of technique that was incredibly well executed but that disrespected the food. It did not particularly taste great, either. In the chef's tasting of about a dozen dishes, there were three that were fantastic. For the others she might as well just taken a dump on the plate. There is just a lot more garbage that tries to pass for great food than great food. It's not too hard to weed out the bad stuff. What is really true is that we eat with all the senses, so you know it's likely to suck when you first see it. If the chef didn't think it was worth the time to make it look decent, why would I consider it decent? As we say in medicine, if it looks like a duck and quacks like a duck, it is probably a duck. Food doesn't go undercover. If you aren't quite sure when you see it, you will definitely know it when you first taste it. What exactly makes it suck can be hard to define because like any art it is intensely personal. However, as you cook, experiment, taste, and educate your palate, you learn what components create a great meal for you. Remember, one man's treasure is another man's trash.

OK, let's get right to it. What makes great food? Because *great* is but a superlative of *good*, as in the accepted definition that *great* is somewhere beyond *very good*, let's start with a more basic premise. What makes good food? Is it just sound nutrition? A bowl of dry oats and unseasoned nuts can be very nutritious, but unless you are the kid who ate the paste in kindergarten, most would agree it needs a bit more in the taste department. Is it just good flavor? But what makes something taste good? That's a bit like trying to define *Art* itself. That discussion has been going on since the dawn of civilization, and I am not smart enough to answer that ancient query. We can, however, probably more uniformly agree on what doesn't taste good: stones and dirt in your beans, sand in your spinach, spoiled meat, mushy gruel thrown into a chipped and broken bowl. The bottom line is that you definitely cannot have good food without good ingredients prepared correctly with care and passion. As the saying goes, you can't make chicken salad from chicken feces. Therefore, if the given standard for good food consists of proper ingredients prepared well with attention to technique, care, and passion, well, what elevates it from that baseline? What takes it from good to great? That's a bit trickier. Everyone has different concepts of what tastes pleasing. A lot of what we consider to be gratifying seems to be formed as we grow up by where we are geographically, socially, and economically. That being said, no one in my family growing up in the urban/suburban east coast of the United States ate a whole lot of sushi back in the day. It was considered bait. However, when I went to Japan for the first time, I had some. I have been in love with it since, something I consider, when done well, a great food.

But why? Trying to answer what makes great food is like trying to answer the Buddhist Koan, "When a tree falls in the forest, if no one is there, does it make a sound?" Does the sound really exist if no one is there to hear it? Can great food exist if there's no one there to eat it? It is not only a subjective analysis but also an analysis that cannot be done without the participants. It is experiential by its very nature. This brings us to the next point: Is great food simply the result of good food and a positive experience? Just how tasty, exactly, is that "death row last meal" when you're really on death row? It must be difficult eating a meal knowing it is your very last on this earth. How could that be a positive experience? Because the experience of the meal really doesn't have time to settle into the long-term memory banks, does it really matter?

It does if, for a few brief moments, it takes you somewhere else. Good food is part of a positive experience. Great food involves you in the process. It combines all those intangibles present and produces a pleasurable encounter of the moment like a perfect communion with the universe, or at least a good orgasm. Good food needs the supporting cast of the ambiance, the company, the place to make a great experience. I think that's why I've never heard anyone in the hospital ask for seconds. I've heard "It's OK" and "It's not that bad," but I've never heard "Oh wow! I've got to have this recipe." Hospitals in general are not places of pleasurable encounters, not to mention the basic food quality and preparation generally sucks.

Great food takes us somewhere else. It can do that all by itself. It is like remembering something lost from your childhood as you walk through a park, catching some unmistakable yet distant floral scent on your nose. In a flash you remember being barely a teenager walking deep in the woods, taking a shortcut across the land with that same scent hanging like a mist in the air. There, with your girlfriend (or boyfriend as the case may be) at your side, you stole your first kiss, something that in the stress and crush of the current Information Age insanity you hadn't thought about in years. But the scent of those flowers brought that memory back faster than a bathroom run after a not-so-Happy Meal. Great food is like that memory because it is involved in the experience of the moment yet transcends that moment. It challenges all our senses with the visual presentation, with taste and smell, with texture and feel. The sounds and other components of the moment are forever an accompaniment to that instant—a lover's laugh and a background babble of street noise in a language you don't understand but as comforting as a babbling mountain brook. It transports us. It takes us to a special place. If good food is like sex, great food is like love with your soul mate. Like love it defies description. You know what it isn't, and you know it when you experience it. And like love, great food is at the same time personal in nature and much better shared than alone.

If great food is an experience in love and love is God, can partaking of manna from heaven bring us closer to God? What is the purpose of food? In the beginning there was food, and food was nutrition, and it was good. Food and medicine long ago served the same purpose: to keep the human animal alive and in optimal functioning capacity. They functioned in synchronicity to keep you whole and well. Food was everyday medicine. Your food was your medicine, and your medicine was your food. Somewhere along the way, at least in the West, medicine became something different. It became something divorced from wellness. It no longer nurtures, no longer suckles us and keeps us from harm. It is harsh and hard, cold and sterile. It exists to repair injury and battle disease, no longer proactive and preventive. Medicine became reactive and left to dwell exclusively in constant battle in the realm of sickness and injury. It became an angry border agent. In ancient China physicians were paid to keep people well; if you got sick, then you stopped paying. In fact, even today, you can go to places in Asia where a practitioner of oriental medicine will diagnose what ails you and the cure is served in a meal prepared with certain items in a definitive way. This type of connection is why we instinctively seek something like Grassroots Gourmet cooking if left to our own devices, away from Madison Avenue, hawkers of expedient, miracle meals and pushers of addictive convenience.

Reestablishing that kind of instinctual relationship is important. I remember one morning it was false dawn, that time at the end of night when the sky starts to lighten. The sun hasn't risen yet, but you know it's coming, truly that veil between the end of the night and dawn of a new day. It is a very brief instance when one thing is ending but the other has not quite begun. As the darkness eases, the stillness retreats. The breeze picks up ever so slightly, and a few leaves fall. It is so quiet you can actually hear it happen.

As I sipped some way-too-early coffee, waiting for the birds to arrive at the feeder and for enough light to see them, I allowed myself to settle into the gentle turning of Earth time. It is not a time of seconds, appointments, and meetings. It is not even a time of minutes, hours, or days. Rather it is a time of seasons, rhythms, centuries, and millennia. It is at once personal and very ancient. In retrospect, it felt really good.

A woodpecker was the first to arrive. Uncharacteristically, he disregarded attacking the tree bark for grubs but snacked on some seeds from the feeder. I wondered why. Maybe he came so early so the other birds wouldn't see this—a woodpecker eating seeds—and ridicule this seed-eating woodpecker. Maybe he was like the guy who runs through the buffet line first so he can grab the quiche and put in on his plate, hide it under the roast beef, and consume it before his buddies can realize what he's done. I felt bad that Woody would be so embarrassed. I had bought top-notch bird seed. I just like to think the woodpecker, like me, felt a gentle nudge of need and responded as any child of nature would. You go after what you must, nothing more or less.

To cook food greatly requires some degree of observance and restraint. It requires understanding that there is something beyond our egos that we can touch when we let go. When we can surrender to that inner higher sublime and subconscious sense, something appears to us as in a vision upon the plate, and then we make it so. Let the rhythms of the seasons, the rhythm of Earth time, reveal itself to you. Let it reveal what is fresh and right. Always allow the ingredients to whisper to you the little techniques, seasonings, and methods they need from you to shine. And always take a little time for yourself to listen to the food, the season, the very harmony of Earth time. I was up early that day, and they say the early bird gets the worm—that of course means the early worm gets eaten. God, Nature, and a great meal are all about Balance.

When I was in college, I took a philosophy course. It was really great. There was this one discussion we had about the existence of absolutes. For example, as I understood it, there existed somewhere out there in the ether a "circleness." All circles participate of this ultimate circle. It is what gives them their "circleness" here in our world, but there is only this one "circle of circleness," one absolute perfect circle. If you're confused, don't feel bad; so was I. Nevertheless the other day, I think maybe I understood this just a little bit better. Let me explain. The other day I went for a hike in the hills of Georgia. It was warm but an otherwise perfect day. The sky was blue with small expanses of soft, incredibly bright, white, billowy clouds. I had walked several miles and stopped to take a break. I sat upon the leaf-littered ground and drank some water. Then I pulled out the peach I had brought along. I had bought it at a roadside farm not hours before. It was fresh from the orchard. It looked perfect. And the smell was the essence of "peachiness." It had ripened on the tree naturally in the sunshine, not picked underripe, shipped, and forced into some unnatural ripening act like some poor altar boy. When I bit into the peach, that perfect "peachiness" is exactly what I experienced. Somehow, alone in the enclave of that forest high in the hills, that peach had connected with that spot somewhere in the universe where "peachiness" comes from, that place where when we think of everything great about a peach—the sight, the smell, the texture, and the taste in its penultimate form—that place is where that comes from. It seemed like an eternity, but I'm sure it was only a moment. But it was one of those rare moments out of time and space. Einstein wrote and proved the space-time concept, but it was this perfect peach connecting to its "peachiness" that pulled me out of both space and time. It allowed me to turn around, dance in the moment, and plunge back. I now know that whenever I cook, think, search for that peach, this is what I will be trying to connect with. I may never again experience it like I did that day. How many life-changing visions does the universe give us anyway? Very few are the answer I would wager on. Nonetheless, I will really enjoy trying, and if I only connect to it in the most infinitesimal way, well, that will bring a smile to my soul. It'd be just, well, peachy.

This was not a religious epiphany. Well, maybe it was, but everyone can relax. I did not see Jesus in my French toast that morning. Let's be clear: We are not talking about faith, which is completely different than organized religion. And we're not really going to discuss organized religion, either. Religion here is used to represent *a specific fundamental set of beliefs and practices involving devotional and ritual observances; particularly any dogmatic, strictly ordered, and intolerant ones*, the sort of fun-sucking, life-draining observances that remind me of, say, life with the ex. This discussion is about God, food, and cooking. What we are talking about is the why behind our practice and procedure.

When the ritual is done for the sake of ceremony, it becomes an empty exercise. An example is when I come across patients receiving an antiquated treatment regimen because "that's the way we've always done it." The original reason for doing things a certain way is lost, and without an understanding of why, empty ritual is promulgated. Ignorant masses performing empty conventions leave an opportunity for self-proclaimed leaders and experts to ascend the pulpit. This is a problem I see creeping into cooking as well as medicine. There seems to be just too much mental masturbation about minutia and not enough focus on simply experiencing the food. These food shows with judges and critics getting all worked up over showing off how much they know—some of these critiques seem to be made more for the critic's benefit to appear erudite than for any actual constructive commentary. Some of these escapades have risen to the level of being critical simply to be critical: one-up-manship and ego domination. What is worse is that there seems to be a trend toward imitation into the general public: an elite group of food snobs and a group of intimidated plebs. The group of elite wannabes act as if food snobbery somehow conferred superior social standing. It reminds of the wine snobbery of decades past. It is a familiar program; a few so-called experts keep the masses intimidated and ignorant. It is only through the experts' graceful and privileged palates that foodie truth can be known. Only they can commune with the universe, and if you're lucky, they'll throw you a bone. Sounds like every dominating, self-serving, secular-focused, organized religion in history. And it sounds a lot like the Soup Nazi.

I am not condemning suitable critique. It is appropriate to be discerning. It is also important to be technically proficient when you are engaging in any task. You have to have it to competently perform whatever task you need to do: heal the sick, perform a martial arts maneuver, or create a delicious meal. But technique only gets you to mediocre—maybe to good. Technique alone can never be great or allow you to see with the eyes of God.

At the other end of the spectrum are less uptight philosophies based on a belief that to know God one must engage in progressive relaxation/receptiveness to achieve an enlightened state. You need to take off your jacket, expose your true self, and generally be fun before any celestial connection can be made. Tension and self-aggrandizement simply serve to mark you as a big fat arse with a big fat ego and in general convey to the universe what an unevolved cretin you really are.

I met a guy who had made several gazillion dollars developing medical devices and selling companies. He told me he had a "no asshole" policy. Simply stated, he had made enough money that he neither needed to work anymore nor put up with assholes. If you were an asshole, he told you within the first five minutes of meeting you to piss off, and

chapter twelve

he was done with you. This makes sense to me. And I can see God having a "no asshole" policy as well; why would any enlightened, all-knowing being want to hang out with a self-important jerk?

Well, what does not being an asshole so you can achieve enlightenment and meet God have to do with cooking? Everything—because if God wants to meet us when we're relaxed, receptive, and happy, then God wants us to be happy cooks and foodies. And what seems to be lurking in the garden is the serpent that is bound to remove that pleasure and passion.

In the martial arts I study, our *soke* has often spoken about the fact that one must perform the *waza* (a series of maneuvers) with feeling. To do it technically correct is not sufficient, for the action must have life and energy if it is to be successful, and that requires an infusion of feeling. The Art of cooking, in a very basic way, is about nourishment. Yet, human beings need more than caloric and nutritional repletion. Those needs are the technical science part of the equation. The other, equally important part of the equation is about the medicine for the soul, that *je ne sais pas* that when you experience it you say, "This was made with love. I can taste it." Across the ocean the indigenous peoples may refer to the fact that the chef has prepared the meal with his or her chi, infusing the meal with that very mysterious, oriental element of life. The execution of the techniques requires that they be made "alive," and without that feeling they are dead, just empty, technical movements, empty ritual. In promoting adherence and devotion to empty ritual, we can lose sight of the very essence of what we sought in the first place. In the martial arts, that is just enough to get you killed. In medicine we may say that a physician has "no bedside manner." He or she may be skilled in the science, and although they may correct a pathological state, they don't heal people. There is a real difference between being a physician and being a healer. And there is a real difference in technical proficiency and food preparation and the Art of cooking.

So no, I didn't find Jesus in my French toast. I didn't find God in a cookbook either. But I did find him in the kitchen. For those of us who seek the kitchen to practice our craft, I find sometimes we do not ask "Why?" and we should. We get caught up in the business of doing instead of being; we focus on the production of product. For me the kitchen is a refuge, a quiet place. It may not necessarily be to others with music blaring and sounds of chopping, blending, and frequently cursing, but within my mind it is a quiet place. As a culinary Artist, this place is my temple. These places are my cathedrals to enter and leave the busy city outside the doors. It is in those hallowed halls that I can shed the cloak of society and let my mind delve into a deeper humanity. It is, for me, a place of meditation. We all have them, and they are as varied as we are individuals. We need to seek them out and practice our crafts, search for our needs, and carry the effects of the experience back with us as we exit the doors and reenter the world outside. The specifics of that experience will be uniquely and personally yours. So where does your pursuit of happiness lead you? Wherever it does, ask "Why?" Then, as Joseph Campbell once said, simply "follow your bliss."

When I am cutting vegetables, preparing meat, and working with grains, I am happy. And that puts me, I believe, a little closer to God. So forget the fear of failure and the constipated critics. Enjoy yourself. Let the anticipation titillate you, the taste satisfy you, and the memory please you. God is the *Art* of cooking—although I swear Mother Mary came to me in the sausage gravy. Pork, after all, is simply divine.

chapter thirteen

why wine?

"We hear of the conversion of water into wine at the marriage in Cana as of a miracle. But this conversion is, through the goodness of God, made every day before our eyes. Behold the rain which descends from heaven upon our vineyards, and which incorporates itself with the *grapes*, to be changed into wine; a constant proof that God loves us, and loves to see us happy."

—BENJAMIN FRANKLIN (1706–1790)

S OME FORM of alcohol is found in every culture throughout the world. That's no coincidence. The history of man (and woman) is inextricably tied to that of alcohol. The exact date Bacchus delivered his gift is unknown and likely tied temporally to the experience of the first hangover. Understanding food and wine is something that in a very real way connects all of us human inhabitants of the planet. There is probably some hardwired aspect of this we have not yet figured out. After fat, the human body consumes alcohol (at 7 kcal/gm) preferentially before using proteins or carbohydrates. Evidence for the consumption of alcoholic beverages goes back more than ten thousand years, with remains of Neolithic beer mugs being identified. Intentional wine making was clearly established by the Egyptians as far back as around 4000 B.C., and it is probably even further back than that date. There is probably some form of an ancestral family connection. Perhaps it is the fact that at one time or another one of our caveman ancestors was holed up in a rehab cave. Wine and all forms of alcohol have a long and storied past with the human race. In days where the water could be dangerous—even lethal—to drink, the natural antibiotic properties of wine provided a source of safe beverage. Since that time wine (and alcohol) has served important nutritional, antiseptic, analgesic, and medicinal roles. The uses have run the gamut from personal to social and gustatory to religious. The mildly pleasing psychotropic effects didn't hurt either. The human race also has a long and ongoing story with mind-altering substances, but that recipe is for another day. Regardless of the reason we began to imbibe, we can draw some power from our long association with all things ethanol.

Along with historical connection, we should seek verification. I am a big believer in verification. As the Buddha said, believe nothing—even if he said it—if it does not agree with your own experience or common sense. Doctors actually telling you that you can/should have a glass or two of vino, as I have been doing for years now, can be a bit controversial. The problem with scientific endeavors is often the fact that if the data doesn't follow conventional wisdom or preconceived notions, it is often just ignored. Slowly, inexorably, the data accumulates like a giant dust bunny in the corner until you have to take notice. This often means years or decades may pass until we get it right, at least right for the moment. Not to say "Well, I told you so," but, well, I told you so. Moderate alcohol consumption has been studied and seems to convey clear cardiovascular benefits such as fewer heart attacks, peripheral vascular disease, and hypertension and perhaps some benefit in terms of a reduction in stroke and a decrease in the incidence of Alzheimer's-related dementia. There also seems to be some potential benefit against developing gallstones, arthritis, osteoporosis, Parkinson's disease, certain forms of cancer, and type-2 diabetes. This may be something you already knew if you listened to grandma as she lived to a healthy and ripe old age by enjoying that glass or two each day. But take note: You may need to educate your personal "health professional." Here I focus on wine as both a complement and a component of a meal.

As a complement to a meal, wine provides opportunity. In this context the wine is an addition to the meal as it is served. You could serve a beer or a coffee as well. The book by Andrew Dornenburg and Karen Page, *What to Drink with What You Eat*, is an absolute bible. People collect hundreds of cookbooks but don't have anything regarding how to balance the meal. The books by Andrea Immer I also find are great resources. Depending on what you are serving, wine or beer or other beverages can reinforce certain flavors found in the food. For example, take a meal with smoked salmon. A wine with smoky characteristics can accentuate the very lightly smoked fish and highlight that particular flavor profile. Conversely, a sharply acidic but balanced wine can offset the fat in the salmon and act to balance the entire presentation as well as refresh the palate. It can bring along some secondary flavors to the party. The right wine can be another tool in your culinary toolbox when you plan your menu.

As a component of the meal, we can look at wine from a perspective of functionality. In this setting the wine is a necessity for the success of the endeavor. You may be using a white wine for a sauce or to deglaze a pan or a red burgundy for beef Bourgogne. We can also use wine as a component of the meal to affect the tempo. Wine served with a meal generally causes us to slow down the eating process. Thus a glass of wine can act as a gentle break on our eatery express; it can help create proper timing for our repast. This pause gives the stomach time to signal the brain when we're full. Along with some water, which should always be served with wine, the additional liquid content again acts to help ding the satiety bell in our heads. I always recommend you drink as much water as wine when dining. Sipping some wine with a meal aids in helping us eat less, loosening the tongue, encouraging conversation, and generally restoring the concept of pleasure in dining versus the "supersize me, eat in two bites while driving in rush-hour traffic and taking phone calls" approach.

Whether it plays a complementary or component role, the inclusion of wine with a meal can not only be a source of gustatory pleasure but also serve an important function toward a more healthy form of dining. Multiple studies have demonstrated the health benefits associated with moderate wine consumption. In population-based studies, those who consume moderate amounts of alcohol live longer and are healthier than either teetotalers or boozehounds. It appears either extreme is detrimental. In most studies, a "glass" of wine is about 5 oz. The definitions vary from study to study, but the range of the healthy benefits and lack of consequences due to overindulgence seem to be associated with about one to three drinks per day. Because there is a mass as well as a genetic component to alcohol metabolism, men are able to consume slightly more wine and retain the benefits of consumption without the complications of excess. Research published in the *Journal of the American College of Cardiology* lends "credence to the idea that light to moderate alcohol intake appears to be good for the heart."[1] In a meta-analysis that combined eight studies encompassing 16,351 people with a history of heart disease, the results showed that the

> cardiovascular mortality showed a J-shaped pooled curve with a significant maximal protection (average 22%) by alcohol at approximately 26 g/day. In the meta-analysis on mortality for any cause, J-shaped pooled curves were observed in the overall analysis (average maximal protection of 18% in the range of 5 to 10 g/day) and in all subgroups according to either the type of patients or the characteristics of the studies. This correlates to about one to three drinks per day.[2]

Some of the largest studies to date have aggregated the results of many smaller trials. One such publication in *The British Medical Journal* examined eighty-four smaller studies that examined the incidence of heart disease and stroke as well as the mortality from both. The results showed "light to moderate alcohol consumption is associated with a reduced risk of multiple cardiovascular outcomes."[3] The risk reduction was between 14 and 25 percent compared to teetotalers. A similar study looking at the markers of heart disease found "favourable [*sic*] changes in several cardiovascular biomarkers . . . [providing] indirect pathophysiological support for a protective effect of moderate alcohol use on coronary heart disease."[4] In particular was an increase in HDL, or good cholesterol. Increasing HDL is very difficult through pharmacologic methods alone.

A very large study out of—surprise—France looked at 149,733 people divided into those who

- never drank (abstainers)
- were low consumers (< 10 g)
- were moderate consumers (10–30 g)
- were heavy consumers (> 30 g)

Ten grams is roughly one drink. Those in the low and moderate categories fared better with respect to overall health than either the heavy drinkers or abstainers. Subjectively, they fared better with respect to physical activity and respiratory function. Objectively, both men and women with increased alcohol intake had higher HDL, or good cholesterol levels. Moderate male drinkers also had a lower risk of cardiovascular disease, lower resting heart rate, less stress and depression, and an overall more favorable (lower) body mass index (BMI), the last being a measure of obesity. Moderate female drinkers had lower blood pressure and smaller waist–hip circumference measurements (another measure of obesity and a potent predictor of cardiovascular events) compared to abstainers.[5] These are important findings for those saying regular alcohol consumption adds pounds and increases blood pressure. The caveat is not to end up in the "heavy" category where those outcomes along with liver disease and general whole-body pickling can result. Then you end up confusing wine-ing (or whining) with winning. For those in the study over thirty, the most common form of alcohol consumed was wine. Interestingly, those French who drank were also more likely to smoke than their abstinent counterparts, yet the health benefits persisted. The conclusion of the study was that compared with abstainers, moderate consumers enjoy a "superior overall health status and a lower risk of (cardiovascular disease)."[6]

Excessive alcohol consumption can cause irreparable heart and liver damage; affect your ability to clot and contribute to other blood disorders; and cause pancreatic damage, gastrointestinal damage, and types of encephalopathy. While wine consumption can reduce the incidence of depression and have a beneficial effect on erectile dysfunction, coyote ugly remains another significant hazard.

It is hard to define the exact causative agent in wine. Some of the beneficial effects of wine have been attributed to their flavonoid content, which may also indicate antioxidant properties. Flavonoid intake has been inversely linked with coronary heart disease. The phenolic substances in red wine inhibit oxidation of human LDL. Flavonoids also have been shown to inhibit the aggregation and adhesion of platelets in blood, which may be another way they lower the risk of heart disease.[7] Wine, like other forms of alcohol, has also been shown to raise HDL levels.[8] Wine contains many other compounds, including a particular polyphenol, resveratrol, which has been shown to have antitumor properties and reduce inflammation. Such effects may lower the incidence of atherosclerosis, the pathologic process involved in heart attacks, strokes, and the development of peripheral vascular disease. There are many complex compounds and innumerable potential interactions to be found in a bottle of wine. Suffice it to say that the current data suggest important potential health benefits with moderate consumption.

As to which is the best, red or white or rosé, still or sparkling, the choice is yours. Experiment and decide what you like. Learning and appreciating wine is like learning and appreciating food. Study and educate your palate. Learn to taste, not just to swill. The important thing is to continue to study and learn. Kevin Zraly's *Windows on the World Complete Wine Course* is an excellent primer. The *Wine Spectator* wine courses are great resources to learn about all aspects of wines, including wine history. Everyone should be a student of history. It's the most economical way to learn. The history of food and wine is the history of man's quest to eat and drink and have a good time along the way. Throw in sex and war, also tied inextricably to food and wine, and you pretty much cover the last five thousand years of civilization. All tribes are concerned with staying alive in the best possible manner, even sometimes at the expense of others. Avoid the snobby pretense and consume what you like, not what somebody tells you to drink.

No matter where you go on this good earth, you can sit among strangers, and if you can share a meal and a glass of wine, you can depart among friends. The corresponding food cultures bind us in a tribal, primal way. Without it, we drift apart like untethered balloons. *In vino veritas.*

past and present

"Enough is as good as a feast."

—JOSHUA SYLVESTER (1563–1618)

GEORGE SANTAYANA wrote in the *Life of Reason* that "when experience is not retained, as among savages, infancy is perpetual. Those who cannot remember the past are condemned to repeat it."[1] It is imperative that, as we seek and follow the path of the Grassroots Gourmet, we understand it is an individual expedition of adventure. All that has been written is to aid as a guideline, not written as a gospel. We must, as the Dalai Lama has remarked, approach all that we are told with a curious skepticism.[2] Not so many years ago, people who survived heart attacks were told they needed to rest in bed for several weeks to recover. In reality we were deconditioning people and delaying, or in some cases thwarting, the very recovery process we sought to facilitate. The element of evolution in understanding and practice is the nature of science and progress, and we must always keep that in perspective. To aid in that endeavor, table 14.1 shows some mostly food-related items with their original recommendations to avoid or use. Remember these when the next set of alarms are raised that seem to contradict direct experience and common sense.

With that list in mind, let's examine some untraditional foods that have been shown to contribute to cardiovascular health. The list contains many items that continue to be

TABLE 14.1. Original Recommendations for Various Foods

Item	Original Recommendation
Eggs	Avoid, high in cholesterol and causes heart attacks
Red Meat	Avoid, high in saturated fat and causes heart attacks
Butter	Avoid, high in saturated fat and causes heart attacks
Avocados	Avoid, high in fat and cholesterol-like compounds
Shrimp	Avoid, high in cholesterol and causes heart attacks
Potatoes	Avoid, high in "bad" carbohydrates
Shellfish	Avoid, high in cholesterol and causes heart attacks
Sugar	Avoid, a source of empty calories; use artificial sweeteners
Cheese	Avoid, high in saturated fat and causes heart attacks
Milk	Avoid, high in saturated fat and causes heart attacks
Nuts	Avoid, high in fat
Chocolate	Avoid, no nutritional value
Wine	Avoid, no nutritional value
Margarine	Use instead of butter (These recommendations were for the trans-fatty-acid–containing margarines.)
Cigarettes	Use, "More doctors smoke Camels than any other cigarette!"[a]

[a] HemeOnc Today (2009)

vilified because of the original page-1 headlines. It seems no one ever reads the retraction on the back pages. There is a world of food to be enjoyed, a vast cornucopia of textures, flavors, spices, and smells to encounter in an equally vast possibility of environs. The prospective experiences are limitless. Use your own common sense to lead you. The Threefold Path of the "Bes," the guidepost for the Grassroots Gourmet's journey to culinary nirvana, is grounded in that reality:

- When we become aware and avoid the call of the junk food/fast food siren, we break the vicious cycle of addiction. We find the path.
- When we learn to be fresh and forsake food adulteration, we reclaim our own palate and all those potential opportunities. We begin to explore the entire gamut of gastronomic possibilities as Nature intended. We walk the path.
- When we find ourselves on time and in proportion, we find ourselves in Balance. We become the path.

From there it is an artisanal journey of discovery. Yet it is a journey always grounded in reason. It is a reason that is based upon direct experience, direct evidence, curious skepticism, and our own common sense. At times you may find yourself in lockstep with the conventional wisdom. At other times you may find yourself in disagreement with the prevailing opinions of the day. That is as it should be. It is your journey and your reality. Keep going.

As an example of such encounters, I have listed some foods about which there seems to be health-oriented confusion and some foods that might not traditionally be considered heart-healthy foods. These things go beyond the usual inane mantra of "eat more fruits and vegetables" because singing that tune is the easy way out. Finding these taste gems are the rewards of seeking. To each his own Buddha, and to each Buddha his own taste. Draw your own conclusions. For me, if someone can find Jesus in a grilled cheese sandwich, I can find enlightenment in a glass of wine and a seared slab of foie gras.

AVOCADOS

Avocados are delicious. I adore them. They are a fantastic fruit, and yes, technically they are a fruit. They can be found in the daily diets of the native peoples of Central America. I found them in everything when visiting the Yucatan Peninsula. They are likewise a staple throughout many regions, where they constitute part of a very healthful diet rich in vegetables and fruits and with a lot of protein consisting of seafood. Yet I am constantly rebuffed in this country by those people who insist that avocados should not be eaten because they are full of fat and contain cholesterol or will increase your cholesterol. Let's dispel some myths. First, avocados contain a relative of cholesterol called phytosterols, not cholesterol. Avocados are a good source of the phytosterol beta-sitosterol. These sterols are a class of compounds related to cholesterol, but they do not act to increase the level of cholesterol in humans. In fact, studies investigating the inclusion of sitosterol and sitosterol-containing compounds in diets found that they acted to lower cholesterol by about 10 percent.[3]

Cholesterol is not metabolized by the body. It is either reabsorbed or excreted from the body through the intestinal tract. Beta-sitosterol and other phytosterols inhibit the absorption of cholesterol. They also act to prevent the reuse (by means of reesterification and incorporation in cholymicrons) of cholesterol and hasten its entry into the intestinal lumen. These compounds also accelerate the enzymes that take cholesterol in circulation and dump it into the intestinal lumen.[4] In other words, these relatives of cholesterol push it out of the way so cholesterol can't get into your body and act to push it out of your body into the intestinal tract where the cholesterol can later be dumped out.

Avocados also contain oleic acid, the main constituent in olive oil. They are rich in potassium, a mineral that is important in the regulation of normal heart rhythm and in the normal functioning of the heart muscle. Folate, which has been studied and prescribed as an adjunctive treatment to aid in the fight against atherosclerosis, is also found in abundance in the avocado. Diets rich in folate have been shown to be beneficial for cardiovascular health. A Japanese study looking at 23,119 men and 35,611 women between ages forty and seventy-nine who completed questionnaires about dietary habits was published in *Stroke: Journal of the American Heart Association* as part of the Japan Collaborative Cohort Study. It was found that higher consumption of folate and B_6 was associated with significantly fewer deaths from heart failure in men. In women they detected significantly fewer deaths from stroke, heart disease, and total cardiovascular deaths. To avoid confounding variables, anyone taking supplements was eliminated from the analysis, thus the findings reflected intake from diet. The protective effects of folate and vitamin B_6 did not change even when researchers made adjustments for the presence of cardiovascular risk factors. The researchers suggest that a diet rich in these compounds help offset dietary intake of other compounds, like homocysteine, or offset genetic predispositions to disease sates.[5] One cup of avocado contains almost 25 percent of the daily recommended intake of these important vitamins. It also contains vitamin E and is a great source of glutathione, lutein, zeaxanthin, and other carotenoids.

BUTTER

I do not know and have never met Paula Deen, but when you're right, you're right. Butter is better. But remember, Paula, more is not always better. Butter got a bad rap on the felony saturated fat charge; a charge that is looking more like a frame-up every day. Everyone was told to bag the butter and eat and cook with hydrogenated, plant-based products like margarine. Those days of artificially produced products that could sit forever on your dairy shelf, my friend, were the halcyon days of trans-fats or trans-fatty acids (TFAs). These are constructs that exist in only trace amounts in nature, found in trace amounts in dairy and bovine stomachs and intestines in such forms as vaccenyl acid. Trans-fats are also extremely atherogenic. They promote plaque buildup in the arteries; in other words, the trans-fatty-acid butter substitutes were far more likely to cause the buildup of atherogenic plaques than the butter it was meant to replace. Governmental studies have noted that substances that contain TFAs pose a "greater risk of coronary heart disease from increases in dietary trans fats than from increases in dietary saturated fats."[6] While the highly processed foods may have little redeeming value besides lower calorie content, natural foods like butter often contain an abundance of macro- and micro-nutrients.

Butter contains vitamins A and D, as well as the other fat-soluble vitamins E and K in an easily absorbable form. It also contains other beneficial substances, such as calcium, phosphorus, and potassium. It has a good amount of sodium and small amounts of fluoride, selenium, zinc, and magnesium (while not a problem in the United States, there exists a form of heart disease that was found in China and believed to be the result of insufficient amounts of selenium in the diet because the soil from that area was particularly deficient in this vital element.)

The fatty acids that are contained within butter are also healthful, unlike the previously discussed TFAs. Conjugated linoleic acid (CLA) in butterfat may afford powerful protection against cancer, as may the fatty acid butyric acid. As in beef, the dairy products from cattle allowed to range naturally and free are much higher in CLA than found in their more confined brethren. Lauric acid, a medium-chain fatty acid, is a potent antimicrobial and antifungal substance. Butter also contains the beneficial omega-3 and omega-6 fatty acids. Certain fats called glycospingolipids aid digestion and protect against gastrointestinal infections.

CHEESE

Cheese, like butter, got a bad rap because of its fat content. Interestingly, cheese was consumed in large amounts as part of the French diet in the French Paradox Study, where diets with lots of cheese produced healthier people. In native populations that consume fresh, unprocessed product, the purported ill effects of cheese and fat do not manifest. A small serving of cheese makes for a perfect appetizer or even a lovely dessert course. It was, after all, what Timer was hankering for all those years. Cheese is rich in calcium, phosphorus, zinc, potassium, and sodium. Cheese is also rich in vitamins A, B_{12}, and riboflavin (vitamin B_2). Diets rich in cheese have been associated with reductions in the risk of osteoporosis, hypertension, tooth decay, and cardiovascular disease. Unlike milk, cheese is low in lactose, and the older the cheese, the less the lactose content (and the stinkier as well).

Regardless of the age, cheese is a great source of bioavailable calcium. It is important to consume foods that are rich in easily absorbable forms of calcium like cheese, as opposed to trying to get the calcium through artificial supplementation. Interestingly, a report on calcium supplementation in the *British Medical Journal* suggests artificial calcium supplementation may increase the risk of a heart attack.[7] The trial was another meta-analysis that looked at data from eleven smaller trials comprising about 12,000 female patients. The data showed that although the total number of women having heart attacks was small (around 1 to 2 percent), among those taking calcium supplements, there was a 31 percent increased risk of having a heart attack. Again, this type of result is correlative, not necessarily causative. Also, supplements with vitamin D were excluded from the analysis. A very remarkable sidenote is that studies that looked at diets rich in calcium did not show any increased cardiac risk.

CHOCOLATE

The benefits of chocolate were known to ancient Mayans possibly as far back as 2,600 years ago.[8] Evidence suggests this food of the gods (the scientific name for the cacao tree is *Theobroma cacao* and means "food of the gods") may actually have been used even further back, dating to the Mayan forebears, the Olmecs. The Olmecs and the Maya inhabited much of what is now Mexico and Central America. In fact, the word *cacao* is from the Olmec language.

Chocolate is made from the fermented, dried, and roasted seeds of the cacao tree. It is a compound, naturally a bit bitter but rich in flavonoids and antioxidants. Antioxidants work to improve cardiovascular health by preventing LDL cholesterol from being oxidized. It is when this type of bad cholesterol is oxidized that it actually becomes "bad," as it is the oxidized form that crosses into the arterial wall and wreaks havoc with the lining of the blood vessels. This leads to an inflammatory response and the formation of plaques, which can ultimately cause heart attacks, strokes, and peripheral arterial disease. A meta-analysis not only reaffirmed the aforementioned benefits but also noted an increase in the levels of HDL, or good cholesterol, as well.[9] The main type of flavonoids in chocolate and cacao are called flavanols, with the highest levels of flavanols found in cocoa. The more a chocolate product is processed, generally the lower the flavanol concentration. The exception is Dutch cocoa, which undergoes an alkali processing step and thus loses some of its flavanol concentration early on. While cocoa contains the highest concentration of flavanols, dark chocolate contains a higher concentration than milk chocolate. Dark chocolate per serving contains about eight times the amount of polyphenol antioxidants than an equivalent serving of strawberries. It appears that different flavanols may produce different results. Several studies utilizing cocoa and the flavanols found within have shown enhanced brain flow in the elderly, enhanced blood flow in postmenopausal women, and mitigating effects on blood clotting.[10]

The fat in chocolate comes from cocoa butter. Cocoa butter contains equal amounts of the fatty acids oleic, stearic, and palmitic acids. Oleic acid is the same beneficial monounsaturated fat found in olive oil. While palmitic acid can cause a rise in cholesterol, stearic acid appears not to affect overall cholesterol levels. In fact some studies have shown that consumption of dark chocolate can reduce LDL cholesterol levels by about 10 percent.[11]

The beneficial compounds found in chocolate may help increase nitric acid production in the blood vessels. This helps them relax and may contribute to the blood pressure–lowering effect observed in people consuming chocolate and cocoa.[12] A meta-analysis measured the blood pressure reduction as a result of ingesting cocoa. Although the number of patients was small (173 patients), the findings revealed a mean reduction of systolic pressure (the top number of your blood pressure) by almost 5 mmHg and the diastolic pressure (the bottom number) pressure by almost 3 mmHG. While that may not seem like a lot, that is actually the range of reduction seen with commonly prescribed antihypertensive medication.[13]

Another study looked at the Kuna Indians, who live near Panama. Hypertension in that population is practically nonexistent; the average blood pressure at age sixty is 110/70 (perfect). Indians who leave the area and subsist on a typical Western diet have the same rate of hypertension as the rest of the Westernized population. This lack of age-related hypertension exists despite the fact that the native Kuna consume more salt than the average American. The secret seems to be in the five cups of cocoa they consume each day. Not only do the Kuna have less hypertension, but also their rates of cardiovascular death, cancer, and diabetes were substantially lower than their mainland brethren (for cardiovascular death, 9.2 versus 83.4; for cancer, 4.4 versus 68.4; and for diabetes, 6.6 versus 24.1; all values per 100,00).[14] Other touted benefits include beneficial effects on platelet function (platelets are the blood agents responsible for clot formation) and reducing insulin resistance. Because of processing and the addition of fats and sugars, discretion must be used in the consumption of chocolate. However, in the recipes that use cocoa, there is less reservation because cocoa contains little sugar and fat.

CRUSTACEANS (SHRIMP, LOBSTER)

Shrimp, lobster, crab, langoustines, and all their kin have gotten a bad cholesterol label. While these shellfish, like eggs, do contain cholesterol, they are incredibly low in fat. It turns out that cholesterol levels are much more dependent on saturated fat intake than ingested levels of cholesterol. Additionally, there may be other compounds within crustaceans that prevent cholesterol uptake when you eat them. Native populations eating a diet rich in fresh mollusks, fish, and shellfish tend to be incredibly healthy. A 3 oz. serving of lobster meat has 83 calories, about 0.5 g of fat, and only about 0.1 g of that is saturated fat. Among crustaceans, shrimp has the highest cholesterol content. A large shrimp contains about 6 calories, about 0.67 g of fat, of which about 0.0001 g are saturated fat, and about 11 mg of cholesterol.

A low-fat diet and high-cholesterol intake (600 mg/day) from shrimps in normolipidemic (those without high cholesterol levels) subjects raised LDL cholesterol by 7 percent but also raised HDL by 12 percent and decreased triglycerides by 13 percent. This change caused the LDL-to-HDL cholesterol ratio to drop (a cardioprotective happening). The end result is a more favorable cardiovascular risk profile. The authors of that study concluded that moderate shrimp consumption in normolipidaemic subjects will not affect overall lipoprotein profiles and can be included in heart-healthy guidelines.[15]

Studies like that one that have been performed since the initial scare showed that shrimp may raise your cholesterol, however, it's your *good* cholesterol that gets the big boost. Population-based studies have found no ill-health effects from diets rich in seafood and shrimp (and squid and other mollusks and crustaceans). According to Professor Elizabeth De Oliveira of Rockefeller University, "consuming shrimp instead of other high fat foods will have beneficial effects."[16]

DUCK

Domestic duck has been around for at least four thousand years. Pekin duck can be traced back to the Mongolian Yuan Dynasty. A lovely duck breast prepared like garbage will taste like greasy garbage. Prepared without the understanding that if it walks like a duck, looks like a duck, and quacks like a duck, it is a duck and not a chicken can lead to a fatty mess. Duck has often been viewed as a fatty type of poultry because of the way the bird distributes the subcutaneous fat, especially around the breast. However, once that layer is removed, the duck itself is a lean bird. Duck fat is mostly unsaturated fat. It contains 35.7 percent saturated, 50.5 percent monounsaturated (particularly high in the monounsaturated linoleic acid), 13.7 percent polyunsaturated fats, and 0.1 percent miscellaneous fats. The polyunsaturated fats contain the omega-6 and omega-3 essential oils. This compares favorably to olive oil, which is 75 percent monounsaturated fat (mostly oleic acid), 13 percent saturated fat, 10 percent omega-6 linoleic acid, and 2 percent omega-3 linoleic acid. Duck fat contains higher amounts of linoleic acid and less polyunsaturated fat than turkey or chicken.[17]

Duck is a great source of iron, phosphorus, zinc, copper, thiamin, riboflavin, niacin, pantothenic acid, vitamin B_6, vitamin B_{12}, and selenium. A skinless duck breast has 40 percent lower fat content than a chicken breast and is an excellent source of protein.

EGGS

The incredible, edible egg. I remember that campaign. Then I remember my delicious eggs being taken away and replaced with something that looked like dried semen and probably tasted worse. Eggs got a bum rap with cholesterol the same way butter did with saturated fats. People have been eating eggs since prerecorded times. Prohibitions regarding egg consumption have focused on potential salmonella infections and their cholesterol content. Chickens that are allowed to range freely and consume a diet as nature intended carry very little risk of salmonella. Salmonella is usually only found in the eggs of ill chickens, and that usually occurs when they are kept overcrowded in the industrial poultry ghettos. Eggs contain essential nutrients; proteins; essential fatty acids;

lutein; zeaxanthin; niacin; riboflavin; biotin; choline; magnesium; fat-soluble vitamins A, D, and E; potassium; phosphorus; iodine; manganese; iron; copper; zinc; sulfur; and vitamin D. Eggs from free-range, vegetarian-fed chickens have higher levels of beneficial omega-3 and omega-6 fatty acids as well conjugated linoleic acids. Although the yolks of eggs do contain cholesterol, studies have shown that moderate egg consumption does not raise blood levels of cholesterol despite the initial warnings. In addition, eggs contain lecithin, which aids in the processing of fats and cholesterol. A study done at Michigan State University found that the cholesterol level among people who ate four or more eggs per week was actually lower than among people who avoided eggs altogether. Additionally, those not consuming eggs were found to be more deficient in vitamin B_{12}, vitamin A, vitamin E, and vitamin C.[18] Other studies have shown no increased rate of cardiovascular risk with moderate egg consumption.[19]

FOIE GRAS

Foie gras (the fatty liver from a goose or duck), is simply the victim of its own provocative tastiness and some bad PR. Let us examine the torchlight of truth.

Foie gras is a natural fat in that it does not contain things like TFAs. Some fat is necessary. Want to know why old people look old? In addition to the breakdown of elastin and collagen as we age, we thin and lose the layer of subcutaneous fat under our skin. That little layer of fat keeps us looking young. More importantly, fat is used:

- as an energy source
- as a transport for fat-soluble necessary vitamins such as A, D, E, and K
- to make products that are used in maintaining normal, healthy cellular function (that is why there are fats known as essential fatty acids. *Essential* as in you need them for life.)

Food cooked in natural fat tastes good to us, 'nuff said.

Foie gras has been around since at least approximately 3000 B.C. in ancient Egypt. The geese there naturally fatten their livers in preparation for their annual migratory journey. In the original French Paradox Study, the area within France with the lowest cardiovascular mortality and highest life expectancy was Toulouse in the Gascony region. In Toulouse they consume insane amounts of foie gras several times a week. At the time of the study, the rate of death for middle-aged men from heart attack in the United States was 315 per 100,000; in France it was 145 per 100,000; in Toulouse it was 80 per 100,000.[20]

Roughly 65 percent of foie gras is unsaturated oleic acid, the same oil that constitutes 60 to 80 percent of olive oil. It also contains omega-3 and omega-6 essential acids. To quote Dr. Renaud, "Goose and duck fat is closer in chemical composition to olive oil than it is to butter or lard."[21]

A native of Gascony, Robert Jacquerez, who lived into his late nineties, remarked that balance is the key: "Always have a salad with your cassoulet, bread with your foie gras. Always drink as much mineral water as wine."[22]

GARLIC

Garlic has been used as both food and medicine in many cultures for thousands of years, dating back to when the Egyptian pyramids were built. In early-eighteenth-century France, gravediggers drank a concoction of crushed garlic in wine, which they believed would protect them from the plague that killed many people in Europe. More recently, during World Wars I and II, soldiers were given garlic to prevent gangrene.[23]

Garlic has one of the highest concentrations of sulfur-containing compounds, more than seventy-five different compounds. One of those compounds, allicin, gives garlic its characteristic pungency. However, allicin is only made available after the garlic is crushed or cut; otherwise it is protected by the cell walls. Once the allicin is released, it is unstable and quickly combines to form many other compounds.[24]

In 2000, the Agency for Healthcare Research and Quality (AHRQ) published an evidence-based "Report on Garlic: Effects on Cardiovascular Risks and Disease, Protective Effects against Cancer, and Clinical Adverse Effects." Here are the main findings:

- In examining thirty-six trials comparing garlic to placebo, it was shown that various garlic preparations demonstrated a small but statistically significant reduction in total cholesterol at one month, with a range of average pooled reductions of 1.1 to 15.8 mg/dL, and at three months with a range of 11.6 to 24.3 mg/dL.
- Eight trials examined outcomes at six months. In these, there were no significant changes in total cholesterol levels, LDL cholesterol levels, HDL cholesterol levels, and triglyceride levels. However, a study from Bastyr College demonstrated that consuming about three garlic cloves per day reduced LDL levels by about 7 percent and increased HDL levels by about 23 percent after one month.[25]
- Twenty-six small, randomized, placebo-controlled trials yielded mixed findings with respect to garlic's effect on blood pressure.
- Twelve small, randomized trials failed to demonstrate a clinically significant effect on blood glucose levels in persons with or without diabetes.
- Two small, short-term trials failed to yield any statistically significant effects of garlic compared with placebo on serum insulin or C-peptide levels.

- Ten small, short-term trials yielded mixed results on garlic's ability to cause or prevent blood clotting.
- There were insufficient data to confirm or refute garlic's ability to prevent heart attacks or atherosclerotic diseases.
- There are some data, primarily from case-control studies, that hint at the fact that dietary garlic consumption may reduce one's likelihood of developing laryngeal, gastric, colorectal, and endometrial cancer and adenomatous colorectal polyps.
- The down sides of garlic consumption include stinky breath and body odor. Other possible side effects include flatulence, esophageal and abdominal pain, small intestinal obstruction, dermatitis, rhinitis, asthma, and bleeding.
- The results suggest the amount needed to reap the health benefits of garlic is about one clove (600 to 900 mg) per day. The results of the meta-analysis were limited by types and compositions of different preparations, sample sizes, and methodologies.

The take-home message appears that it aids in reducing total cholesterol, LDL (bad) cholesterol, and triglycerides in the short term (three months). Long-term benefit is unclear. Garlic has been shown to decrease levels of homocysteine and C-reactive protein, therefore it may be useful in reducing cardiovascular risk factors.[26]

MOLLUSKS (CLAMS, OYSTERS, SQUID, OCTOPUS, ETC.)

Despite the hysteria to the contrary at various times, I cannot find any problem with any of the delicious food that comes out of the sea as long as the product hasn't been made toxic by us. Mercury may be the messenger to the gods, but we need to keep him out of our seafood. Many mollusks contain cholesterol, like crustaceans and eggs, that led to advisements to forgo these delicious denizens of the sea for fear of cardiovascular problems. The heart is a muscle, and like any muscle it needs iron to bring it oxygen. Three ounces (about nine small clams) contains about 24 mg of iron. The recommended daily allowance is 18 mg for premenopausal women and 8 mg for men and postmenopausal women. Clams are also a good source of phosphorus, potassium, zinc, copper, manganese, and selenium. Clams contain both taurine and coenzyme Q_{10}. They are a good source of vitamins A and B_{12}. That same 3 oz. serving of clams also contains about 140 mg of omega-3 fatty acids. The 3 oz. you eat also has almost 12 g of protein, less than 65 calories, and less than 1 g of fat.

The cholesterol found in such mollusks as clams has not been shown to raise cholesterol levels in people who consume them, much like the story with crustaceans and eggs.

In fact, epidemiological studies looking at diets rich in seafood, including things like clams, have consistently shown low levels of cardiovascular events. It may have to do with the very low levels of fat in clams. In small studies looking specifically at clams and other shellfish, consumption of a diet rich in clams has been shown to raise HDL, the good cholesterol. This effect may also have to do with the other types of marine sterols found in clams having an inhibitory effect on cholesterol absorption. Cholesterol absorption from the human digestive tract has been shown to be decreased by clam consumption.[27] A study looking at the effect of eating shellfish compared to chicken found that there was no significant difference in total cholesterol or LDL cholesterol.[28]

The same story holds for oysters. What had originally been assumed to be cholesterol in oysters was actually other types of sterols that turned out to be beneficial. The skinny on oysters is that they have the best profile of shellfish in terms of calories, fat, saturated fat, and cholesterol. Researchers at the Yale/New Haven Connecticut Nutrition Center report that up to six medium oysters have only 50 calories, 2 g of fat, and about 0.5 g of saturated fat.[29] For squid and octopus, it's the same story without the shell.

MUSHROOMS

Mushrooms have been used medicinally and as a food source for thousands of years. They are mostly (80 to 90 percent) water and are thus very low in caloric value. They are an excellent source of potassium and fiber. In addition to important cardiovascular elements like potassium, mushrooms are rich in copper, riboflavin, niacin, and selenium. Niacin is used to lower bad cholesterol (LDL) and raise good cholesterol (HDL). Some mushrooms even contain vitamin D. Lentinan, a compound found in shiitake mushrooms, has been shown to positively stimulate the immune system.

NUTS

Nuts got the bad fat rap we've seen before. Many nuts are high in fat and thus were placed on the *verboten* list. However, it turns out that consuming nuts on a regular basis can lower bad cholesterol levels and reduce the overall risk of heart disease. A meta-analysis out of Loma Linda University and published in the *Archives of Internal Medicine* pooled data from twenty-five smaller studies. The nuts under examination included almonds, hazelnuts, pecans, pistachios, walnuts, and macadamia nuts. It also included peanuts, even though the peanut is *not* a nut; it is a legume. Daily consumption was 67 g, or about 2.4 oz., and the study examined both men and women of varying cholesterol levels, but none were on medication. LDL, or bad cholesterol, was reduced by more than 7 percent, and there were other health benefits. Among some other groups, those consuming a

Western diet benefited the most, and "increasing consumption of nuts as part of an otherwise prudent diet can be expected to favorably affect blood lipid levels (at least in the short term), and have the potential to lower coronary heart disease risk."[30]

RED MEAT (BEEF, LAMB, AND PORK)

For as long as I can remember, the conventional wisdom in medicine has been to tell people to avoid red meat because it is high in saturated fat, but like many of our approaches, we are learning this may be an oversimplification. A meta-analysis from the Harvard School of Public Health and published in *Circulation* suggests that the cardiovascular risk associated with red meats comes primarily from the highly processed and chemically treated varieties, such as bacon, sausage, hotdogs, and other processed lunch and deli meats. The nonprocessed meats examined were beef, lamb, and pork (not poultry).

While both contain fat, cholesterol, and saturated fat, the processed choices are much higher in salt, preservatives, and additives. The analysis combined data from twenty different studies involving more than 1.2 million people worldwide. The findings revealed that daily consumption of about 2 oz. of processed meat was associated with a 42 percent increased risk of heart disease and a 19 percent increased risk of diabetes. Conversely, a 4 oz. daily serving of red meat from beef, pork, lamb, or game did not increase the risk of heart disease nor did it significantly increase the risk of diabetes. The rates of smoking, exercise, and other risk factors were similar between the two groups.

The study concluded people, especially those already at risk of heart problems or with high blood pressure, should consider reducing consumption of bacon, processed ham, hotdogs, and other packaged meats that have a high salt and nitrate content. The heavily processed choices had four times the amount of sodium and 50 percent more nitrates than their unprocessed counterparts. I would add to that the processed versions also contain high levels of additional compounds and preservatives. This combination is what may have led to an unintended consequence in the effort to keep food preserved. The levels of saturated fat and cholesterol were roughly equivalent between the highly processed and unprocessed meats. To reduce your risk of harm from consuming red meat, it is recommended to stick with unprocessed meats and to prepare all meats from scratch.[31]

That study does not even address the option of using what I advocate, which is natural (hormone and antibiotic free) beef that is allowed to roam free and consume natural grasses. Cattle, lamb, and the like are herbivores; feeding them high-protein pellets made from ground-up bits of other animals just is not their natural diet. Cramming them in feedlots and pens where they cannot move, let alone get any exercise, may increase yields but decreases potential health benefits. These are the animals whose conditions are so poor they need prophylactic antibiotics. The average store-bought beef you find in the super-chain mega-marts is often chock full of antibiotics and hormones. Wild-animal fats are different from both farm-animal fats and processed fats, claims Eric Dewailly, a professor of preventive medicine at Laval University in Quebec.[32] Farm animals, cooped up and stuffed with agricultural grains (carbohydrates), typically have lots of solid, highly saturated fat.[33] When the animals are allowed to thrive naturally, we find things like beneficial omega-3 fatty acids in the red meat. Omega-3 fatty acids are beneficial and essential fatty acids with a plethora of healthy benefits. Animals with natural diets are lower in overall saturated fatty acids, which are generally bad, and higher in polyunsaturated fatty acids, which are generally good. Products from grass-fed animals have increased conjugated linoleic acid, also good, by 50 percent and omega-3 fatty acids by 40 percent. The animals allowed to move about naturally are also lower in overall fat and higher in vitamin E, a natural antioxidant. The beauty of consuming these natural, grass-fed products is that they simply taste better. They have a delicious flavor you want to savor.

In fact, it may not even be what we worry about in the meat, the saturated fat, that is the causative problem. Another meta-analysis published in March 2010 involving twenty-one different studies found that intake of saturated fat wasn't linked to a statistically significant increased risk of heart disease, stroke, or cardiovascular disease. While food for thought, these studies do not establish a cause-and-effect relationship; they are correlative. Recent data have suggested that the genesis of many chronic disease states are not just a result of low omega-3 fatty acid intake but a more complex relationship related to a ratio of omega-6 to omega-3 fatty acids.[34] The grass-fed free-range beef have a much more favorable profile of omega-6 to omega-3 compared to grain-fed feedlot offerings.

SEA URCHIN ROE

The sea urchin is a member of the echinoderm clan and a relative of starfish and sea cucumbers. The roe is the part of the sea urchin that is consumed. Roe is a rich source of vitamins A and D, very-long-chain fatty acids, and zinc.[35] Sea urchins also contain anandamide, a euphoria-causing chemical found in the roe that has also been shown to be involved in working memory.[36] Endogenous anandamide is present at very low levels, has a very short half-life, starts working faster than its marijuana-derived counterpart THC, but is more quickly destroyed by the body. The substance may affect the endocannabinoid system, which partially controls pleasure and pain signals, but it doesn't produce a perpetual natural high. Anandamide, also found in chocolate, is important in the regulation of feeding behavior and the neural generation of motivation and pleasure.[37] So even though there are no clear cardiovascular benefits, sea urchin roe is a food that makes you happy, and that just cannot be a bad thing.

but doc, i can't
common myths and misconceptions

"Do or do not. There is no try."

—YODA

WHY ARE you reading this book? It's probably because you would like to eat healthier and feel better. It's also because you probably like to eat things that taste good. It's no doubt that you are confused about how to accomplish this. You are lost and alone in this crazy carny. You can hear those freaky clowns outside the funhouse whispering your name. Or are they inside? How did you lose your way and arrive at these crossroads? Experts describe a myriad of causes, including fast food, insufficient exercise, lack of sleep, increased work-related stress, urbanization, and Western cultural influence all as contributors to our current lackluster condition.[1] One of the problems, as Daniel Epstein of the World Health Organization notes, is that "people fill up on things that have high caloric value but little nutritional value."[2] So people eat more because their body is not getting what it needs from what it is taking in, malnutrition standing in the midst of plenty. As we eat more refined sugar, fat, and salt, we crave more, and the vicious cycle continues. The world's 1.6 billion overweight adults are estimated to grow by 40 percent over the next decade, and every guilty individual has his or her share of convenient excuses. I had mine as well. As an interventional cardiologist, I know the outcomes of these poor decisions. I see it every day. I hear the excuses every day as well. It seems that we can talk the talk but can't walk the walk because we can only waddle along.

We have discussed the keys to success to break this stranglehold. This is at its heart a book about food because Americans love to eat. I love to eat. We can eat fresh and delicious, but we must educate our palates and break the addictions so we recognize what fresh and delicious really is all about. We can eat fresh and delicious if we educate ourselves so we know what we're getting, how to get it, and how to prepare it—Grassroots Gourmet cooking. We can eat fresh and delicious if we understand quality and quantity, and every now and then we can go to the pantry, lock the door, and indulge our food-driven fantasies in a guilt-free orgy of mastication. However, the luxury of vacation presupposes that we actually work at something. This requires actively engaging the program steps. Yet before we can seriously embark on anything, the time for excuses has got to end. People have a number of excuses as to why they haven't, can't, or won't change their habits, all of which I will try to address.

I'VE TRIED BREAKING THE JUNK FOOD AND FAST FOOD ADDICTION BEFORE, AND I JUST CAN'T DO IT

First, eliminate *can't* from your vocabulary. It seems a small thing, but when we reinforce ourselves in the negative, we just serve to initiate a negative self-fulfilling prophecy. This is not a book about daily positive affirmations, but we must believe we can achieve self-control before we can actually obtain it. No successful athlete enters into a competition thinking "I can't win this."

In speaking with my many patients over the years, breaking the fast food and junk food addiction bears a lot of similarity to quitting smoking, and there seems to be some consistent themes I've noticed when looking at people who are successful at quitting smoking. The successful types seem to have a lot of friends and family urging them to quit. They put themselves in an environment conducive to reinforcing what they wish to accomplish. The unsuccessful people are surrounded by, or they surround themselves with, people who continue to smoke. As mentioned in an earlier chapter, at a martial arts seminar one time, a person asked about the "best techniques to use in a bar fight." The instructor didn't hesitate: "Don't go to bars." If you want to avoid fast food, don't pull in or go through the drive-through. People trying to quit smoking who can find other forms of enjoyment, such as sports or eating (hence the oft-cited weight gain while attempting to quit smoking), seem to be successful. Those who use smoking as a form of stress relief are not so successful. Some have success cold turkey, some need to wean off, some need adjunctive medications, some need combinations of all available therapies and some don't need any of these. So although there are consistent general themes for those who successfully quit smoking, the exact methodologies are very individualized. You need to personally examine not only what you eat but also where you eat and why. Are you eating at the fast food joint? Are you bringing it home from the drive-through because it's convenient? Are you eating because you think it's time to eat, because you're bored, or because you're lonely? I think every individual needs to look at their own circumstances, including emotional connections to eating. Once you have the knowledge of the hows, whys, wheres, whats, and whens you eat, you can begin to address each. Sun Tzu wrote more than two thousand years ago in his classic *The Art of War* that to know neither your enemy nor yourself was to lose one thousand battles. Know your enemy but not yourself, and five hundred you shall win, and five hundred you shall lose. Know both your enemy and yourself, and one thousand battles you shall surely win. Knowledge is power.

I HATE TO EXERCISE

I do, too. However, the fact of the matter is that exercise is good for a number of reasons. There are plenty of books and programs on fitness and exercise. This isn't one of them. But you need to do it, even if it is a walking program. It is good for the entire cardiovascular system. It allows your body to positively channel the stress hormones we release while confronting our everyday world. Having observed patients who have had junk food diets with no exercise and had heart trouble, there is an interesting phenomenon they often describe after a few weeks of cardiac rehabilitation. They often tell me that, after exercising regularly for a few weeks, they no longer crave the fast food or junk food. They start to crave other things like salads or fruit. Although not a double-blind, randomized, placebo-controlled trial, I think it does lend some empirical evidence to the fact that, to increase your chances of long-term success, some form of exercise needs to be included.

I'M UNDER STRESS; I'VE GOT
TOO MUCH ON ME RIGHT NOW

I hear that one all the time. Let me let you in on a little secret they taught us in our residency regarding permanent stress relief. It's called death; that's when all the daily stress and strife will end. So be happy because now you know all stress eventually resolves. However, until you take the long dirt nap, it's going to be around, and subsequently what you need to do is deal with it. Find some form of stress relief, even if it just wearing big-girl panties. But two pints of Ben and Jerry's and a nap on the couch doesn't count as an effective stress program. The Buddha noted that all life is suffering. We will have good times and bad times, just like Led Zeppelin promised. Enjoy the contrast and the good times, reflect, and learn in the valleys. And always, always, keep going. As I just mentioned, exercise can be an excellent form of stress relief. You can use meditation, yoga, prayer, or massage. Find what works for you and incorporate it into your routine. Excessive eating, smoking, drinking, and drug abuse are choices that are best left to professionals.

I CAN'T COOK

Phooey. Everyone can cook utilizing a few simple techniques. Is Rachael Ray some closet neurosurgeon? If she can approximate cooking, there is no doubt you can succeed. As in the martial arts, a few basic techniques will cover 90 percent of your needs. And as in the martial arts, what often appears to be a very complex maneuver can often be broken down into several basic techniques joined together. There are a few exceptions, but they are the exceptions. You may not be able to execute a lozenge cut, but in all reality, you will probably never have the occasion to need to execute it. The Grassroots Gourmet cooking recipes in this book don't require a culinary degree. Most recipes don't. There are innumerable resources available in the form of video, books, and Internet blogs (like www.whatscookingwithdoc.com) that can ease any angst. What you need to cook well is passion. Be passionate about what you're preparing and serving, and take delight in the taste and the compliments you will receive. Take pride in what you accomplish.

I CAN'T GET THOSE INGREDIENTS

Double phooey. In these recipes there is room, purposefully, for substitution. The reason is simple. What you want to get is the quality ingredients that are available fresh. That is one of the tenets of Grassroots Gourmet cooking. The underlying theme of this book is simple and fresh. Learn some basic techniques, flavor combinations, and recipes and create from there. Stock up on staples (flours, grains, spices, etc.). But stop by the fresh markets, farmers' or otherwise, and see what produce, fresh meats, and seafood is available on a frequent basis. Then purchase what you'll use in the next few days. Stay away from the canned, processed, and overly refined stuff as much as possible. If you are lucky enough to have a neighborhood butcher and/or fishmonger, be his or her new best friend. You won't have a better resource for poultry, meats, and fish. And there is this little thing called the Internet. Many of the quality vendors provide some of the harder-to-find items or even the common items at reasonable prices and delivered to your door. It doesn't get much more convenient than that. For special occasions, or to get that really good truffle oil, one can also order online and have the little treasures in time to cook.

I COOK THE MEALS, BUT I'M NOT LOSING WEIGHT, SO I MIGHT AS WELL JUST EAT WHAT I WANT

Well, this is *not* a weight loss book. If your current diet consists of the average American slop, you will probably shed some pounds. But do not forget that it is not only what you eat but also how you eat, especially as in how much is on your plate. So if you have the Fat Albert buffet plate, even if it is a healthfully constructed meal, you will not trim the waistline. To lose weight, ultimately you need to burn more calories than you take in. There are many weight loss books and programs around. If you need to lose weight, find what works for you and do it. The key to keeping the weight off is what happens after you finish the weight loss program. Many, many people and many of my patients over the years lost weight over several months. They successfully sprinted. But a lifetime of eating is a marathon event. They did not know what to do when they didn't want or need to be on a weight loss diet anymore. This is the point where many weight loss regimens fail in the long term. This book is about the marathon part, the part to help you for the rest of the journey after you're at a weight you want to stay. This is about preparing and eating great food that's great for you for the rest of your life.

I DON'T HAVE TIME

No one does. The very pace of our current society is one of the contributors to our current crisis. It is the fast-paced, on-the-go, already-late frenzy that we call our daily life that has created an opportunity for overprocessed, readily available McMortems to be made so ubiquitous. The daily rush fosters us to embrace the easy path. That path is lemming made and leads over the cliff. Sometimes when life gives you lemons, you just have to suck 'em.

Yet if we really drill it down, though, for the most part, it is not really an issue of enough time. It is an issue of priority. If this is important, you will find the time. You can prepare many things ahead, so it may take some weekend or weeknight time here and there. If you spend fifteen minutes in a drive-through and go ten minutes out of your way to get there, you could drive straight home and make a meal. If you like/need to spend time with family or friends, make your cooking part of the process. Share trips to get ingredients, and visit while you cook. If you need alone time, tell them to all bugger off and seek the monastic refuge of your kitchen and cook. Like the ad says, "Just do it."

techniques, tips, and other tasty bits

NOTES ON PREPARATION

It does no good to bypass the fast food joints; purchase wholesome, fresh ingredients; portion them out; and construct a menu only to dump them in oil and attempt a deep fry because that is the only way you know how to cook. It's a bit like buying Dom Pérignon and using it for a mimosa. We need to know some basic kitchen skills so we can cook appropriately. Technique may not be everything, but it is the foundation upon which something sits. This is nothing more than having the right set of "culinary tools" to pull out of your "culinary toolbox" for the job at hand. You do not have to go to culinary school to learn these. There are great resources in books and videos and on the Internet. I have a whole series of three- to five-minute instructional videos called *Code Delicious* (free to view, as always) on my website, What's Cookin' with Doc (www.whatscooking withdoc.com). The videos walk you through everything from basic knife skills to making homemade stocks to stuffing chicken breasts. As for these basics, most people actually already have them or can quickly learn them. Once you are comfortable with the basics, you can move onward and upward to more challenging techniques and foods. With your foundation knife skills and a well-stocked pantry and freezer full of staples, you have a great underpinning upon which to construct almost any dish. Add in the knowledge of how to sauté, fry, roast, grill, broil, boil, poach, simmer, braise, and bake, and you are able to prepare most any dish. These are skills most anyone can learn and accomplish with adequate competency. Before you try to master the skills, a few helpful definitions should make the learning process that much easier.[1]

MISE EN PLACE

I am often asked what is needed to get started cooking delicious food. Do we need posh gadgets, expensive chef's knives, and twelve pounds of foie gras? My first response is that to cook successfully we need to have good basics and good fundamentals and our technique must be sound. To that end I respond that we need *mise en place. Mise en place* (meez ahn plahs) is the French term that literally means "everything in its place" or "to put in place." When we get ready to do a coronary intervention in the cardiac catheterization laboratory, we must first make sure we have *mise en place*. We must make sure that all the possible supplies we need are readily available. The ones that we know we are going to need are at hand and ready to go in an instant. All the setting up that can be done in advance has been done. This is the same mentality I take into the kitchen. It means all my prep work that can be done ahead of time has been done. Items are properly weighed and measured. All the tools and equipment that I need to work with have been identified and laid out. Ovens are preheated. Ice baths are ready. The work space I am going to utilize is clean, clear, and ready. This is done every time, the same way, and the same basic checklist. When you are finishing your roux is not the time to start chopping onions. I encourage you to take the time to prepare your *mise en place*. If you do this, you will find your enjoyment level rises as your stress level decreases. That's the first step to happy food.

The best way to get a sense of what constitutes *mise en place* is to work through an example. As far as the minimal equipment you need to start, it is really just a good chef's knife. It is versatile, and almost any kitchen task required can be done with the eight- to ten-inch bladed jewel. A good chef's knife can be had from a variety of makers. It will likely cost you a couple hundred dollars, but it should last you a lifetime. It is your samurai sword, so I recommend you go test drive a few before you purchase. Make sure the grip, weight, and balance are comfortable. Once you know what you want, you can purchase or shop online. I cooked for a long time with some cheap knives. That's where I got all my serious injuries. A cheap knife will quickly lose its edge and become dull. They are often not properly balanced. This creates a situation where you have to exert more force to get the job done. You end up tearing through the product and giving yourself a jagged cut.

I also recommend good, individual cutting boards. I have plastic, dishwasher-safe boards separately labeled for meat, poultry, and fish. I recommend that your cutting boards be individualized and dishwasher safe. Using these types helps prevent cross-contamination and is just good cleanliness. I have a bamboo board for breads, vegetables, and fruits. The final necessity is a good fire extinguisher. It is the piece you never want to use, but if you need it, you'll be damn glad you have it.

With a quality chef's knife, some cutting boards, and the extinguisher, we can look to an example of preparing a fall feast featuring barbecue pork with pan-simmered apples and napa cabbage, roasted corn with cilantro-lime butter, and apple pie granita for dessert. To emphasize the process, we will use a week-long preparation strategy for the fall feast. Obviously, for a meal to be done in a single day or evening, just compress the process.

DAY 1: SHOPPING

The best way to get organized for a specific task, in this case preparing a food and feast gathering, is to make sure you have what you need before you start. Sounds simple, but I think we've all been there when, in the midst of undoubtedly the most critical time period, we look around to say, "Damn, I'm out of that." This method avoids that problem.

1. Gather all the recipes you will use.
2. Make a master inventory list of all the ingredients, including quantities.
3. Make sure you list each ingredient under the proper recipe heading, that way if you can't get something, you know which recipe you have to change.
4. Check off which items are already in your kitchen. Do not forget to check dates of expiration and for spoilage. For example, check the dates on baking soda or eggs if you have to use them. Make sure you have the quantities needed; if you need two cups of milk, make sure it's not gone sour and there's enough.

Here's an example list for our fall feast:

- Wild Game Brine
  3 c. pickling salt
  1 c. brown sugar
  1 orange, quartered
  1 lemon, quartered
  4 sprigs of thyme
  2 sprigs of rosemary
  4 cloves of garlic, smashed
  1 jalapeño or other hot pepper, sliced lengthwise with membrane intact
  1 onion, quartered
  3 ribs of celery, roughly chopped
  3 carrots, roughly chopped

⅓ c. apple cider vinegar

1 can of Guinness beer

4–5 quarts water

- Pork Barbecue

  Charcoal or gas for grill/smoker

  Wood chips for smoking

  1 pork butt (6–8 lbs.)

- Basic Pork Barbecue Rub

  1 tsp. cumin seed

  1 tsp. fennel seed

  1 tsp. coriander seed

  ¼ tsp. garlic powder

  ¼ tsp. cayenne pepper

  ¼ tsp. dried oregano

  ¼ tsp. dried thyme

  ¼ tsp. onion powder

  1 tsp. smoked paprika

  1 tsp. dried chipotle chili pepper

- Western North Carolina–Style Barbecue Sauce

  4 tbsp. butter or Smart Balance substitute

  1½ c. onion, finely chopped

  4 cloves of garlic, chopped

  ½ tsp. garlic powder

  ½ tsp. cayenne pepper

  ½ tsp. dried oregano

  ½ tsp. dried thyme

  ½ tsp. onion powder

  2 tsp. smoked paprika

  2 tsp. dry mustard

  1 tsp. cayenne pepper

  ½ tsp. ground black pepper

  6 oz. tomato paste

  1½ c. water

  ¾ c. apple cider vinegar

  2 tbsp. honey

- Roasted Corn with Cilantro-Lime Butter

  1 ear of corn per guest

  8 oz. (equal to 2 sticks) butter or Smart Balance substitute

2 limes

¼ c. cilantro, finely chopped

- Pan-Simmered Apples and Napa Cabbage

  2 Granny Smith apples

  2 oz. (4 tbsp.) butter or Smart Balance substitute

  ¼ c. apple cider vinegar

  ¼ c. apple juice

  1 lemon

  1 head of napa cabbage, thinly sliced

  1 tbsp. shallot, finely chopped

  1 tbsp. olive oil

  1 tsp. cinnamon, freshly ground

  ¼ tsp. allspice, freshly ground

  1 clove, freshly ground

  ½ c. light chicken stock

- Apple Pie Granita

  ⅓ c. natural organic sugar or Splenda/Truvia (use proper sweetness conversion)

  3 c. apple juice

  1 lime

  2 tbsp. apple pie spice

  6–8 oz. vanilla yogurt

- Apple Pie Spice

  4 tbsp. ground cinnamon

  2 tbsp. ground nutmeg

  1 tbsp. ground allspice

  1 tbsp. ground cardamom

After we see what we have in the kitchen and what we need to get, we can purchase the necessary items. Once we have all the items in the kitchen, we make a quick prep list. We don't want to have to do everything at once at the last minute, so we do as much ahead of time as possible while preserving the integrity of fresh, Grassroots Gourmet cooking. Here's an example for our fall feast prep list, with Monday being the day we make our inventory list, check the stock in our kitchen, and shop. Saturday is the day to feast.

Table 16.1 outlines very quickly what we need to do each day. Monday we plan our menu, collect recipes, make a complete inventory list, check the stock, and get the ingredients we need. Tuesday we make the rub and apple pie spice mixtures and so on down the week. When Saturday, the feast day, arrives, we need only smoke the pork, roast the corn, and cook the cabbage, all very simple tasks. When we go to cook each

TABLE 16.1. Fall Feast Prep List

To Make	Mon.	Tues.	Wed.	Thur.	Fri.	Sat.
Brine	—			X		
Pork	—				X	Put on smoker
BBQ Sauce	—		X			X
Cabbage	—					X
Corn	—					
Cilantro-Butter	—		X			
Rub	—	X				
Apple Pie Spice	—	X				
Granita	—				X	

individual recipe, we apply the same *mise en place* principle on an individual recipe scale. A great example is the Pate a Choux video in the "Recipe Video Demos" section at www.whatscookingwithdoc.com. Everything we need is premeasured and located within easy reach. For example, with the apple pie granita, we would have our metal nine- or ten-inch baking dish ready and next to our blender. Our apple pie spice was already made, and we have two tablespoons measured and ready to be dumped into the blender. Our lime juice, apple juice, and sugar or substitute are also measured and ready to go. Then it is one simple step to properly combine our ingredients and finish the recipe. It is neat and efficient in a quick but not rushed manner. It should resemble a well-executed basketball play or offensive drive in football, a methodical, organized, and effective march up the court or field resulting in a perfect score.

SEASONING

Always season as you cook. The simplest way to ruin a meal is to over- or underseason it. Seasoning as you cook brings out the flavors at each level of preparation. Adding seasoning, salt, and pepper as you cook during each phase of the dish preparation allows you to build layers of flavor. Be careful in adding the salt, but don't refrain from seasoning because you can't just add seasoning at the end if you've underseasoned during the cooking process. That never works. If you wait until it is done, the food will be bland. Then when you try to get the seasoning level right, it will just taste salty. You need to taste, season, and taste throughout. I am constantly tasting and adjusting the seasoning as I cook so that the food is properly seasoned at completion. Also, I use kosher salt when I say *salt*, unless otherwise noted.

There are two important exceptions to this seasoning golden rule. Whenever reducing anything, such as pan juices, liquids, and stocks, do not season to taste at that point. As the liquid evaporates, the salt will remain, and the dish will become too salty. For that reason, when I make my stocks, I do not add any salt because in the vast majority of cases I am reducing the stock. The reduction will cause the salt to concentrate and will ruin everything.

THE SPICE(S) OF LIFE

I think spices are incredibly important in cooking. Great food is all about flavor. One of the things that can also give food its flavor in addition to spices is fat. Combined with a great flavor profile, a little fat like olive oil can carry all those flavors of the dish. It can transport flavor because a lot of flavor compounds are fat soluble. Many flavor compounds from the dish's main ingredients, flavors from the fat itself, and any additional flavors from spices and seasonings can only be carried by fat molecules. Some foods, like tomatoes, require a fat like olive oil to release some of their more healthful compounds. The fat can also add what the Japanese call *umami*. Often referred to as the "fifth taste," it refers to that pleasing mouth-feel. It's why toast and fresh-baked bread taste better with butter, although not everything does. This action of fat allows the dish to become more flavorful. If something like olive oil is used with proper restraint, the meal can also be made healthier. Unfortunately, currently in the United States, I think we have abandoned careful flavor preparation in favor of a big wallow in the fat pond. Using just primarily fat does add some flavor and texture, and it's easy. It's the lazy way to cook. As David Kessler, former head of the Food and Drug Administration, mentions in his book *The End of Overeating*, our fast food nation has hooked folks onto craving that fat and especially fat with salt. The more of it you eat, the more you crave. Morgan Spurlock experienced that firsthand in his movie *Supersize Me*, where he started becoming addicted to the fat and salt.

So how does one break that vicious cycle? Why, by fighting fire with fire, of course, or flavor with flavor in this case. First and foremost, our food has to taste great. We can do that through judicious use of carriers like fat, spices, and seasonings. We build flavor profiles and combinations to challenge and delight the palate. We use sugar, salt, and fat the way a surgeon wields a scalpel: maximum effect with minimal use. Using the fat as a contributor and as a carrier as opposed to the end product of the meal creates great taste with less fat. You'll actually have people tasting your food, not just gorging on fatty brains like zombies from *Dawn of the Dead*.

To execute this palate-awakening maneuver, I turn to my martial arts experience. In our particular martial art, we have a series of exercises and drills that have a practical application but also serve to teach some fundamental principles. We call these *hon waza*. Once the basic form is mastered, then diverse variations, often referred to as *henka*, are practiced. Often, I see those with huge egos and little skill screwing up the *hon waza* and deflecting their inadequacies with an "Oh, I was doing a *henka*." No, you were screwing up the basic. In medicine every patient is different and requires a personally tailored regimen, but the basic algorithms of treatment success are derived from the congregated data of large clinical trials. These guidelines form the basics from which the individual needs are adjusted. When physicians ignore these standards of practice, they are negligent. A culinary equivalent occurred when I was going to a restaurant, a rather expensive bistro, and ordered the ostrich entree. It sounded intriguing and interesting if prepared correctly. I've had ostrich before, and it's a delicious lean meat. This one came with a vanilla sauce. I know what you're thinking, and you're right: It definitely did not work. But it could have if prepared differently. The chef really did not have a good grasp of a basic flavor profile, a basic guideline, principle, or *hon waza*, before he went out to experiment, so it was a disaster. The restaurant closed shortly thereafter.

What I might suggest as a start is to work with some familiar profiles. A great resource that every kitchen should have is *Ethnic Cuisine: The Flavor-Principle Cookbook* by Elisabeth Rozin. In her most excellent book, she notes that different cultures tend to "combine a small number of flavoring ingredients so frequently and so consistently that they become definitive of that particular cuisine."[2] I've included a few here from her outstanding resource. This is by no means a definitive list but merely a good primer and starting-off point:

- Central Asia: cinnamon, fruits, and nuts
- China (General): soy sauce, rice wine, and ginger
- Mandarin/Peking (Northern China): miso, garlic, and sesame
- Szechuan (Western China): sweet, sour, and hot flavors like sugar, vinegar, and Szechuan peppers
- Cantonese (Southern China): black beans and garlic
- Eastern Europe (Semitic): onion and chicken fat
- Eastern/Northern Europe: dill, caraway, allspice, and paprika; often with sour cream
- France (General): olive oil, garlic, basil, wine, herb butter, wine or stock with cheese
- Provence: thyme, rosemary, marjoram, sage, and tomato
- Normandy: apple, cider, and calvados
- Greece: olive oil, tomato, lemon, cinnamon, and oregano
- India (General): curries and turmeric
- Northern India: cumin, ginger, and garlic
- Southern India: mustard seed, coconut, tamarind, and chilies
- Italy (General): olive oil, garlic, and basil

- Northern Italy: wine vinegar
- Southern Italy: parsley, anchovy, and tomato
- Japan: shoyu (soy sauce), sake, and sugar
- Mexico: tomato, lime, and chilies
- North Africa: cumin, coriander, cinnamon, ginger, onion, tomato, and fruit
- Spain: olive oil, garlic, nuts, onions, peppers, and tomato
- Thailand: fish sauce, curries, and chilies
- West Africa: peanut, chilies, and tomato

This is a *hon waza* of basic flavor profiles. Play with these. Once you're comfortable with them, then you can start to pull necessary components from each profile as you need to get the results for your dish. This is one of the fundamental principles in my use of fusion cuisine.

BASICS

I have tried to include a number of "basics" in both chapters 17 and 18. These are basic recipes. Once you are comfortable with these and the basic cooking principles they embody, then add your own unique twists and variations. For example, after you master the basic pasta dough, you can add fresh basil, mushrooms, or sun-dried tomatoes. Once you have perfected the basic risotto, add lobster, truffles, oven-roasted tomatoes, or saffron and spices, whatever you like. Have fun because, when you are having fun doing something you care about, then you become passionate. If you become passionate about what you are putting into yourself and your loved ones, then you have put healing medicine into your food.

GRILLING 101: KNOW YOUR BUTT FROM YOUR BRISKET

It amazes me that so many professionals, in any field, never really get a good grip on the basics. I believe that to achieve competence at any level you must have a solid grasp of the fundamentals. This knowledge foundation is what allows you to derive great technique. On the shoulders of knowledge and technique sits Art. That's where greatness lives no matter what you do. So to take some activity, vocation, or endeavor to that level, you have to do your homework. I saw on an episode of a cooking show how these professional chefs who wanted to run a major operation couldn't even identify where the different cuts of beef came from. So to save face at the Labor Day grill-out, we'll cover some basic beef knowledge. Even if you can't grill, if you stand there and spout this off to the unsuspecting, you'll sound like a genius.

First off, most of your beef will come from steers. Steers are male cattle castrated prior to maturity. These bovine eunuchs are then processed into four pieces, or quarters.

There are two forequarters and two hindquarters. These are then processed into primal cuts. They are the chuck, brisket and shank, rib, short plate, short loin, sirloin, flank, and round (see figure 16.1). These are different areas of the animal, and thus these cuts differ in flavor and tenderness. They also favor different methods of preparation.

The chuck represents the animal's shoulder region. It is flavorful but tough. The cuts derived from this primal are cross-rib pot roast, chuck short ribs, cube steak, stew meat, and ground chuck.

The brisket and shank come from the forequarter below the chuck. This area contains the animal's breast (brisket) and the foreshank. The ribs and breastbone are removed from the brisket. Nonetheless, it remains a tough piece of meat but is well suited to simmering, braising, or pickling, as in corned beef. The shanks are often used for stocks or consommés.

The rib, not surprisingly, contains six to twelve ribs as well as a portion of backbone. This cut produces roast prime rib of beef. The prime here does not refer to grade; rather it reflects the fact that this cut contains the majority of the primal meat. If the eye muscle (center portion) is removed from the ribs, then you get a boneless rib eye roast. This can be cut into rib eye steaks. The separated rib bones are beef barbeque ribs. The ends of the rib bones trimmed off this primal are the beef short ribs.

The short plate is directly below the rib primal on the forequarter. This primal yields short ribs and skirt steak. These are flavorful but tough cuts. They are suitable for simmering, braising, or marinating and grilling. Fajita meat is often skirt steak. Some portions of the short plate may be used in ground beef.

Moving onto the hindquarters, there is the short loin. It is the front of the back, if you will. The short loin contains one rib, the thirteenth, and a portion of the backbone. Some

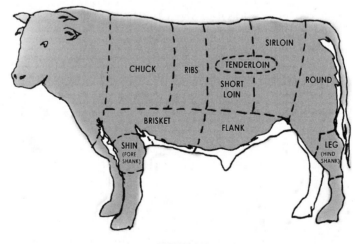

FIGURE 16.1

chapter sixteen

of the most tender (and expensive) cuts come from this primal. The loin eye is a continuation of the rib eye muscle. This runs along the top of the T-shaped backbone. If the loin eye meat is removed from the bone, you get the boneless strip loin, from which boneless strip steaks are cut. Below the loin eye muscle on the other side of the backbone lays the most tender cut of all, the beef tenderloin. Cutting the short loin crossways with the bone in, from front to back, produces club steak with no tenderloin, T-bone steaks with a small portion of tenderloin, and Porterhouse steaks with large portion of tenderloin. The entire tenderloin contains the section in the short loin known as the short tenderloin as well as a portion that extends into the next primal, the sirloin, known as the butt tenderloin. If the entire tenderloin is removed, it can be cut into chateaubriand, filet mignon, and tournedos.

The sirloin, into which the tenderloin extends, lies between the short loin and the round. It contains hip and backbone. This primal produces bone-in or boneless roasts and steaks, which, while flavorful, are generally not as tender as those from the strip loin.

The flank lies directly below the loin primals. It is to the rear of the short plate and is a boneless cut. This primal produces the flank steak, or London broil. The meat may also be used in ground beef. There is a small cut from this area known as the hanging tenderloin, which is very tender and delicious.

The final primal is the round. It contains the hind leg and can be quite large. It provides a variety of cuts, including top round, outside round, bottom round, knuckle, and shank. This primal also provides the steamship round cut.

GRILLING 102: FROM SNOUT TO TAIL

Pork

For Americans, the history of pork is tied to the history of Uncle Sam. During the War of 1812, the U.S. government shipped pork to soldiers in barrels. These barrels were stamped with the letters *U.S.* and the name of the meat packer, Sam Wilson. The soldiers referred to the barrels as "Uncle Sam's meat." Thus we have pork to thank for the national icon Uncle Sam.

Pork is also divided into primal sections (see figure 16.2). The hogs, following slaughter, are dived into two lengthwise halves. The primal cuts are derived from these. The primals are the shoulder, Boston butt, belly, loin, and ham. The ham should not be confused with the picnic ham. The term *picnic ham* actually refers to the primal shoulder. This is the lower portion of the foreleg. It is one of the less tender areas of the hog. These cuts can be smoked (the aforementioned picnic hams), cut into shoulder butt steaks, or cut into smaller stewing pieces. Many pit masters in the South use whole pork shoulder as the preferred barbecue cut. The shoulder hock is the foreleg portion of this primal. It is almost always smoked and used for flavorings in soups, stews, and braised dishes.

The Boston butt is not a butt at all. It is the square cut directly above the shoulder primal. It is a very meaty and tender cut. It can be cut into steaks or chops. When it is smoked, it is sometimes referred to as a "cottage ham." It is also a favorite for barbeque.

While the Boston butt is not a butt at all, the pork belly is actually the belly. This primal is located directly below the loin. It is from this region that the pork spareribs come from. The nonsparerib portion of the belly can be used to produce bacon.

The loin contains the highest-quality portion of the hog, and the most expensive cuts are derived from this primal. This primal is located directly behind the Boston butt and includes the entire rib area. The pork loin comes from this primal; it consists of a very tender, single eye muscle. It is actually a very lean cut of meat. The pork tenderloin is located on the inside of the rib bones. As the name implies, the tenderloin is the most tender cut of pork. The ubiquitous pork chop can be derived from the entire loin primal. The most-highly-prized chop is the center cut, just after the blade bone at the front and the portion at the rear are removed. Smoked boneless pork loin is also known as Canadian bacon. The rib bones from this primal are known as pork back ribs. Fatback, although not technically part of the primal, comes from this region.

The primal ham is the hog's hind leg. As the name implies, this cut is often smoked or cured to produce various hams. The shank portion of the ham is called the ham hock. It is used in an analogous fashion to the shoulder hock.

Seafood

There are some basic tips and things to look for when picking out seafood to assure freshness. The following are some general criteria for determining the freshness of fish and shellfish:

- Smell: Fresh seafood should have no odor or a slight smell of the ocean.
- Eyes: They should be clear and full. Avoid product with cloudy or sunken eyes.

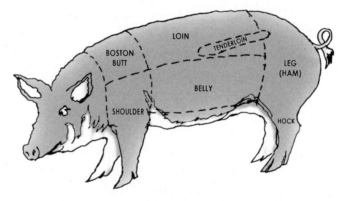

FIGURE 16.2

- Gills: The gills should be intact and bright red. Avoid brown discoloration.
- Texture: Fresh fish should have a firm, not mushy, texture.
- Fins and Scales: They should be moist. Avoid product with dried-out scales and fins.
- Appearance: The fish should appear moist and shiny.
- Live: If purchasing live, the product should show vigorous movement. Crustaceans should move. Clams, mussels, and oysters should close if partially opened when examined. The exceptions are geoducks and razor and steamer clams.

When purchasing seafood, the following are some additional seafood terminology you may come across:

- Whole or Round: caught intact
- Drawn: viscera removed
- Dressed: viscera, gills, fins, and scales removed
- Pan-Dressed: viscera, gills, and scales removed; fins trimmed; head may be removed
- Butterflied: a pan-dressed fish that is boned and opened like the wings on a butterfly; sides are attached by the spine or skin
- Fillet: side of a fish removed intact
- Steak: a cross-section cut

ON SELECTING PROTEINS

By consuming insane amounts of overprocessed fast and junk foods, we incur the negative effects of too much cholesterol, salt, fat, and sugar. These manipulations often seem to involve the protein portion of our meals. It is a double-edged sword because, not only do we reap negative effects, but also we miss the beneficial effects of fresh, natural alternatives. This includes the delicious bounty from the sea. The Institute of Medicine notes that:

> Seafood is a widely available, nutrient-rich food that provides high quality protein, low in saturated fat and rich in polyunsaturated fats, and particularly the omega-3 fatty acids eicosapentaenoic acid (EPA) and docosahexaenoic acid (DHA). Research conducted over the past several years suggests that there are benefits linked to eating seafood that include the dietary advantages associated with consuming a low-fat protein source and possible additional benefits linked to brain and visual system development in infants and reduced risk for certain forms of heart disease.[3]

Omega-3 fatty acids are polyunsaturated fatty acid (PUFA), a good type of fat. They are essential for growth and good health. Many studies have shown that a diet rich in omega-3 fatty acids may help lower triglycerides and increase HDL cholesterol, the good cholesterol. Even though their diet was high in fat, because it was primarily derived from seafood and contained omega-3s, the Inuit people were found to have reduced triglycerides, heart rate, blood pressure, and atherosclerosis. That's good for my heart patients. Omega-3 fatty acids may also act as an anticoagulant to prevent blood from clotting and may help lower high blood pressure. That's also good for my heart patients. In addition, these compounds have been shown to potentially protect against Alzheimer's disease, Parkinson's disease, and rheumatoid arthritis and improve immune function. A specific omega-3 PUFA, docosahexaenoic acid (DHA), may reduce inflammation while preserving infection-fighting abilities of white blood cells. A recent animal study out of Spain suggests that these compounds may increase insulin sensitivity. Decreased sensitivity to insulin, or insulin resistance, is a major problem associated with metabolic syndrome and type-2 diabetes. Future investigations will look into using these compounds in conditions like asthma. That's good for everyone. One of the best sources of these omega-3s are cold-water, oily fish, such as salmon, and to a lesser degree fish like tuna. The bottom line is that seafood is very good for you, but it is important to make sure what you get is reliably fresh. Processing can remove goodness and taste and add unwanted flavors, textures, and mystery compounds.

Overprocessed food and altered animal products are not what I recommend. It's not what I eat. To me, these are not healthy choices. A great example of another good protein choice is found in natural, grass-fed beef that is hormone and antibiotic free. These are beef cattle that are allowed to roam free and consume natural grasses. These animals are herbivores; feeding them high-protein pellets made from ground-up bits of other animals just is not their natural diet. I don't want to eat animals stressed out because they are subject to unnatural acts. We have taken something natural and beneficial and made it unhealthy. When the animals are allowed to thrive naturally, we find things like beneficial omega-3 fatty acids in the red meat. Animals with natural diets are lower in overall saturated fatty acids (bad) and higher in polyunsaturated fatty acids (good). Products from grass-fed animals have increased conjugated linoleic acid by approximately 50 percent and omega-3 fatty acids by approximately 40 percent. Both of these things are good. The animals allowed to move about naturally are also lower in overall fat and higher in vitamin E, a natural antioxidant. They also tend to have lower ratios of omega-6 to omega-3 fatty acids. Higher ratios found in the typical Western diet have been suggested as a contributor to such chronic diseases as diabetes and heart disease.

A word here about chickens and breasts: I highly recommend buying whole chickens and butchering them yourself. It only takes a few minutes, and there are a number of good reasons to do it. First, you pay significantly less per pound than buying the same grade of bird precut. Second, you get to use the whole chicken, including the carcass for things like homemade stock. You get the thighs and drumsticks to cook as well. Third, the longer the chicken is whole, the fresher the meat. And speaking of whole, look for free-range organic birds. Like beef, they have a superior nutrition profile. Not only are there the aforementioned benefits, but I've done a number of taste trials, and often these more humanely raised birds flat out taste better. Stressed-out birds make for lousy meat, and if you really want to see stressed-out birds, then just visit an overcrowded poultry farm.

Yet, none of these health benefits means anything if people won't eat it. As a chef I know people won't eat any of the food if it doesn't taste good. It has to taste good. If it doesn't taste good but is good for you, it's not food; it's just medicine. The beauty of consuming these products fresh from the sea or the farm is that they simply taste better. They all have a delicious flavor you want to savor. Fresh product like this is what I use when I do my Grassroots Gourmet cooking. It is what I use to cook with and serve because it is what I want to eat. It is a pleasure. As a chef, for me, it is all about taste. As a physician I know it's the right prescription to make my food healthful. Translation: It's great-tasting food that's great for you. And that's culinary nirvana, my friend.

MORE TOYS

The array of gadgets and equipment for the kitchen is endless. And unless you have an endless supply of money, you need to be selective as to what you purchase. Even if your cash is endless, you kitchen space probably isn't. If you clutter your work area with unused appliances, pots, pans, and the latest mini-burger grill pan, you will be violating the first rule of *mise en place*: a concise, organized, and clean work area. As previously mentioned all you really need to start, aside from some pots and pans, is a good chef's knife. You will want to acquire more tools as your experience, repertoire, curiosity, and desire grow. I am a big fan of Alton Brown's rule of utility: Always go for the multitasker when you have the option. Here are a few, not necessarily expensive, items you should consider.

Thermometer

I highly recommend several types of thermometers. If you are going to deep fry in a Dutch oven or other pot, you need a thermometer that reaches up to 375 degrees Fahrenheit. A good candy thermometer that can clip onto the pot and reach the bottom is a good choice and a necessity if you plan to work with sugar and sweets. You should have a meat thermometer so you can check the internal temperature of meats you cook. It can prevent not only overcooked food and ruined meals but also undercooked food and illness as well. I use an instant-read meat thermometer as well as one with a probe that I can place with food in the oven. It has a temperature alarm so I can set it to go off when food reaches the desired temperature. As you get busy preparing the other items while food cooks in the oven, this can be a lifesaver.

Timer

Another inexpensive little lifesaver is a simple timer. When simply cooking one or two things, you may not need it. However, when you have three or five things going at once as you bring the meal together, this will remind you to remove that en croute appetizer from the oven before all you have left is a lump of coal.

Mixer

If you are planning to do any baking whatsoever, and I suggest you do, you will need a good stand mixer. It is indispensible when mixing batters or whipping egg whites. I make all my bread and do all my kneading with my mixer and dough hook. It takes only a few minutes with my mixer to make bread or pasta dough. I don't use a bread machine because, with the dough I make in the mixer, I can make regular loaves in a loaf pan, French bread, pizza, round loaves, rolls, and the list goes on. I have attachments for my mixer so I use that not only to make pasta dough but also to roll out sheets, form noodles, and grind meat.

Mandolin

You can and should practice your cutting with your chef's knife and be able to obtain uniform pieces. However, when I need a lot of thin slices or strips, the mandolin is the way to go. Make sure you get one that is sturdy and won't slide. Always, always use the hand guard. If you do not and you slip, it can remove digits as quickly as it can make coleslaw.

Scale

I would consider this essential, especially when you want to portion out the measurements and servings. I use it whenever I can, simply because mass measurements that you get from a scale are more accurate then volume measurements. A cup of flour may vary as to how many ounces are in it due to weather (e.g., during times of high humidity versus low humidity). Conversely the weight may vary depending on how tightly you pack the measuring cup. If you use the weight, the weight will always be the same; twelve ounces will be twelve ounces. This makes the recipes reproducible, precise, and accurate. That is exactly what you must have to properly perform any kind of baking. I have several scales, one being a precision scale for smaller measures and one for everyday use. I have digital scales that can flip between U.S. and metric measures. Make sure you have at least one good, quality scale.

Food Processor

This is another appliance I would consider essential. Make sure you get one that will hold adequate amounts to accommodate your cooking. The extra attachments that grate cheese and so on are nice, but a powerful basic processor with some sharp blades is the most important criteria.

Blenders

Although you can use a processor or a regular blender to puree, blend, or otherwise liquefy, I love my immersion blender. I do a lot of sauces and soups. If you plan to do the same, you will find a good, powerful immersion blender an indispensible ally. Beware of cheap ones with small motors (underpowered) and plastic blades with a small working area. You want something you can stick on the back of your boat and power off to your favorite fishing hole with.

Pizza Stone

Nothing fancy here. You can even go extra cheap and get some unglazed stone from a home supply store. I like to make a lot of pizzas and breads. These stones really do make a difference. You can't make a decent loaf of French bread on a metal pan; at least I can't. They also help your oven perform better by absorbing the heat and serving as a heat sink so temperatures are less variable when you add food.

Sieves/Strainers

Again nothing fancy, but you need some sieves with different sizes. I always strain anything that needs to have a smooth, uniform consistency. Even after using my immersion blender, there can be unrecognized chunks, so if I need it smooth or something like custard, I always strain. It is one small step that pays huge dividends at service.

Deep Fryer

This one is a bit of a luxury. You can use a Dutch oven, oil, and thermometer. Yet if I am going to deep fry, I want to do it right. A good deep fryer will help you hold the oil temperature where you set it. I find I have a much easier time, greater control, and precision using the deep fryer's temperature setting than I do over the stovetop. A correct, consistent oil temperature means the food deep fries correctly. When food is deep fried correctly, it actually absorbs very little oil. When oil temperature is too low, that is when food absorbs the oil, resulting in greasy, unpleasant, and unhealthy food.

Scoops and Ladles

Once again, it need not be anything fancy or expensive. It is important, especially when determining serving sizes, to be able to deliver the proper amount. It is a good idea to have several sizes of scoops and ladles properly marked.

Graters and Zesters

I have two graters of differing size that I use for both grating and zesting. There are many different types and sizes. I think a few that work for you are all you need, but it is a good idea to have at least one. You will find you use it more than you think, zesting citrus rinds or small amounts of cheese or nutmeg and such to complete a presentation.

A WORD ON RECIPES

There are well over a hundred recipes in this book. You may cook them all a thousand times; you may only cook them once. Depending on your culinary skill, you may vary the recipes from the very first time around. All of that is perfectly fine. This not a collection of recipes to make you a celebrity chef clone, especially because I am not a celebrity chef.

The recipes here represent a wide range of flavors, techniques, and applications. They were chosen this way on purpose. The idea is to use this collection of recipes as your "kitchen training manual." In the martial arts, we often practice a series of moves referred to as a *waza* or *kata*. The idea behind this is to learn a certain principle. You simply cannot train for every potential combination of events you may encounter; the world of combat is too wide. What I teach is a principle. We learn a technique, what it embodies, and where and how it applies. We learn when to use it and when not to use it. These recipes are your kitchen *waza*. Each one teaches you a method of preparation and how to work with a different ingredient or application of flavor profiles. I have traveled broadly and eaten broadly and at times expanded broadly. There are flavors and methods from Asia, India, Africa, Central and South America, the Middle East, and Europe. There is regional cuisine like Southern American fare and universal basics. When you finish these recipes, you will have been exposed to many techniques and flavor profiles. Your toolbox, your personal repertoire, will be filled with useful items. When you move on to creating your personal culinary artistry, which is the goal of every Grassroots Gourmet, you have the tools to do it. In medical school you learn algorithms and data. In the real world, you learn every patient is unique and requires a customized approach within the framework of scientifically sound, outcomes-based medicine. In the same way, let these recipes be your Grassroots Gourmet cooking textbook so that when you finish you can pick up any cookbook or check out any Web-based recipe or video, and know you are ready for the creative challenge to make that experience personally yours. You will have gone from eater to taster, from simple cook to chef. You will have transformed into a Grassroots Gourmet and are on your way to becoming your own culinary Buddha.

firsts (recipes)

IT'S TIME to get down to the food. The firsts discussed here go by a number of other names: starters, appetizers, small plates, tapas, and so on. The names are not important, but the portion size and timing are. This is a part of the meal, not *the* meal. The amount you serve will vary, but ultimately it should sit on a small plate and make a small snack. But do not confuse this with a snack. Do not place everything out in one bowl and let everyone help themselves, endlessly munching. That defeats the idea. Here is what we want to accomplish with this service:

- Serve this course fifteen to twenty minutes before you serve the main course.
- Either before or during, serve an eight-ounce glass of water to accompany the course.
- This is one appetizer portion; no seconds or thirds on the plate.
- Serve only one first course.
- The first items can be used as sides (in appropriate first-sized portions) and served with mains to form a complete dinner-sized meal.

Firsts can be expanded to become a main. For example, you can take the Mediterranean roasted tomato salad, add a four-ounce grilled chicken breast, and have that as a meal. As with all the recipes, if not specifically noted, season with salt and pepper to taste.

SALSA

WHAT CAN I say? There's a reason this is the world's most popular condiment. I like some heat in my salsa, so feel free to vary
it. I like it fresh and a bit chunky so it's on the pico de gallo
side of the equation. It's a great topping for meats, especially
fish. I especially like to change the flavors by adding a seasonal
or fresh fruit, like crisp apples, mangoes, or Asian pears, to this
basic recipe. It's great on chopped vegetables or homemade
baked tortilla or pita chips. If you like it hot, keep the jalapeño
with the seeds. For a milder version, remove the seeds before
adding the pepper.

Nutrition Facts		
Serving Size 2 oz (57g)		
Servings Per Container 16		
Amount Per Serving		
Calories 15	Calories from Fat 0	
		% Daily Value*
Total Fat 0g		0%
Saturated Fat 0g		0%
Trans Fat 0g		
Cholesterol 0mg		0%
Sodium 125mg		5%
Total Carbohydrate 3g		1%
Dietary Fiber 1g		4%
Sugars 1g		
Protein 0g		
Vitamin A 8%	• Vitamin C 20%	
Calcium 0%	• Iron 0%	

* Percent Daily Values are based on a 2,000
calorie diet. Your daily values may be higher
or lower depending on your calorie needs.

		Calories	2,000	2,500
Total Fat	Less than	65g	80g	
Sat Fat	Less than	20g	25g	
Cholesterol	Less than	300mg	300mg	
Sodium	Less than	2,400mg	2,400mg	
Total Carbohydrate		300g	375g	
Dietary Fiber		25g	30g	

Calories per gram:
Fat 9 • Carbohydrate 4 • Protein 4

3–4 pounds Roma tomatoes, seeded and chopped
¾ bunch fresh cilantro, chopped
2 lemons, juiced
1 lime, juiced
¼ tsp. of lemon zest
½ red onion, chopped
½ green pepper, chopped
1 small jalapeño or chipotle pepper, chopped, and/or 1 tbsp. adobo sauce
    (optional; add more if you like it hot)
2 garlic cloves, finely chopped
Salt and pepper to taste

Combine all the ingredients except cilantro in the food processor. Pulse for 8–10 seconds. Add cilantro and pulse for 3–5 more seconds. Allow to come to room temperature
to serve.

healthy bytes "Hot peppers," like chili peppers or the jalapeño peppers used in this recipe,
are members of the capsicum species of plants. It is believed that the active ingredient in these
peppers, capsaicin, may actually protect the stomach lining from damage by killing bacteria
and stimulating the protective stomach secretions. These peppers have also been used as a
digestive aid and as an appetite stimulant. They can also produce endorphins, the body's natural pain blockers. Capsaicin, when applied topically, is a vasodilator and enhances circulation,
leading to a warm feeling and pain relief. But I recommend you eat it instead of rubbing it all
over, at least if there's company present.

GUACAMOLE SALAD

THIS IS ONE of my most favorite firsts. I call this guacamole salad because I like it with little more than just smashed avocados. It is a delightfully tasty, healthy treat. One of my favorite memories of this little guacamole salad was when I was vacationing in Merida, Mexico, with some good friends. We walked down to the local open-air market. Using our best broken Spanish, we were able to buy the ingredients we needed as well as a pile of fresh corn tortillas. We went back to the hotel and mixed up the guacamole poolside with a bowl, a spoon, and a pocket knife. We squeezed some fresh lime juice for margaritas and made a meal of it. Muy bien!

Nutrition Facts		
Serving Size 2 oz (57g)		
Servings Per Container 20		
Amount Per Serving		
Calories 50	Calories from Fat 45	
		% Daily Value*
Total Fat 5g		8%
Saturated Fat 0g		0%
Trans Fat 0g		
Cholesterol 0mg		0%
Sodium 50mg		2%
Total Carbohydrate 2g		1%
Dietary Fiber 5g		18%
Sugars 0g		
Protein 1g		
Vitamin A 0%	•	Vitamin C 15%
Calcium 0%	•	Iron 2%

* Percent Daily Values are based on a 2,000 calorie diet. Your daily values may be higher or lower depending on your calorie needs.

	Calories	2,000	2,500
Total Fat	Less than	65g	80g
Sat Fat	Less than	20g	25g
Cholesterol	Less than	300mg	300mg
Sodium	Less than	2,400mg	2,400mg
Total Carbohydrate		300g	375g
Dietary Fiber		25g	30g

Calories per gram:
Fat 9 • Carbohydrate 4 • Protein 4

3 avocados (preferably Haas), roughly mashed
½ bunch fresh cilantro, chopped
1 lemon, juiced
2 limes, juiced
¼ tsp. of lemon zest
¼ c. red onion, chopped
¼ c. red pepper, chopped
1 small jalapeño, chopped, and/or 1 tbsp. adobo sauce (add more if you like it hot)
1 Roma tomato, seeded and finely chopped
2 garlic cloves, finely chopped
½ tsp. cumin
Salt and pepper to taste

Pour the citrus juice over the avocados to help prevent them from turning brown. Combine all the ingredients except the cilantro in the food processor. Pulse for 8–10 seconds, add the cilantro, and pulse for 3–5 more seconds. Serve immediately or cover the top directly with plastic wrap to prevent the guacamole from discoloring and refrigerate. Allow to come to room temperature to serve.

healthy bytes Avocados are super rich in oleic acid, omega-9 fat, and monounsaturated fat. The monounsaturated fats are believed to actually lower cholesterol. In studies examining this, "bad" cholesterol (known as LDL) and triglycerides both went down. The HDL, or "good," cholesterol went up. Another substance that is thought to lower total cholesterol is beta-sitosterol. Beta-sitosterol was shown to reduce cholesterol in sixteen human studies as noted in the *American Journal of Medicine*.[1] Monounsaturated fat like that found in avocados

---

has also been linked to a reduced risk of cancer and diabetes. These fats are a key component to the Mediterranean diet, which in many studies, has lowered the risk of heart disease and diabetes. Avocados also contain lutein, a natural antioxidant that helps your eyes stay healthy and maintains healthy skin. Avocados are also a great source of fiber, with an average of eleven to seventeen grams of fiber per avocado. When you shop, realize that there is a difference between California and Florida avocados. A California avocado has 20 percent fewer calories (approximately 289 calories as compared to 365 for the Florida variety). California avocados also have approximately 13 percent less fat, 60 percent less carbohydrates, and more lutein than their Floridian brethren. However, Florida avocados have roughly 20 percent more potassium.

BLUE CHEESE DIP

THIS IS A great snack in small quantities. It is very rich, so a little can go a long way. I like it with cut vegetables, like carrots, celery, peppers, or bok choy. It is also delicious drizzled over some garden-fresh tomatoes and used like a salad dressing.

½ c. Greek-style yogurt
1 lemon, juiced
4 oz. crumbled blue cheese
1 tsp. garlic, finely chopped
1 tbsp. apple cider vinegar
Approximately ¼ c. cilantro leaves
½ c. good-quality olive oil

Combine all the ingredients in a food processor and blend. Refrigerate and serve chilled.

healthy bytes Cilantro is also known as coriander. Coriander is believed to come from the Greek word *koris*, meaning "bedbug," as it was said they both emitted a similar odor. The herb is also known as Chinese parsley. The ancient Chinese believed it provided immortality and also used the herb in love potions, due to its supposed aphrodisiac qualities. The herb is mentioned in the book *The Arabian Nights* (also known as *One Thousand and One Nights*), which is over one thousand years old. It grows wild in southeast Europe and has been long cultivated in Egypt, India, and China. It was brought by the Spanish to Mexico and Central and South America, where it is now part of the native cuisine. Cilantro was used by the ancients as an "appetite" stimulant and continues to serve that function today; it is considered an aid to the digestive system. As an appetite stimulant, cilantro

Nutrition Facts		
Serving Size 2 Tbs (30g)		
Servings Per Container 20		
Amount Per Serving		
Calories 50	Calories from Fat 35	
		% Daily Value*
Total Fat 4g		6%
Saturated Fat 1.5g		7%
Trans Fat 0g		
Cholesterol 5mg		2%
Sodium 160mg		7%
Total Carbohydrate 3g		1%
Dietary Fiber 0g		0%
Sugars 1g		
Protein 2g		
Vitamin A 2%	•	Vitamin C 2%
Calcium 4%	•	Iron 0%

* Percent Daily Values are based on a 2,000 calorie diet. Your daily values may be higher or lower depending on your calorie needs.

	Calories	2,000	2,500
Total Fat	Less than	65g	80g
Sat Fat	Less than	20g	25g
Cholesterol	Less than	300mg	300mg
Sodium	Less than	2,400mg	2,400mg
Total Carbohydrate		300g	375g
Dietary Fiber		25g	30g

Calories per gram:
Fat 9 • Carbohydrate 4 • Protein 4

aids in the secretion of gastric juices. A poultice of coriander seed can be applied externally to relieve painful joints and rheumatism. Some sources even report that the seeds can be mixed with violets as a remedy for a hangover.

GAZPACHO

I LOVE THIS soup. It's something you can make ahead of time, and it gets better as the flavors slowly meld together. In the summertime down South, you get these delicious, fresh vegetables at the farmer's market or roadside stands. The roasted corn adds a crunchy sweetness that elevates this cool, refreshing soup.

Nutrition Facts		
Serving Size 8 fl oz (244g)		
Servings Per Container 10		
Amount Per Serving		
Calories 60	Calories from Fat 5	
		% Daily Value*
Total Fat 0.5g		1%
Saturated Fat 0g		0%
Trans Fat 0g		
Cholesterol 0mg		0%
Sodium 530mg		22%
Total Carbohydrate 14g		5%
Dietary Fiber 3g		11%
Sugars 6g		
Protein 2g		
Vitamin A 170%	•	Vitamin C 80%
Calcium 4%	•	Iron 6%

* Percent Daily Values are based on a 2,000 calorie diet. Your daily values may be higher or lower depending on your calorie needs.

	Calories	2,000	2,500
Total Fat	Less than	65g	80g
Sat Fat	Less than	20g	25g
Cholesterol	Less than	300mg	300mg
Sodium	Less than	2,400mg	2,400mg
Total Carbohydrate		300g	375g
Dietary Fiber		25g	30g

Calories per gram:
Fat 9 • Carbohydrate 4 • Protein 4

5–6 lbs. fresh tomatoes, skins removed and seeded
    (½ the tomatoes finely chopped)
3 cucumbers, peeled and seeded (1 finely chopped)
2 carrots, peeled (1 finely chopped)
3 celery stalks (1 finely chopped)
1 red pepper (½ finely chopped)
2 ears of corn, roasted
1 garlic clove
2 tbsp. fresh lemon juice
1 tbsp. hot sauce
1 tbsp. Worcestershire sauce
Salt to taste
Pepper to taste
½ tsp. fat-free sour cream and chives for garnish

Combine the finely chopped ingredients and roasted corn in a large bowl. Place the remaining vegetables in a food processor until you have a fine puree. Add to the chopped vegetables along with the remaining ingredients. Stir and chill for at least 1 hour.

healthy bytes Celery in Asia is used as a base for juices containing fruit (remember, tomatoes are actually a fruit by scientific classification). Celery is terrific for appetite control and can be used to curb carbohydrate cravings. Chewing celery stimulates saliva production and will aid in the digestive process. Celery has been recommended in traditional Chinese medicine as a treatment for high blood pressure for centuries. The phytochemicals, called phthalides, are what are believed to produce this effect. Studies have shown that they work by relaxing the muscle tissue in artery walls and also act to increase blood flow. Phthalide also is believed to lower the level of stress hormones.

Celery is also a source of silicon, which is getting renewed attention in terms of good bone health. The silicon content in celery can help renew joints, bones, arteries, and connective tissue. Celery also contains an ingredient called acetylenics, which have been shown to slow the growth of cancer cells. It also contains phenolic acids, which block the action of prostaglandins, some of which are thought to encourage growth of cancerous tumors.

MEDITERRANEAN ROASTED TOMATO SALAD

THIS IS A great "base recipe." From this salad you can add grilled chicken, shrimp, or other roasted or grilled veggies to create an amazing summer salad entrée. If you can get garden-fresh grape tomatoes, all the better. The fresher the tomatoes, the sweeter they will be after the roasting process. I prefer the grape tomatoes because you can keep them whole after roasting them and because of their natural sweetness.

10 oz. grape tomatoes
2 tbsp. good-quality olive oil
1 tsp. salt + additional kosher salt
2 cucumbers
4 oz. feta cheese (fat free if desired)
1 lemon, juiced
1 tbsp. dried oregano
1 tbsp. dried basil
1 tbsp. dried thyme
1 bunch (approximately ½ c.) of fresh basil
½ tsp. freshly ground pepper

Nutrition Facts		
Serving Size 4 oz (113g)		
Servings Per Container 6		
Amount Per Serving		
Calories 100	Calories from Fat 60	
		% Daily Value*
Total Fat 6g		**10%**
Saturated Fat 3g		**14%**
Trans Fat 0g		
Cholesterol 15mg		**5%**
Sodium 200mg		**8%**
Total Carbohydrate 8g		**3%**
Dietary Fiber 2g		**10%**
Sugars 2g		
Protein 4g		
Vitamin A 25%	•	Vitamin C 15%
Calcium 25%	•	Iron 30%

* Percent Daily Values are based on a 2,000 calorie diet. Your daily values may be higher or lower depending on your calorie needs.

		Calories	2,000	2,500
Total Fat	Less than		65g	80g
Sat Fat	Less than		20g	25g
Cholesterol	Less than		300mg	300mg
Sodium	Less than		2,400mg	2,400mg
Total Carbohydrate			300g	375g
Dietary Fiber			25g	30g

Calories per gram:
Fat 9 • Carbohydrate 4 • Protein 4

Place the tomatoes in a roasting pan large enough for them to lie in one layer. Drizzle with olive oil and salt and place in a 325° F oven for approximately 25 minutes. The skins should just be starting to turn brown and split. Remove from the oven and cool to room temperature. While the tomatoes are roasting, peel the cucumbers and split lengthwise into equal halves. Using a teaspoon, scoop out the seeds, cover with kosher salt and let stand for approximately 15 minutes to draw out some of the cucumbers' moisture. Using a paper towel, wipe off the salt mixture from the cucumbers (it will be a wet, salty sludge). Rough chop the cucumbers and place in a bowl with the feta, lemon juice, and dried herbs. Rolling the basil leaves together into a cigar shape, cut strips across the short axis—a chiffonade cut. Add the basil and cooled tomatoes to the bowl. Drizzle good-quality olive oil over the salad and lightly toss. Salt and pepper to taste.

healthy bytes Cooked tomatoes, especially those cooked with olive oil, are a rich source of the carotenoid lycopene. Because carotenoids are fat-soluble nutrients, you get maximum absorption if you eat them with fat or consume them with fat-rich foods, such as avocado and olive oil. There are numerous studies on the properties of lycopene that have shown that, in addition to reducing and protecting against prostate cancer, it protects against lung cancer and stomach cancer. There is also preliminary research that shows potential protection against pancreatic, oral, breast, and cervical cancers. In addition to cancer protection, lycopene can also protect the heart against oxidative damage, which is believed to play a role in atherosclerosis and heart attacks. Tomatoes offer benefits in reducing other heart attack–associated risk factors. One study published in *The American Heart Journal* showed that treatment with antioxidant-rich tomato extract can reduce blood pressure in patients with hypertension.[2] Tomatoes that are store bought are often "ripened" with ethylene gas, which may make them look good but give them a suboptimal taste—*caveat emptor*!

PESTO

THIS IS ANOTHER incredibly versatile topping. It is great on bread or crackers, with vegetables, or mixed in pasta. It is also part of a great main. Add a few slices of bread, some thin slices of dried meats, and cheese and enjoy that with a glass or two of wine. It is a completely satisfying main to unwind with after a long day. As a starter it can be served a variety of ways and really sets the tone for a Mediterranean-style or pasta main. It is also another great "base recipe." Once you've got this classic version down, you can add many different herbs, nuts, or whatever you like.

1 c. fresh basil
1 garlic clove, chopped
¼ c. pine nuts, toasted
½ c. fresh parmesan cheese, grated
Approximately ½ c. good-quality olive oil
1 tsp. salt
½ tsp. fresh-cracked black pepper

Nutrition Facts		
Serving Size 1 oz (28g)		
Servings Per Container 10		
Amount Per Serving		
Calories 150	Calories from Fat 130	
		% Daily Value*
Total Fat 14g		**22%**
Saturated Fat 3.5g		18%
Trans Fat 0g		
Cholesterol 10mg		**3%**
Sodium 440mg		**18%**
Total Carbohydrate 2g		**1%**
Dietary Fiber 1g		2%
Sugars 0g		
Protein 5g		
Vitamin A 4%	•	Vitamin C 2%
Calcium 15%	•	Iron 2%

* Percent Daily Values are based on a 2,000 calorie diet. Your daily values may be higher or lower depending on your calorie needs.

	Calories	2,000	2,500
Total Fat	Less than	65g	80g
Sat Fat	Less than	20g	25g
Cholesterol	Less than	300mg	300mg
Sodium	Less than	2,400mg	2,400mg
Total Carbohydrate		300g	375g
Dietary Fiber		25g	30g

Calories per gram:
Fat 9 • Carbohydrate 4 • Protein 4

CONTAINS: Milk, Nuts

Place all the ingredients except olive oil in a food processor. Drizzle in the olive oil as the mixture is processing, stopping as needed to scrape down the sides. Stop when desired consistency is reached; I like a thin, pastelike consistency. Reseason with salt and pepper if needed.

healthy bytes Basil has been shown in research to have unique health-protecting effects in two basic areas: basil's flavonoids and volatile oils. The unique array of active constituents called flavonoids found in basil provides protection at the cellular level. In studies on human white blood cells, these compounds act to protect cell structures, including chromosomes, from radiation and oxygen-based, free-radical damage. Basil's volatile oils have been shown to block the activity of an enzyme in the body called cyclooxygenase, or COX (many anti-inflammatory medications like aspirin and ibuprofen also block this enzyme). This is responsible for the anti-inflammatory effect of basil. Because the oils in basil are highly volatile, it is best to add the herb near the end of the cooking process so it will retain its maximum essence and flavor.

OVEN-ROASTED ROSEMARY POTATOES

POTATOES ARE delicious and provide a hearty, filling starch accompaniment to any main dish. I really like these sometimes as a first all by their lonesome. The trick is not to ruin the natural benefits of the potato by adding things like butter, sour cream, bacon, and cheese. They are easy to prepare, and the leftovers, if you have any, can be chopped and reheated in a pan with onions for a quick stovetop serving of hash browns.

Nutrition Facts		
Serving Size 9 oz (255g)		
Servings Per Container 8		
Amount Per Serving		
Calories 480	Calories from Fat 250	
		% Daily Value*
Total Fat 28g		43%
Saturated Fat 7g		37%
Trans Fat 0g		
Cholesterol 155mg		52%
Sodium 310mg		13%
Total Carbohydrate 10g		3%
Dietary Fiber 1g		5%
Sugars 2g		
Protein 47g		
Vitamin A 10%	•	Vitamin C 15%
Calcium 6%	•	Iron 45%

* Percent Daily Values are based on a 2,000 calorie diet. Your daily values may be higher or lower depending on your calorie needs.

	Calories	2,000	2,500
Total Fat	Less than	65g	80g
Sat Fat	Less than	20g	25g
Cholesterol	Less than	300mg	300mg
Sodium	Less than	2,400mg	2,400mg
Total Carbohydrate		300g	375g
Dietary Fiber		25g	30g

Calories per gram:
Fat 9 • Carbohydrate 4 • Protein 4

4 tbsp. olive oil, divided in half
4–6 sprigs rosemary
1–1½ lbs. fingerling or small new potatoes
1 tsp. salt
½ tsp. fresh ground pepper
1 tsp. lemon juice
¼ tsp. lemon zest

Preheat the oven to 350° F. Using a dish just big enough to hold the potatoes without having them sit on top of each other, place some olive oil in the bottom. Break or cut half of the rosemary sprigs into several 1 in. pieces and place in the roasting pan with the oil. (The idea here is to allow the rosemary to subtly flavor the oil.) Heat in the oven for 15 minutes. Remove the pan, remove the rosemary if you like or leave it on the bottom, and add the potatoes. Toss them around the dish, adding additional oil, salt, and pepper. After they have been tossed, drizzle the lemon juice and zest over the top and lay the remaining sprigs of rosemary on top. Cook for 30–45 minutes or until done. Remove the sprigs, reseason if necessary, and serve.

healthy bytes Rosemary has several healthy components, two of which are caffeic acid and rosmarinic acid. These two are anti-inflammatory in nature. These compounds may aid in such conditions as asthma, liver, and heart disease. Rosemary also contains vitamin E; many additional flavonoids thought to help in the prevention of other conditions; and compounds that prevent the breakdown of acetylcholine, a vital neurotransmitter in the brain that is needed to promote healthy memory. Studies are being done to see how rosemary impacts conditions like Alzheimer's disease. It is interesting to note that the ancient Greeks considered rosemary vital to memory and wisdom.

PAN-SIMMERED APPLES AND NAPA CABBAGE

THIS DISH just reminds me of fall. The smell of cinnamon and apples brings back memories of my mom's apple pies. We would take family outings to the orchards and pick our own apples. We got them by the bushel, but somehow no matter how many she cooked, I never got tired of those pies. This is a healthy alternative, creating a sweet, succulent side dish that is perfect for pork or veal. You can use any apple you like; I prefer the firm tartness of Granny Smith.

2 oz. butter or Smart Balance substitute
1 tbsp. olive oil, divided
2 apples, peeled, cored, and sliced
¼ c. apple cider vinegar
¼ c. apple juice
1 lemon, juiced
1 tsp. fresh ground cinnamon
¼ tsp. fresh ground allspice
1 clove, ground
1 tbsp. shallot, finely chopped
1 head of Napa cabbage, thinly sliced
½ c. light chicken stock (see recipe in chapter 19)

Nutrition Facts		
Serving Size 8 oz (227g)		
Servings Per Container 6		
Amount Per Serving		
Calories 110	Calories from Fat 80	
		% Daily Value*
Total Fat 9g		**14%**
Saturated Fat 2.5g		**11%**
Trans Fat 0g		
Cholesterol 5mg		**1%**
Sodium 90mg		**4%**
Total Carbohydrate 7g		**2%**
Dietary Fiber 0g		**0%**
Sugars 2g		
Protein 2g		
Vitamin A 8%	•	Vitamin C 20%
Calcium 6%	•	Iron 8%

* Percent Daily Values are based on a 2,000 calorie diet. Your daily values may be higher or lower depending on your calorie needs.

	Calories	2,000	2,500
Total Fat	Less than	65g	80g
Sat Fat	Less than	20g	25g
Cholesterol	Less than	300mg	300mg
Sodium	Less than	2,400mg	2,400mg
Total Carbohydrate		300g	375g
Dietary Fiber		25g	30g

Calories per gram:
Fat 9 • Carbohydrate 4 • Protein 4

CONTAINS: Fish

Heat a medium saucepan over medium heat. Melt the butter or Smart Balance with ½ tsp. of olive oil. Add the apples, apple cider vinegar, apple juice, lemon juice, cinnamon, allspice, and clove. Cook until the liquid has reduced by about half. Meanwhile, in another saucepan heat the remaining olive oil over medium heat, and cook the shallots for about 1 minute. Add the cabbage and the chicken stock, and cook, stirring occasionally, until the cabbage is tender with just a little crunch left. Drain in a colander and combine with the apple mixture.

healthy bytes Apples have many, many health benefits besides keeping doctors away. Apples are high in flavonoids, phytochemicals, and antioxidants. They are thought to inhibit the growth of cancer cells and reduce "oxidative stress" on DNA; both are factors related to heart disease and many forms of cancer. A little-known fact is that apples are one of the best dietary sources of boron, which is a mineral essential to strong, healthy bones and therefore may be of use in osteoporosis prevention.

ROASTED CORN WITH CILANTRO-LIME BUTTER

THIS IS A very simple dish and very versatile. Do not let that fool you. This recipe is another "basic." Perfect grilling and roasting of all different kinds of veggies is a skill to master; here we use corn on the grill. If you like to use an alternative when making the compound butter, I have found Smart Balance works well, and you can get it with additional omega-3s. It doesn't seem to detract from the taste, especially when you add additional flavors. Cilantro, lime, and corn are a classic flavor profile, but feel free to vary. These butters are great ways to add secondary, subtle flavors to meals and really elevate the entire dish. They are easy to make and can be made ahead and frozen for several months as well.

8 oz. butter or Smart Balance substitute
1 tbsp. lime juice
2 tbsp. chopped cilantro
As many ears of corn as guests, allowing 1 ear per person

Nutrition Facts		
Serving Size 3 3/4 oz (106g)		
Servings Per Container 6		
Amount Per Serving		
Calories 160	Calories from Fat 90	
		% Daily Value*
Total Fat 10g		16%
Saturated Fat 3g		14%
Trans Fat 0g		
Cholesterol 5mg		1%
Sodium 110mg		5%
Total Carbohydrate 18g		6%
Dietary Fiber 2g		10%
Sugars 3g		
Protein 3g		
Vitamin A 0%	•	Vitamin C 10%
Calcium 0%	•	Iron 2%

* Percent Daily Values are based on a 2,000 calorie diet. Your daily values may be higher or lower depending on your calorie needs.

	Calories	2,000	2,500
Total Fat	Less than	65g	80g
Sat Fat	Less than	20g	25g
Cholesterol	Less than	300mg	300mg
Sodium	Less than	2,400mg	2,400mg
Total Carbohydrate		300g	375g
Dietary Fiber		25g	30g

Calories per gram:
Fat 9 • Carbohydrate 4 • Protein 4

CONTAINS: Fish

Allow the butter or butter substitute to soften to room temperature. Using a wooden spoon or electric mixer, cream the butter. Mix in the lime juice and cilantro. Place in some plastic wrap. If you have a bamboo mat (used for rolling sushi), place the plastic wrap over the mat. Roll the plastic wrap over the butter mixture to form an even log, about 1 inch in thickness. Twist off the ends to seal, and refrigerate until needed.

To roast the corn, allow the ears to soak submerged in water for at least 30 minutes. Remove from water, and grill the whole ears for several minutes. Remove the surrounding leaves and silk, allowing the kernels to slightly brown on the grill, and serve.

healthy bytes Lime came into fashion as the citrus of choice of maritime explorers on long sea voyages. Magellan lost 80 percent of his crew to scurvy, a vitamin deficiency disease due to inadequate vitamin C in the diet. This disease presents with black skin and ulcers and difficulty breathing, and it can lead to death. In the 1790s British sailors in the Royal Navy were given rations of lime, and to this day Brits are known as "limeys." In addition to vitamin C, limes contain other beneficial compounds, including citrate and vitamin A. The peels of lemon and limes contain limonene, which has been found to be high in anticancer properties. And of course, you just can't make a decent margarita without limes.

COLD SOBA NOODLES

DURING MY first trip to Japan, I had just enough money for my martial arts training, so there was a lot of eating on a budget. That meant a lot of cold soba noodles. Soba are a Japanese buckwheat noodle. It was served cold with a seasoned broth, filling and satisfying—especially on a warm, humid day. Even though I lived off that for three weeks, I still love it, and it makes a great appetizer or side. If you can't find soba, you can use other Japanese-style noodles, like udon or somen. Serving the whole thing warm and adding some veggies with chicken, shrimp, or pork converts this from a summertime refresher to a year-round treat.

2 c. dark chicken or meat stock (see recipe in chapter 19)
1 tbsp. salt
6 oz. soba noodles
1 tbsp. miso paste
1 tbsp. sesame oil
1 tbsp. rice wine vinegar
1 tsp. garlic puree
1 tsp. fresh cilantro, finely chopped
½ tsp. sriracha sauce
4 tsp. scallion or green onion, finely chopped

Nutrition Facts		
Serving Size 4 3/10 oz (122g)		
Servings Per Container 6		
Amount Per Serving		
Calories 90	Calories from Fat 30	
		% Daily Value*
Total Fat 3.5g		5%
Saturated Fat 0.5g		3%
Trans Fat 0g		
Cholesterol 0mg		0%
Sodium 610mg		25%
Total Carbohydrate 11g		4%
Dietary Fiber 0g		0%
Sugars 2g		
Protein 4g		
Vitamin A 2%	•	Vitamin C 2%
Calcium 0%	•	Iron 2%

* Percent Daily Values are based on a 2,000 calorie diet. Your daily values may be higher or lower depending on your calorie needs.

		Calories	2,000	2,500
Total Fat	Less than		65g	80g
Sat Fat	Less than		20g	25g
Cholesterol	Less than		300mg	300mg
Sodium	Less than		2,400mg	2,400mg
Total Carbohydrate			300g	375g
Dietary Fiber			25g	30g

Calories per gram:
Fat 9 • Carbohydrate 4 • Protein 4

Heat a medium saucepan over high heat. Bring the stock and salt to a boil. Reduce the heat, and add the noodles. Cook until slightly al dente. Drain the noodles, reserving the stock. Add the remaining ingredients, except the onion, to the warm stock and cool. Refrigerate the noodles. Serve the cold noodles topped with the green onion, with some of the flavored stock as a dipping sauce.

healthy bytes Buckwheat, which are soba noodles, is not a cereal grain; it is actually a fruit seed that is related to rhubarb and sorrel. It makes a wonderful substitute for people who are sensitive to wheat or other grains that contain glutens. Buckwheat's beneficial effects are due in part to its rich supply of flavonoids, particularly rutin. These compounds contribute to buckwheat's lipid-lowering activity and ability to help maintain blood flow, keep platelets from clotting excessively, and protect LDL from free-radical oxidation (which contributes to athero-sclerosis). All these actions help to protect against heart disease.

CORN TORTILLAS

TORTILLAS ARE indispensible. They taste great and are culinary multitaskers. They are great for holding taco fillings. They can be fried or baked into chips for snacking with guacamole or salsa. Stale, they become a soup ingredient. The list goes on. On a recent trip to Mexico with friends, we went to the open-air town market. We had some fresh tortillas that were still warm when we walked back to the hotel. I can taste the warm corn tortilla filled with the fresh guacamole salad we made poolside. Or maybe it was just the tequila in the margaritas!

12 oz. masa flour
½ tsp. salt
12 oz. warm water

Nutrition Facts		
Serving Size 2 oz (57g)		
Servings Per Container 12		
Amount Per Serving		
Calories 100	Calories from Fat 10	
		% Daily Value*
Total Fat 1g		2%
Saturated Fat 0g		0%
Trans Fat 0g		
Cholesterol 0mg		0%
Sodium 100mg		4%
Total Carbohydrate 22g		7%
Dietary Fiber 3g		11%
Sugars 0g		
Protein 3g		
Vitamin A 0%	•	Vitamin C 0%
Calcium 4%	•	Iron 10%

* Percent Daily Values are based on a 2,000 calorie diet. Your daily values may be higher or lower depending on your calorie needs.

	Calories	2,000	2,500
Total Fat	Less than	65g	80g
Sat Fat	Less than	20g	25g
Cholesterol	Less than	300mg	300mg
Sodium	Less than	2,400mg	2,400mg
Total Carbohydrate		300g	375g
Dietary Fiber		25g	30g

Calories per gram:
Fat 9 • Carbohydrate 4 • Protein 4

Preheat a griddle to 350° F. Combine salt and flour. Add the water a little at a time and incorporate fully. The dough should come together in a firm, moist way without cracking into crumbs. Roll out the dough into approximately 2 oz. patties.
Place the patties on a tortilla press covered with parchment paper or other nonstick sur-face on the bottom and the top (the person who taught me used Walmart bags cut into circles). Press down firmly. Remove the tortilla by peeling the nonstick covering back. Place on the preheated griddle. Once the edges start to lift and you can grasp the tortilla

without it tearing, flip it over. Push the edges back onto the griddle with your fingertips. Once the tortilla starts to puff, flip it over for another 1 to 2 minutes, and then remove.

`healthy bytes` Masa flour is made by a high-temperature alkaline cooking procedure called nixtamalization. This lime-cooking technique releases all the healthy substances in corn more effectively than any other process. Masa provides potassium, calcium, and fiber. It is low fat and low sodium also.

TORTILLA SOUP

THIS IS A variation based on a regional favorite from the Yucatan region of Mexico. I had this type of soup when we visited the area. It was made with fresh ingredients, and it was delicious! This version combines the traditional flavors of this soup with a tang of sour. If you like the soup a little on the spicier side, leave some or all of the seeds and membranes of the jalapeño. This is where most of the heat of the pepper resides.

1 tbsp. olive oil
2 skinless chicken breasts
Vegetable oil or cooking spray
4 corn tortillas
1 c. chopped onion
Salt
Freshly ground pepper
2 tsp. garlic, freshly minced
½ tsp. dried oregano, preferably Mexican
½ jalapeño (remove seeds and membrane)
1 c. fresh Roma tomatoes, peeled, seeded, and chopped
¼ c. fresh lime juice
2 tsp. adobo sauce
4 c. light chicken stock (see recipe in chapter 19)
¼ c. seasoned rice wine vinegar
1 bay leaf
¼ c. fresh cilantro, finely chopped
Avocado, thinly sliced lengthwise
Lime, cut into wedges
Mango or papaya, chopped
Flat-leaf parsley

Nutrition Facts

Serving Size 8 oz (227g)
Servings Per Container 8

Amount Per Serving	
Calories 210	Calories from Fat 80

	% Daily Value*
Total Fat 9g	13%
Saturated Fat 1.5g	8%
Trans Fat 0g	
Cholesterol 40mg	13%
Sodium 600mg	25%
Total Carbohydrate 13g	4%
Dietary Fiber 1g	6%
Sugars 4g	
Protein 18g	

Vitamin A 6%	•	Vitamin C 30%	
Calcium 4%	•	Iron 6%	

* Percent Daily Values are based on a 2,000 calorie diet. Your daily values may be higher or lower depending on your calorie needs.

		Calories	2,000	2,500
Total Fat	Less than		65g	80g
Sat Fat	Less than		20g	25g
Cholesterol	Less than		300mg	300mg
Sodium	Less than		2,400mg	2,400mg
Total Carbohydrate			300g	375g
Dietary Fiber			25g	30g

Calories per gram:
Fat 9 • Carbohydrate 4 • Protein 4

Preheat an oven to 400° F. Heat a medium saucepan over medium heat. Add a little olive oil and brown the chicken breasts; they do not need to be fully cooked (they'll finish cooking in the soup). Remove from the heat, let cool, and dice into bite-sized chunks. Cut the tortillas into thin strips. Spray a baking pan lightly with neutral oil, like vegetable oil. Lay the strips on the pan, and spray the exposed sides of the strips with the oil. This way both sides cook. Place in the oven for 10 to 12 minutes or until browned and crisp. Remove and set aside. In a medium stockpot over medium heat, add some olive oil and sauté the onions with salt and pepper until soft. Add garlic, oregano, jalapeño, chicken, and tomatoes. Stir for another minute. Then add lime juice, adobo sauce and half of the tortilla strips, crushed. Stir another minute to combine. Reseason if necessary. Add the chicken stock, and bring to a boil. Reduce the heat, and add the vinegar, bay leaf, and cilantro. Simmer 30 to 45 minutes. To serve, remove the bay leaf, portion each bowl, then divide the remaining tortilla strips on top. Garnish each bowl with a quarter of the avocado, a lime wedge, 1 tsp. of mango or papaya, and ½ tsp. of parsley.

healthy bytes   Oregano is rich in calcium, magnesium, zinc, potassium, copper, boron, manganese, vitamin C, vitamin A, and niacin. Studies like the one from the *Journal of Agricultural and Food Chemistry* show oregano is the herb with the highest antioxidant activity.[3] In fact it is believed to have forty-two times more activity than apples and up to four times as much as blueberries. The medicinal part of oregano is in the oil from the leaves and the fresh plant itself. The plant contains thymol, which has strong antifungal, antibacterial, and antiparasitic properties and is especially useful against the fungus *Candida albicans*, which can cause infections.

ZUCCHINI STUFFED WITH HERBED CHÈVRE

THIS IS A delicious cold appetizer or accompaniment to a dish like gazpacho. The herbed chèvre itself can be spread like butter on a slab of hot bread.

    ½ c. pine nuts
    4 oz. chèvre, room temperature
    2 tsp. shallot, finely chopped
    1 tsp. truffle oil
    ¼ tsp. freshly ground pepper
    1 tsp. fresh thyme, finely chopped
    1 tsp. fresh basil, chopped
    1 tsp. flat-leaf parsley, finely chopped

Approximately 3½ tbsp. good-quality olive oil, divided
Approximately 2 tsp. salt
1 small to medium green zucchini

Place a small nonstick pan over medium heat. Allow the pan to heat, and add the pine nuts. Keep the pan moving, and gently toast until the pine nuts turn a light brown. The nuts have a tendency to burn, so don't leave the pan unattended. When toasted, remove from heat, transfer to a container, and allow to cool. In a small mixing bowl, fold into the chèvre the pine nuts, shallot, truffle oil, pepper, thyme, basil, and parsley, being careful not to overmix or the cheese may break. Return to the refrigerator. Drizzle approximately 2 tbsp. of olive oil on a baking sheet. Lightly season with salt and pepper. On a cutting board, cut off the stem end of the zucchini. Cut a small section lengthwise so the zucchini will sit flat on the cutting board, stem end pointing away from you. Holding the zucchini firmly, press down with a vegetable peeler, and cut approximately ⅛ to ¼ inch slices lengthwise. Alternatively you can use a mandolin or cut very carefully with a knife. As each thin strip is cut, lay it on the baking pan. When the pan is full or all the zucchini has been cut, drizzle the remaining 1½ tbsp. of olive oil over the slices. Taste one for seasoning, and adjust accordingly. Retrieve the chèvre, and place a generous amount at the end of the strip closest to you. Roll the zucchini away, and place on a tray standing on end. If you have difficulty lifting the zucchini to roll, use the tip of a knife to lift the edge closest to you. Serve immediately or refrigerate for several hours.

healthy bytes Goat milk cheese, when compared to cow milk cheese, is lower in fat, calories, and cholesterol. It is good for those who may be lactose intolerant. The fat particles in goat milk are close in size to those in mother's milk. Goat milk products are said to be "naturally homogenized" and therefore easier to digest for the lactose intolerant. Goat cheese is high in calcium and amino acids and a good source of protein.

BABY SPINACH AND SAUTÉED MUSHROOMS

THIS IS AN example of an incredibly versatile first. Serve it as a side, or cool the mushrooms, add other accoutrements and a warm dressing, and it is a wilted spinach salad for a main. It is a two-part construction but worth the little bit of extra effort.

1 lb. fresh white button mushrooms (the smaller the size, the better)

2 tbsp. olive oil

1 tsp. salt

½ tsp. freshly ground pepper

1 shallot, chopped thinly lengthwise

Approximately ¼ c. white wine vinegar

1 bunch fresh baby spinach

2 oz. butter or Smart Balance substitute

1 tbsp. fat-free sour cream

Approximately 1 tsp. balsamic vinegar

Nutrition Facts		
Serving Size 4 oz (113g)		
Servings Per Container 6		
Amount Per Serving		
Calories 40	Calories from Fat 20	
		% Daily Value*
Total Fat 2.5g		**4%**
Saturated Fat 0g		**0%**
Trans Fat 0g		
Cholesterol 0mg		**0%**
Sodium 210mg		**9%**
Total Carbohydrate 3g		**1%**
Dietary Fiber 4g		**15%**
Sugars 0g		
Protein 3g		
Vitamin A 4%	•	Vitamin C 15%
Calcium 4%	•	Iron 15%

* Percent Daily Values are based on a 2,000 calorie diet. Your daily values may be higher or lower depending on your calorie needs.

	Calories	2,000	2,500
Total Fat	Less than	65g	80g
Sat Fat	Less than	20g	25g
Cholesterol	Less than	300mg	300mg
Sodium	Less than	2,400mg	2,400mg
Total Carbohydrate		300g	375g
Dietary Fiber		25g	30g

Calories per gram:
Fat 9 • Carbohydrate 4 • Protein 4

CONTAINS: Milk

Clean the mushrooms, and cut any large ones in quarters. Heat a medium saucepan over medium heat. Add a little olive oil, and heat until the oil just starts to smoke. Add the mushrooms. They will sizzle; if they don't, remove and heat the pan further. It is important that they sauté and brown. Add salt, pepper, and the shallot. Keep tossing and cooking until the mushrooms assume a golden-brown color. Pour the white wine vinegar around the edge of the pan. Cook for another 1 to 2 minutes, and remove from heat. Make sure the spinach has been properly washed, cleaned, and dried. Add the spinach and butter or Smart Balance to the heated pan. You may need to add the spinach in quick batches, depending on the size of the pan. The spinach will quickly reduce. When the spinach has reduced, pour off the excess moisture and then add the sour cream. After the sour cream is mixed in, remove from the heat. Combine spinach and mushrooms. Drizzle a little balsamic vinegar on top, and serve.

healthy bytes Spinach contains thirteen flavonoids with anticancer properties active against such malignancies as prostate, skin, colon, and bone cancers. It is considered a brain food and is believed to reduce neurological damage after strokes, which may be due in part to its anti-inflammatory action. Spinach has four natural ACE inhibitors (it blocks a specific enzyme) to reduce blood pressure. It is also a great source of iron and vitamin K.

TRUFFLED AND SMASHED ROOT VEGETABLES

I LIKE SMASHED root vegetables because I like the vegetables to be a little chunky, country style. If you like a finer mash, mash away to your liking, but avoid beating the potatoes or putting them in a food processor, as this can make them a bit gluey. The addition of parsnip and carrot add a subtle sweetness to the dish that allows for a reduction in the amount of butter needed or the addition of heavy sweet cream.

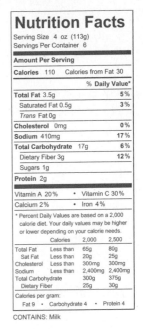

Nutrition Facts

Serving Size 4 oz (113g)
Servings Per Container 6

Amount Per Serving	
Calories 110	Calories from Fat 30

	% Daily Value*
Total Fat 3.5g	5%
Saturated Fat 0.5g	3%
Trans Fat 0g	
Cholesterol 0mg	0%
Sodium 410mg	17%
Total Carbohydrate 17g	6%
Dietary Fiber 3g	12%
Sugars 1g	
Protein 2g	

Vitamin A 20%	•	Vitamin C 30%
Calcium 2%	•	Iron 4%

* Percent Daily Values are based on a 2,000 calorie diet. Your daily values may be higher or lower depending on your calorie needs.

	Calories	2,000	2,500
Total Fat	Less than	65g	80g
Sat Fat	Less than	20g	25g
Cholesterol	Less than	300mg	300mg
Sodium	Less than	2,400mg	2,400mg
Total Carbohydrate		300g	375g
Dietary Fiber		25g	30g

Calories per gram:
Fat 9 • Carbohydrate 4 • Protein 4

CONTAINS: Milk

½ carrot, peeled and cut into chunks
1 parsnip, peeled and cut into chunks
1 lb. potatoes, like Yukon golds, peeled and cut into chunks
2 oz. butter or Smart Balance substitute
1 tsp. salt
½ tsp. freshly ground pepper
2 tbsp. fat-free sour cream
1 tbsp. truffle oil
1 tsp. chives, chopped

Place the carrot and parsnip in a large pot with salted water. Add the potatoes, bring to a boil, and cook all the vegetables until fork tender. Remove and strain the vegetables in a colander. Place back in the pan for about another 30 seconds to remove any remaining moisture. Place in a bowl, and using a masher, smash the vegetables with butter or Smart Balance. Add salt, pepper, truffle oil, and sour cream. Taste and reseason with salt and pepper if needed. Serve garnished with chives.

healthy bytes Parsnips are rich in folate, calcium, potassium, and fiber. They are a member of the umbelliferous vegetable group, which the National Cancer Institute has identified as having qualities that protect against cancer. Parsnips contain phthalides, a phytochemical group that provides benefits by stimulating good enzymes and inhibiting inflammatory ones.

COCONUT VEGETABLES

THE ORIGINS of this dish are Caribbean inspired. I can recall my first visit to the island of Providenciales, part of the British West Indies in the Turks and Caicos chain. The airport was a strip; there was one barely paved road, one Club Med, and one hotel, along with a few bungalows. Nothing like that remains of that simple time; progress can be relentless. Then, we knew all the islanders and ate with the locals. I still don't think I've ever had a better conch, turtle, or island-cooked vegetables than that night at Henry's Road Runner. Sadly, that island treasure closed, but this recipe serves as a great reminder of a great time. (My brother also found out he was allergic to turtle that night. I don't think he's forgotten the evening either.)

Nutrition Facts

Serving Size 4 1/2 oz (128g)
Servings Per Container 12

Amount Per Serving

Calories 120   Calories from Fat 70

	% Daily Value*
Total Fat 8g	12%
Saturated Fat 7g	33%
Trans Fat 0g	
Cholesterol 0mg	0%
Sodium 30mg	1%
Total Carbohydrate 11g	4%
Dietary Fiber 2g	9%
Sugars 2g	
Protein 3g	

Vitamin A 40%	•	Vitamin C 50%
Calcium 2%	•	Iron 10%

* Percent Daily Values are based on a 2,000 calorie diet. Your daily values may be higher or lower depending on your calorie needs.

		Calories	2,000	2,500
Total Fat	Less than		65g	80g
Sat Fat	Less than		20g	25g
Cholesterol	Less than		300mg	300mg
Sodium	Less than		2,400mg	2,400mg
Total Carbohydrate			300g	375g
Dietary Fiber			25g	30g

Calories per gram:
Fat 9 • Carbohydrate 4 • Protein 4

1 tbsp. butter or Smart Balance substitute
1 c. onion, chopped
1 tsp. fresh garlic, finely chopped
1 tsp. fresh ginger, finely grated
1 tsp. fresh thyme, finely chopped
1 serrano green chili or other hot chili (leave seeds and membrane intact for extra spice), split lengthwise
1 medium potato, parboiled, peeled, and cut into chunks
2 carrots, peeled and cut into chunks
1 can (14 oz.) coconut milk
1 c. broccoli florets
1 c. cauliflower florets
Salt to taste
Pepper to taste

In a medium saucepan, melt the butter or Smart Balance, and cook the onions until translucent. Add the garlic, ginger, thyme, chili, potatoes, and carrots, along with the coconut milk. Bring to a boil, reduce the heat, and cook for about 10 minutes. Add the broccoli and cauliflower florets, and cook for another 5 minutes. If the sauce thickens too much, add 1 to 2 tbsp. of water. Serve when the broccoli and cauliflower are cooked but still crisp. Remove the split chili prior to serving, and season as needed.

healthy bytes Coconuts are full of fiber, potassium, and magnesium, but they do have some saturated fat. The saturated fats in coconut are the medium-chain triglyceride type. These are very different from the dreaded "long-chain fat" found in typical industrial mega-market meat. They are easier to metabolize, and they are almost exclusively used for energy and not stored. These fats contain a particular fatty acid called lauric acid. More than 50 percent of the fat in coconuts is lauric acid. Lauric acid is antiviral and antimicrobial, thus it helps boost immunity.

GRILLED ASPARAGUS WITH TRUFFLED VINAIGRETTE

THIS IS A fabulous dish that can function as a side or all alone. This dish can also be chilled and served cold as part of an antipasto. Don't forget to cut the stems back on the asparagus. I also like to peel the stem end of anything other than a very fresh young shoot, as these tend to get a bit woody. If the asparagus gets a little limp before you grill, place them in an ice bath for about 20 minutes. It's like veggie Viagra. The truffled vinaigrette can be used as a dressing for a number of other dishes or salads as well.

Nutrition Facts		
Serving Size 3 oz (85g)		
Servings Per Container 6		
Amount Per Serving		
Calories 50	Calories from Fat 35	
		% Daily Value*
Total Fat 3.5g		6%
Saturated Fat 0.5g		3%
Trans Fat 0g		
Cholesterol 0mg		0%
Sodium 100mg		4%
Total Carbohydrate 4g		1%
Dietary Fiber 2g		7%
Sugars 1g		
Protein 2g		
Vitamin A 10%	•	Vitamin C 8%
Calcium 2%	•	Iron 10%

* Percent Daily Values are based on a 2,000 calorie diet. Your daily values may be higher or lower depending on your calorie needs.

	Calories	2,000	2,500
Total Fat	Less than	65g	80g
Sat Fat	Less than	20g	25g
Cholesterol	Less than	300mg	300mg
Sodium	Less than	2,400mg	2,400mg
Total Carbohydrate		300g	375g
Dietary Fiber		25g	30g

Calories per gram:
Fat 9 • Carbohydrate 4 • Protein 4

1½ tbsp. champagne vinegar
1 tbsp. shallot, finely minced
¼ c. vegetable oil
2 tbsp. truffle oil
1 tsp. salt
½ tsp. white pepper
1 bunch asparagus, trimmed and peeled
1 tbsp. olive oil

In a mixing bowl, combine the vinegar and shallot. Whisk in the vegetable and truffle oils. Salt and pepper to taste, and set aside. Rub the asparagus spears lightly with olive oil and place on the grill. If you do not have access to a grill, heat a medium pan with a little olive oil and cook in the pan, turning frequently. Place the asparagus on a serving tray and drizzle the vinaigrette on top.

healthy bytes Asparagus is one of the only plants that have distinct male and female versions. The males are skinny, and the females are fatter. There are two parts to asparagus, the root and the stalk. In ayurvedic medicine, the root is used as a diuretic and to strengthen the female reproductive system. Chinese medicine also uses the root for medicine. In addition to its medicinal use, asparagus is believed to have aphrodisiac qualities. In India it is called *shatavari*, which means "she who possesses one hundred husbands." Asparagus contains potassium, folate, vitamin K, and also many more flavonoids and antioxidants.

ROASTED CORN AND BLACK BEAN SALAD

THIS IS A great way to use some leftover roasted corn. Soak the onion in an ice bath for about 15 minutes to help remove any of the bitter, raw–red onion flavors. The jicama adds a subtle but nice crunch.

2 limes, juiced
2 ears of roasted corn, kernels removed from the cob
1 can (15 oz.) of black beans, rinsed and drained
¼ c. red onion
Approximately ¼ tsp. hot sauce
2 tbsp. freshly cilantro, chopped
¼ c. jicama, thinly sliced
1 tsp. salt
½ tsp. freshly ground pepper

Nutrition Facts		
Serving Size 4 1/2 oz (128g)		
Servings Per Container 6		
Amount Per Serving		
Calories 130	Calories from Fat 10	
		% Daily Value*
Total Fat 1g		**1%**
Saturated Fat 0g		**0%**
Trans Fat 0g		
Cholesterol 0mg		**0%**
Sodium 390mg		**16%**
Total Carbohydrate 26g		**9%**
Dietary Fiber 7g		**30%**
Sugars 3g		
Protein 8g		
Vitamin A 2%	•	Vitamin C 10%
Calcium 2%	•	Iron 10%
* Percent Daily Values are based on a 2,000 calorie diet. Your daily values may be higher or lower depending on your calorie needs.		

		Calories	2,000	2,500
Total Fat	Less than		65g	80g
Sat Fat	Less than		20g	25g
Cholesterol	Less than		300mg	300mg
Sodium	Less than		2,400mg	2,400mg
Total Carbohydrate			300g	375g
Dietary Fiber			25g	30g

Calories per gram:
Fat 9 • Carbohydrate 4 • Protein 4

In a mixing bowl, combine all the ingredients. Toss and season with salt and pepper.

healthy bytes Jicama is a root vegetable that is originally from South America, where it is served as a street food. Jicama is a bit bland by itself, but it has the ability to take on other flavors, much like tofu. It is low calorie, low fat, and high in fiber. Jicama also contains calcium, magnesium, potassium, vitamin C, vitamin A, and beta-carotene.

SWEET POTATO FRIES

I WAS NOT a big sweet potato person until I had these. If you're looking for a delicious snack, these are them. The heat and spice provide a contrast for the natural sweetness. These fries are done in the oven. A slightly less healthy but scrumptious alternative allows you to cook them at the last minute by cooking them like regular fries. Season them as soon as they come out of the oven or fryer and serve.

2 large sweet potatoes, peeled and cut into strips
2 tsp. salt
½ tsp. pepper

¼ tsp. ancho chili powder
1 tsp. garlic powder
¼ tsp. chipotle chili powder
2 tbsp. olive oil

Place all ingredients in a sealable plastic bag, and toss. Rest in the refrigerator at least 4 hours or overnight. To cook, preheat oven to 450° F. Remove the bag from the refrigerator, and empty the fries onto a sheet pan. Bake for 15 minutes, flip the fries, and cook for another 10 minutes (or a little longer if deeper color/char is desired). Season with additional salt and pepper.

healthy bytes Sweet potatoes are not really related to the potato. They are a member of the morning glory family and are believed to have been around since prehistoric times. They are loaded with fiber, mostly in the skin; antioxidants; beta-carotene; vitamin A; and potassium.

Nutrition Facts	
Serving Size 3 oz (85g)	
Servings Per Container 4	
Amount Per Serving	
Calories 140	Calories from Fat 70
	% Daily Value*
Total Fat 8g	13%
Saturated Fat 0.5g	3%
Trans Fat 0g	
Cholesterol 0mg	0%
Sodium 40mg	2%
Total Carbohydrate 16g	5%
Dietary Fiber 2g	10%
Sugars 3g	
Protein 1g	
Vitamin A 220% • Vitamin C 4%	
Calcium 2% • Iron 4%	

* Percent Daily Values are based on a 2,000 calorie diet. Your daily values may be higher or lower depending on your calorie needs.

	Calories	2,000	2,500
Total Fat	Less than	65g	80g
Sat Fat	Less than	20g	25g
Cholesterol	Less than	300mg	300mg
Sodium	Less than	2,400mg	2,400mg
Total Carbohydrate		300g	375g
Dietary Fiber		25g	30g

Calories per gram:
Fat 9 • Carbohydrate 4 • Protein 4

REFRIED BLACK BEAN FOUR-LAYER DIP

THIS IS AN incredibly versatile dish that is a quick and easy preparation. The refried beans themselves make a great side topped with sour cream or crème fraiche and chopped tomato or, even better, some fresh salsa. A great appetizer or lunch can be made from layering the beans in individual 8 oz. ramekins or baking dishes and making small servings of the four-layer dip for one or two. The base with beans can be made ahead and kept in the refrigerator. When you need a serving, simply top with cheese, pop under the broiler, remove, top, and serve. If you don't have the dried beans to reconstitute yourself, use a can of prepared, no-fat refried black beans. You can also convert the four-layer dip to seven-layer dip simply by adding a layer of guacamole, salsa, and the optional sour cream.

16 oz. dried black beans, rinsed and rehydrated in water
    overnight
1 bay leaf

Nutrition Facts	
Serving Size 4 oz (113g)	
Servings Per Container 12	
Amount Per Serving	
Calories 220	Calories from Fat 80
	% Daily Value*
Total Fat 9g	14%
Saturated Fat 3.5g	17%
Trans Fat 0g	
Cholesterol 15mg	5%
Sodium 1380mg	57%
Total Carbohydrate 26g	9%
Dietary Fiber 6g	23%
Sugars 2g	
Protein 10g	
Vitamin A 60% • Vitamin C 15%	
Calcium 45% • Iron 60%	

* Percent Daily Values are based on a 2,000 calorie diet. Your daily values may be higher or lower depending on your calorie needs.

	Calories	2,000	2,500
Total Fat	Less than	65g	80g
Sat Fat	Less than	20g	25g
Cholesterol	Less than	300mg	300mg
Sodium	Less than	2,400mg	2,400mg
Total Carbohydrate		300g	375g
Dietary Fiber		25g	30g

Calories per gram:
Fat 9 • Carbohydrate 4 • Protein 4

CONTAINS: Milk

1 yellow onion, divided
2 garlic cloves, peeled and smashed
2 tsp. salt
4 tbsp. good-quality olive oil, divided
¼ tsp. fresh ground cumin
¼ tsp. oregano, Mexican if available
1 tbsp. chipotle pepper, chopped
1¾ to 2 c. light chicken stock (see recipe in chapter 19)
¼ c. cheddar and pepper jack cheeses, shredded (use soy cheese if desired)
⅓ c. lettuce, shredded
⅓ c. medium tomatoes, seeded and chopped
1 tbsp. fat-free sour cream (optional)
Guacamole and salsa (optional)

Place the rehydrated beans in a medium saucepan with enough cold water to cover by 1 to 2 inches. Bring to a boil for 10 minutes, then drain in the sink in a colander. Wash the beans to remove any scum. Return to a medium saucepan and use enough fresh water to cover by 1 to 2 inches. Bring to a boil, then reduce heat to simmer. Add the bay leaf, 2 onion quarters, and the smashed garlic. Simmer for 30 to 45 minutes, or until the beans are tender. Add the salt and cook until the beans are very tender, an additional 15 to 30 minutes. Drain the beans in a colander set in the sink like before. Discard the bay leaf, onion quarters, and garlic. In a medium skillet, heat 3 tbsp. olive oil over medium-high heat. Add the remaining onion, chopped, and cook until soft, about 4 to 5 minutes. Add the minced garlic, cumin, and oregano and cook for an additional minute. Add the beans and 1 c. of the chicken stock, and using a potato masher, mash the beans until chunky-smooth. Add the chipotle pepper and ¾ c. more of the stock, and cook, stirring, until the beans are very thick and flavorful, about 10 minutes. If it becomes too thick, simply add more of the stock. When the beans have reached the desired consistency, stir in 1 tbsp. olive oil. To make the layer dip, place a layer of the beans in the bottom of the serving dish, approximately ½ inch in depth. For individual or smaller portions, you can use smaller (8 oz.) baking dishes. Preheat the broiler on high. Place a layer of cheese on top, and place under the broiler on high for 1 to 3 minutes, until cheese is melted and golden brown. Remove from the oven. Place a layer of lettuce, then a layer of tomato, and an optional layer of sour cream on top. To make seven-layer dip, place salsa then guacamole on top of the cheese, and continue to dress as mentioned.

healthy bytes Black beans are an excellent source of fiber. If you are sensitive to sulfites, black beans may help. They are an excellent source of the trace mineral molybdenum, which is an integral component of the enzyme sulfite oxidase. This enzyme is responsible for detoxifying sulfites. Black beans and other beans are useful foods for people with irregular glucose metabolism, such as diabetics and those with hypoglycemia, because beans have a low glycemic index rating. This means that blood glucose (blood sugar) does not rise as high after eating beans as it does when compared to, for example, white bread.

TUSCAN ITALIAN WHITE BEAN SOUP

THIS SOUP IS just perfect on a fall or winter day. You can start it and let it cook in the crockpot if you have to go off to work or away for a few hours. This soup makes a great meal by itself, served with some olives, grilled vegetables, crusty bread, and olive oil. If you don't have the dry beans, you can use a 14 oz. can. Just pick up the recipe where the beans are tender. Top with a little freshly ground Asiago or parmesan cheese if desired.

Nutrition Facts		
Serving Size 8 oz (227g)		
Servings Per Container 24		
Amount Per Serving		
Calories 100	Calories from Fat 30	
		% Daily Value*
Total Fat 3.5g		5%
Saturated Fat 1g		4%
Trans Fat 0g		
Cholesterol 5mg		2%
Sodium 230mg		10%
Total Carbohydrate 12g		4%
Dietary Fiber 3g		12%
Sugars 4g		
Protein 5g		
Vitamin A 40%	•	Vitamin C 40%
Calcium 4%	•	Iron 6%

* Percent Daily Values are based on a 2,000 calorie diet. Your daily values may be higher or lower depending on your calorie needs.

		Calories	2,000	2,500
Total Fat	Less than		65g	80g
Sat Fat	Less than		20g	25g
Cholesterol	Less than		300mg	300mg
Sodium	Less than		2,400mg	2,400mg
Total Carbohydrate			300g	375g
Dietary Fiber			25g	30g

Calories per gram:
Fat 9 • Carbohydrate 4 • Protein 4

8 oz. kidney beans, rinsed and rehydrated in water overnight.
8 oz. cannellini beans, rinsed and rehydrated in water overnight.
3 tbsp. olive oil
¼ c. pancetta, diced
¼ c. prosciutto, diced
2 c. yellow onions, diced
1 c. celery, diced
1 c. carrots, diced
4 garlic cloves, sliced
Salt
Freshly ground black pepper
10 oz. grape or cherry tomatoes
2 qts. light chicken stock (see recipe in chapter 19)
2 sprigs rosemary
3 sprigs thyme
1 sprig oregano
1 bay leaf
1 tsp. red pepper flakes
2 heads cabbage, large ribs removed and cut into bite-sized pieces
Freshly ground Asiago or parmesan cheese (optional)

Place the rehydrated beans in a medium saucepan with enough cold water to cover by 1 to 2 inches. Bring to a boil for 10 minutes, then drain in the sink in a colander. Wash the beans to remove any scum. Return to a medium saucepan and use enough fresh water to cover by 1 to 2 inches. Bring to a boil, then reduce heat to simmer. Simmer for another 30 to 45 minutes until tender. In a large pot, heat the olive oil over medium heat. Add the pancetta, and cook until slightly crispy, about 3 minutes. Add the prosciutto, and cook an additional minute. Sauté the onion, celery, carrot, and garlic for 3 to 4 minutes. Season with salt and freshly ground black pepper. Add the tomatoes, the cooked and drained kidney beans and cannellini beans, and the chicken stock. Using an herb sack or piece of cheesecloth, place the rosemary, thyme, oregano, and bay leaf inside, close the pouch, and place in the pot. Season with the red pepper flakes, salt, and pepper. Cook for 15 minutes, and then add the cabbage. Continue cooking until the beans are completely tender.

healthy bytes   Cabbage is probably one of the most important vegetables by virtue of its nutritional and cancer-fighting benefits. The cancer-fighting phytochemicals in cabbage are called indoles. These indoles increase "good" estrogen to help fight the "bad" estrogen that has been implicated in some forms of breast cancer. Cabbage is a great source of everyday vitamins and minerals. It contains calcium, magnesium, potassium, vitamin C, vitamin K, beta-carotene, carotenoids, lutein, and zeaxanthin. Red or purple cabbage is not just a pretty addition; they also offer a wonderful source of anthocyanins. This is the same class of pigment molecules that are found in blueberries. These flavonoids act as powerful antioxidants that fight free-radical damage in cells.

SUCCOTASH

THIS IS A great summertime dish when the corn and beans can be bought fresh. You can grill the corn for just a few minutes to add a slight char. This gives the dish a whole extra flavor dimension.

    2 tbsp. olive oil
    1 shallot, finely chopped
    ¼ c. onion, chopped
    3 garlic cloves, chopped
    3 ears of corn, grilled and kernels removed from cob
    1 lb. butter or lima beans
    Approximately 1 c. tomatoes, seeded and chopped
    1½ c. chicken stock (see recipe in chapter 19)
    2 tbsp. lime juice

Heat oil in a large saucepan. Add shallots, onion, and garlic, and cook until translucent, approximately 2 minutes. Add the corn and beans, and cook an additional 1 to 2 minutes. Add the tomatoes and stock. Bring to a boil, reduce, and simmer to reduce stock by ⅓ to ½. Add the lime juice prior to serving.

healthy bytes Shallots are in the same family of vegetables as leeks and onions. They are very high in vitamin C, potassium, fiber, folic acid, calcium, and iron. Shallots are also a good source of protein. They contain two types of sulfur-containing compounds, allypropyldisulphine (APDS) and flavonoids, such as quercetin. Flavonoids have been shown to be useful compounds in fighting cancer, heart disease, and diabetes and have potent antioxidant properties. Shallots also contain saponins, which may also have cancer-fighting abilities. Shallots have an added benefit in that they are also anti-inflammatory, antiviral, and antiallergenic. In holistic circles, shallots are used as a liver-detoxifying agent.

Nutrition Facts
Serving Size 8 oz (227g)
Servings Per Container 6

Amount Per Serving	
Calories 200	Calories from Fat 45

	% Daily Value*
Total Fat 5g	8%
Saturated Fat 1g	4%
Trans Fat 0g	
Cholesterol 0mg	0%
Sodium 25mg	1%
Total Carbohydrate 34g	11%
Dietary Fiber 5g	21%
Sugars 7g	
Protein 9g	

Vitamin A 10%	•	Vitamin C 35%
Calcium 4%	•	Iron 15%

* Percent Daily Values are based on a 2,000 calorie diet. Your daily values may be higher or lower depending on your calorie needs.

		Calories	2,000	2,500
Total Fat	Less than		65g	80g
Sat Fat	Less than		20g	25g
Cholesterol	Less than		300mg	300mg
Sodium	Less than		2,400mg	2,400mg
Total Carbohydrate			300g	375g
Dietary Fiber			25g	30g

Calories per gram:
Fat 9 • Carbohydrate 4 • Protein 4

OPEN-FACED GOUGÈRE MINI-BLTS

THESE ARE a favorite of mine when stuffed with fresh shredded lettuce, fresh chopped garden tomatoes, a few pieces of crispy bacon (lardon style), and a bit of Greek yogurt on top. Serve with a bowl of roasted corn and tomato soup—truly a code delicious!

24 gougères (see recipe in chapter 19)
1½ lbs. bacon, cut lardon style
Approximately 1 c. tomato, chopped
Approximately 1 c. lettuce, shredded
4 tbsp. Greek yogurt

Assemble the cut gougères by layering from the bottom up: shredded lettuce, chopped tomato, and bacon. Top with ½ tsp. of Greek yogurt.

healthy bytes Yogurt has many health benefits. It is made with live active cultures, or probiotics, which is good bacteria that can help keep your digestive system working properly. Yogurt is also

Nutrition Facts
Serving Size 1 1/5 oz (34g)
Servings Per Container 24

Amount Per Serving	
Calories 150	Calories from Fat 130

	% Daily Value*
Total Fat 15g	23%
Saturated Fat 5g	25%
Trans Fat 0g	
Cholesterol 15mg	6%
Sodium 20mg	1%
Total Carbohydrate 2g	1%
Dietary Fiber 0g	0%
Sugars 0g	
Protein 1g	

Vitamin A 4%	•	Vitamin C 2%
Calcium 2%	•	Iron 0%

* Percent Daily Values are based on a 2,000 calorie diet. Your daily values may be higher or lower depending on your calorie needs.

		Calories	2,000	2,500
Total Fat	Less than		65g	80g
Sat Fat	Less than		20g	25g
Cholesterol	Less than		300mg	300mg
Sodium	Less than		2,400mg	2,400mg
Total Carbohydrate			300g	375g
Dietary Fiber			25g	30g

Calories per gram:
Fat 9 • Carbohydrate 4 • Protein 4

CONTAINS: Milk

high in calcium and a great source of protein. Greek yogurt is thicker and creamier than regular yogurt, is lower in carbohydrates and sodium, and contains more protein than regular yogurt.

ROASTED CORN AND TOMATO SOUP

TOMATOES ARE available year round, but I really consider this a seasonal dish. The store-bought nuggets with the taste and texture of a tennis ball cannot compare to fresh-out-of-the-garden tomatoes one gets in season. It is these succulent, sweet flavor bombs that make all the difference in this soup.

2½ lbs. garden tomatoes
1 tsp. salt
2 tbsp. olive oil + additional for garnish
2 carrots, finely chopped
2 ears corn, roasted
2 garlic cloves, finely chopped
1½ tsp. ground fennel seed, freshly roasted
2 tsp. fresh oregano
2 tsp. fresh thyme
2 tbsp. dried basil
1½ tsp. dried tarragon
1 bay leaf
1 sprig fresh mint
1 jalapeño, cut lengthwise
½ tsp. freshly ground black pepper
1½ c. chicken stock (see recipe in chapter 19)
1 tbsp. parmesan cheese, finely grated
Truffle oil

Nutrition Facts		
Serving Size 8 oz (227g)		
Servings Per Container 8		
Amount Per Serving		
Calories 70	Calories from Fat 10	
		% Daily Value*
Total Fat 1.5g		2%
Saturated Fat 0g		0%
Trans Fat 0g		
Cholesterol 0mg		0%
Sodium 300mg		13%
Total Carbohydrate 14g		5%
Dietary Fiber 3g		13%
Sugars 6g		
Protein 4g		
Vitamin A 50%	•	Vitamin C 35%
Calcium 4%	•	Iron 6%

* Percent Daily Values are based on a 2,000 calorie diet. Your daily values may be higher or lower depending on your calorie needs.

	Calories	2,000	2,500
Total Fat	Less than	65g	80g
Sat Fat	Less than	20g	25g
Cholesterol	Less than	300mg	300mg
Sodium	Less than	2,400mg	2,400mg
Total Carbohydrate		300g	375g
Dietary Fiber		25g	30g

Calories per gram:
Fat 9 • Carbohydrate 4 • Protein 4

Preheat the oven to 350° F. Place the tomatoes in an oven-proof roasting pan, and season lightly with salt and 1 tbsp. olive oil. Roast the tomatoes for 20 to 30 minutes. The tomatoes will just start to split and brown when done. While the tomatoes are roasting, heat some olive oil on medium heat. Place the carrots and corn in a sautoir (straight-sided saucepan), and cook until soft (about 5 to 10 minutes). Add the garlic, fennel, oregano, thyme, basil, tarragon, bay leaf, mint, and jalapeño, and cook for several more minutes, allowing flavors to combine. Add the tomatoes, pepper, and chicken stock. Bring to a boil, reduce heat, and simmer for 20 minutes. Remove the bay leaf, mint sprig, and jalapeño. Use an immersion blender to puree, or process in small batches in a food processor or blender. Season with salt and pepper as needed. Place in a bowl, drizzle with a few drops of olive or truffle oil, and sprinkle cheese on top. Garnish with a small mint leaf.

healthy bytes Fennel's dried fruit contains an essential oil, anethole, which gives it the licorice flavor, as well as limonene, a phytochemical, and quercetin, an anti-inflammatory flavonoid. It is believed that fennel counteracts spasms of the smooth muscle in the stomach, relieving gas and cramps.

FETA POTATO LEEK SOUP

I CAN REMEMBER watching Julia Child make potato leek soup. It has probably been around in one form or another as long as people have been cooking. You can blend the soup entirely smooth or leave some chunks if you like it that way. I love the tang and additional creaminess that the feta cheese adds, and you can use fat-free feta if you like.

Nutrition Facts		
Serving Size 8 oz (227g)		
Servings Per Container 12		
Amount Per Serving		
Calories 160	Calories from Fat 60	
		% Daily Value*
Total Fat 7g		**10%**
Saturated Fat 4g		**19%**
Trans Fat 0g		
Cholesterol 20mg		**7%**
Sodium 370mg		**15%**
Total Carbohydrate 18g		**6%**
Dietary Fiber 2g		**8%**
Sugars 3g		
Protein 7g		
Vitamin A 8%	•	Vitamin C 25%
Calcium 10%	•	Iron 8%

* Percent Daily Values are based on a 2,000 calorie diet. Your daily values may be higher or lower depending on your calorie needs.

	Calories	2,000	2,500
Total Fat	Less than	65g	80g
Sat Fat	Less than	20g	25g
Cholesterol	Less than	300mg	300mg
Sodium	Less than	2,400mg	2,400mg
Total Carbohydrate		300g	375g
Dietary Fiber		25g	30g

Calories per gram:
Fat 9 • Carbohydrate 4 • Protein 4

CONTAINS: Milk

2 leeks, white and light green parts, leaves discarded
1½–2 lbs. potatoes (like Yukon golds)
2 tbsp. butter or Smart Balance substitute
3 garlic cloves, chopped
6 c. chicken stock (see recipe in chapter 19)
6 oz. feta cheese
1 tsp. salt
½ tsp. white pepper

Finely dice the leeks, and wash them thoroughly, as they are grown in sand. Peel and cut the potatoes into large chunks and set aside. In a large soup pot, sauté the leeks in butter or Smart Balance over medium heat until translucent, about 3 to 5 minutes. Add the garlic, and stir for another minute. Add the chicken stock and potatoes. Simmer for about 30 minutes until the potatoes are fork tender. Using an immersion blender (or in small batches in a blender), blend the mixture. Once everything is smooth, add the crumbled cheese and season with salt and white pepper.

healthy bytes Leeks are a great source of two very important carotenoids for eye health: lutein and zeaxanthin. It is thought that these two carotenoids have the ability to help prevent macular degeneration. Leeks are also high in fiber, calcium, iron, vitamin K, and vitamin A.

FRIED RICE

THIS IS AN easy, healthy, and filling preparation. You can add all sorts of seasonal vegetables, and turn the whole thing into a main by adding a little meat or fish. If you can use day-old rice that has dried out a bit, it will absorb the flavors and cook crispier in the oil. For a dramatic look, I use black Chinese rice.

1–2 tbsp. peanut or other oil
1 hot pepper, sliced lengthwise
1 tsp. ginger, finely chopped
1 tsp. garlic, finely chopped
1 tbsp. onion, finely chopped
1 egg, beaten
2 c. cooked rice
2 c. mixed vegetables (I like a combination of peas, water chestnuts, bamboo shoots, carrots, baby corn, and napa cabbage or bok choy)
1 tbsp. soy sauce
Scallion or cilantro, chopped

Nutrition Facts		
Serving Size 6 oz (170g)		
Servings Per Container 4		
Amount Per Serving		
Calories 200	Calories from Fat 70	
		% Daily Value*
Total Fat 8g		**12%**
Saturated Fat 1.5g		**8%**
Trans Fat 0g		
Cholesterol 50mg		**17%**
Sodium 50mg		**2%**
Total Carbohydrate 27g		**9%**
Dietary Fiber 4g		**14%**
Sugars 0g		
Protein 5g		
Vitamin A 70%	•	Vitamin C 10%
Calcium 2%	•	Iron 6%

* Percent Daily Values are based on a 2,000 calorie diet. Your daily values may be higher or lower depending on your calorie needs.

	Calories	2,000	2,500
Total Fat	Less than	65g	80g
Sat Fat	Less than	20g	25g
Cholesterol	Less than	300mg	300mg
Sodium	Less than	2,400mg	2,400mg
Total Carbohydrate		300g	375g
Dietary Fiber		25g	30g

Calories per gram:
Fat 9 • Carbohydrate 4 • Protein 4

CONTAINS: Eggs, Peanuts

Heat the oil in a deep pan or wok until smoking. Add the hot pepper and cook for about 1 minute to season the oil. Remove the pepper; add the ginger, garlic, and onion; and cook for about 1 minute. Add the egg and scramble. Add the rice and then the vegetables, tossing quickly until the vegetables and rice are slightly crispy and browned. The exact time will vary depending on the veggie types and amounts. Do not add too much volume to the wok or you risk steaming and boiling instead of frying quickly over high heat. Add the soy sauce, quickly toss, and remove from heat. Garnish with chopped scallion or cilantro.

healthy bytes Brown rice is more nutritious than white, as the bran layer is left intact. It is high in fiber, niacin, vitamin B_6, magnesium, manganese, and selenium and contains some vitamin E. The fiber content in brown rice lowers the glycemic index.

LATKES

TO THIS DAY I am not really sure what the difference between a latke, a hash brown, and a potato pancake really is. Because it is so darn delicious by any name, I don't really care. This version fries up nice and crisp as long as you remember two important rules: keep the oil hot and don't overcrowd the pan. Placing food into hot oil drops the temperature. Too many latkes in the pan will mean they sit in oil, which has to get back up to frying temperature. The result is that the latkes absorb a lot of oil and come out greasy and unpleasant.

2 lbs. potatoes, grated
¾ c. onion, finely chopped
1 shallot, halved and sliced
3 eggs
1 tsp. lemon juice
1 tbsp. garlic, finely chopped
2 tbsp. rice flour
1 tbsp. all-purpose flour
1 tsp. salt
½ tsp. freshly cracked black pepper
Oil for frying (such as canola)
Sour cream
Applesauce

Grate the potatoes, and set aside in some cold water. Combine all the other ingredients except for the oil, sour cream, and applesauce. Drain the potatoes, and place them in a clean tea towel or dish rag. Squeeze the water out by twisting the ends of the towel and wringing. Add the potatoes to the mix. Heat a neutral oil (like canola) in a pan over medium heat. Take a handful of the mixture, squeeze out any additional liquid you can, and place into the pan. Fry until golden brown and delicious (GB&D!) on one side, flip, and finish on the other. Serve with sour cream and apple sauce

healthy bytes Potatoes are a very good source of vitamin C, vitamin B$_6$, copper, potassium, manganese, and dietary fiber. They also contain a variety of phytonutrients that have antioxidant activity. Among these important health-promoting compounds are carotenoids, flavonoids, and caffeic acid. Potatoes also contain unique tuber storage proteins, such as patatin, which exhibit activity against free radicals. These help promote cardiovascular well-being and are potential cancer-fighting compounds.

PUMPKIN CORNBREAD

CORNBREAD IS good any time of year, but this particular version shines around Thanksgiving. You can, of course, make a basic version, leaving out the pumpkin and pumpkin pie spice. You can add some sausage, jalapeños, and many other items to this versatile staple. If it gets stale, use it for a fantastic stuffing for pork or poultry dishes. It is especially tasty used in a stuffed pork chop or even served as a main with just some beans.

¼ c. vegetable oil
1 c. yellow cornmeal
½ c. all-purpose flour
½ c. canned pumpkin
1 ear corn, roasted and kernels removed (approximately $1/3$–½ c.)
2 tsp. baking powder
½ tsp. baking soda
1 tsp. salt
1 tbsp. pumpkin pie spice
¼ tsp. cayenne pepper
¼ tsp. freshly ground black pepper
1½ c. buttermilk
1 large egg, lightly beaten
3 egg whites

Nutrition Facts		
Serving Size 1 3/10 oz (37g)		
Servings Per Container 24		
Amount Per Serving		
Calories 50	Calories from Fat 10	
		% Daily Value*
Total Fat 1g		2%
Saturated Fat 0g		0%
Trans Fat 0g		
Cholesterol 10mg		3%
Sodium 200mg		8%
Total Carbohydrate 8g		3%
Dietary Fiber 1g		2%
Sugars 1g		
Protein 2g		
Vitamin A 15%	•	Vitamin C 0%
Calcium 2%	•	Iron 2%

* Percent Daily Values are based on a 2,000 calorie diet. Your daily values may be higher or lower depending on your calorie needs.

	Calories	2,000	2,500
Total Fat	Less than	65g	80g
Sat Fat	Less than	20g	25g
Cholesterol	Less than	300mg	300mg
Sodium	Less than	2,400mg	2,400mg
Total Carbohydrate		300g	375g
Dietary Fiber		25g	30g

Calories per gram:
Fat 9 • Carbohydrate 4 • Protein 4

CONTAINS: Eggs

Preheat the oven to 425° F. Place the vegetable oil in a 9-inch baking pan or cast iron skillet, and place in the oven to heat. Combine the cornmeal, flour, pumpkin, corn, baking powder, baking soda, salt, pumpkin pie spice, cayenne, and black pepper, and mix well. In a small bowl, combine the buttermilk and whole egg. Add to dry ingredients, and stir just to combine. Whip the egg whites to soft peaks and gently fold into the mixture. Remove the hot pan from the oven, drain excess vegetable oil so the pan is lightly coated, and pour the cornmeal batter into the skillet. Bake for 25 to 30 minutes, or until firm and golden brown on top.

healthy bytes Pumpkin is very high in potassium, beta-carotene, and vitamin A. Pumpkin is considered by some a for-your-eyes-only food, but it is good nutrition for the whole body. It contains the carotenoids lutein and zeaxanthin and more than 12,000 IU of vitamin A. The pumpkin seeds also have great value as they contain beta-sitosterol, a phytosterol that is believed to have a benefit in treating benign prostate hyperplasia, or BPH, which may be a precursor to prostate cancer. Beta-sitosterol is also thought to help reduce blood cholesterol levels.

SMOKED SALMON "PIZZA" WITH LEMON-CURRY HOLLANDAISE

FOLLOW THE directions for either the basic bread dough or basic pizza dough recipes in chapter 19. If you have premade crusts, you can use those. The lemon-curry hollandaise is a basic hollandaise sauce recipe. This version uses olive oil instead of butter. Any item you wish to use as a topping is fine. I like the flavor profile of the smoky and fatty (with good omega-3s) smoked salmon with the citrus and spice of the lemon-curry sauce. The chèvre adds an extra tang and richness. This is perfect with a wine such as a chenin blanc or champagne (which, let's face it, is about perfect with everything).

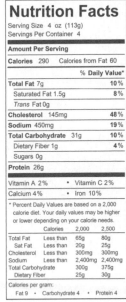

Nutrition Facts

Serving Size 4 oz (113g)
Servings Per Container 4

Amount Per Serving

Calories 290   Calories from Fat 60

	% Daily Value*
Total Fat 7g	10%
Saturated Fat 1.5g	8%
Trans Fat 0g	
Cholesterol 145mg	48%
Sodium 450mg	19%
Total Carbohydrate 31g	10%
Dietary Fiber 1g	4%
Sugars 0g	
Protein 26g	

Vitamin A 2%	•	Vitamin C 2%
Calcium 4%	•	Iron 10%

* Percent Daily Values are based on a 2,000 calorie diet. Your daily values may be higher or lower depending on your calorie needs.

	Calories	2,000	2,500
Total Fat	Less than	65g	80g
Sat Fat	Less than	20g	25g
Cholesterol	Less than	300mg	300mg
Sodium	Less than	2,400mg	2,400mg
Total Carbohydrate		300g	375g
Dietary Fiber		25g	30g

Calories per gram:
Fat 9 • Carbohydrate 4 • Protein 4

CONTAINS: Eggs

½ c. olive oil (not extra virgin)

2 lemons, juiced

3 egg yolks

1 tsp. curry spice

Basic Bread or Pizza Dough (1 dough recipe makes approximately 3 pizzas; see chapter 19)

4 oz. chèvre

Capers

4 oz. good-quality smoked salmon

¼ tsp. salt

¼ tsp. white pepper

Additional toppings, such as tomato, dill, and basil

Heat the oil and lemon juice over medium heat. Do not let the oil get too hot, or when you add the eggs, you will end up with scrambled eggs. Place the egg yolks in a metal bowl you can place over a pot with simmering water (a double boiler, which you can remove as needed from heat). When the oil mixture is warm, gently add ¼ to ⅓ of it to the eggs and whisk to temper the egg mixture. After incorporation, gently add the remaining oil mixture. Heat the mixture over the simmering water and whisk until it is light and frothy. Remove from the heat as the sauce starts to thicken. Add the curry spice, and set aside.

Preheat your oven to 550° F. Stretch the dough out into desired pizza sizes; I recommend 8 to 12 inches, which yields about three pizzas from the basic dough recipe. Place the thin layer of sauce on the dough along with some chèvre and some capers, if you like. Bake for about 10 minutes, until the crust is golden brown. Remove and top with the smoked salmon, season with salt and pepper (I also like a little fresh tomato, dill, and basil), and enjoy.

healthy bytes Salmon is rich in omega-3s, which are the polyunsaturated fatty acids (PUFA) found in some plants; grass-raised, free-range, natural and game meats; and in fatty fish like salmon. These compounds have shown some potential anticancer effects as well as the potential to help prevent Parkinson's and Alzheimer's diseases. Omega-3s have been shown to reduce the rate of heart attacks and strokes, reduce blood pressure, and reduce atherosclerosis. The American Heart Association (AHA) now recommends people consume fatty fish like salmon twice a week.[4] The benefits keep rolling in. An animal study out of Spain suggests that these compounds may increase insulin sensitivity.[5] Decreased sensitivity to insulin, or insulin resistance, is a major problem associated with metabolic syndrome and type-2 diabetes. A specific omega-3 PUFA, docosahexaenoic acid (DHA), may reduce inflammation while preserving infection-fighting abilities of white blood cells. Future areas of investigation may look into using these compounds in conditions like asthma.

REFRIED BEANS

BEANS ARE one of the staple foods worldwide. They are low in fat, high in protein, and incredibly versatile. You can make a meal with some veggies and cheese piled high on a fresh corn tortilla. You can have them as a side with some queso fresco; add a slice of corn bread, and you have another delicious encounter. If you want to make some quick but have not soaked the beans, use some from a can.

16 oz. dried kidney beans, soaked overnight
2 tbsp. olive oil
1 c. yellow onions, chopped
1 tbsp. garlic, minced
1 tbsp. dried red chili pepper, minced, or 1 tsp. cayenne pepper
3 tbsp. chili powder
1 tbsp. ground cumin
1 tsp. salt
1 tbsp. chopped oregano
6 oz. queso fresco, chopped
½ c. vegetable nage or chicken stock (see recipes in chapter 19)
2 tbsp. adobo sauce

In a large pot, add the presoaked beans and enough water to cover by 1 to 2 inches. Bring to a boil, then simmer uncovered for about 2 hours, adding more water as necessary to keep the beans covered. The beans should be very tender. Drain the beans, then mash them, and set aside. In a large, heavy skillet, heat olive oil over medium-high heat. Add the onions and cook for about 2 minutes. Add the garlic, dried red chili pepper or cayenne, chili powder, cumin, salt, and oregano, and cook another 1 to 2 minutes. Add the beans, cheese, nage, and adobo sauce, and cook for another 5 to 10 minutes or until it thickens.

healthy bytes Cumin is also known as "black seed" or *Nigella sativa*. In many Arabian, Asian, and African countries, it is used to reduce allergy symptoms. Cumin also contains limonene, which is believed to block some cancers. It is thought to help digestion and reduce heartburn.

Nutrition Facts

Serving Size 4 oz (113g)
Servings Per Container 12

Amount Per Serving

Calories 220   Calories from Fat 80

	% Daily Value*
Total Fat 9g	**14%**
Saturated Fat 3.5g	**17%**
Trans Fat 0g	
Cholesterol 15mg	**5%**
Sodium 1380mg	**57%**
Total Carbohydrate 26g	**9%**
Dietary Fiber 6g	**23%**
Sugars 2g	
Protein 10g	

Vitamin A 60%	•	Vitamin C 15%
Calcium 45%	•	Iron 60%

* Percent Daily Values are based on a 2,000 calorie diet. Your daily values may be higher or lower depending on your calorie needs.

	Calories	2,000	2,500
Total Fat	Less than	65g	80g
Sat Fat	Less than	20g	25g
Cholesterol	Less than	300mg	300mg
Sodium	Less than	2,400mg	2,400mg
Total Carbohydrate		300g	375g
Dietary Fiber		25g	30g

Calories per gram:
Fat 9 • Carbohydrate 4 • Protein 4

CONTAINS: Milk

ROASTED BUTTERNUT SQUASH AND POMEGRANATE

THIS IS A dish to convert those who are not big winter squash fans. I know; I was one of them. Once again, by cooking for others and through properly tasting the food as we cook, we can become fans of things we thought we hated. I now love winter squash in all its forms: stuffed in raviolis, in soup, and, in particular, this dish. The pomegranate seeds add a hint of sweet crunch and a visually pleasing dab of color.

1 butternut squash (1–2 lbs.), peeled, seeded, and rough chopped
3 tbsp. olive oil, divided
1 tsp. salt
½ tsp. freshly ground black pepper
2 tbsp. shallot, finely chopped
1 pomegranate, seeded
2 tbsp. cream
2 tbsp. butter or Smart Balance substitute

Nutrition Facts

Serving Size 4 oz (113g)
Servings Per Container 12

Amount Per Serving

Calories 120   Calories from Fat 70

	% Daily Value*
Total Fat 8g	**12%**
Saturated Fat 3g	**14%**
Trans Fat 0g	
Cholesterol 10mg	**4%**
Sodium 420mg	**17%**
Total Carbohydrate 12g	**4%**
Dietary Fiber 3g	**13%**
Sugars 6g	
Protein 1g	

Vitamin A 80%	•	Vitamin C 15%
Calcium 2%	•	Iron 2%

* Percent Daily Values are based on a 2,000 calorie diet. Your daily values may be higher or lower depending on your calorie needs.

	Calories	2,000	2,500
Total Fat	Less than	65g	80g
Sat Fat	Less than	20g	25g
Cholesterol	Less than	300mg	300mg
Sodium	Less than	2,400mg	2,400mg
Total Carbohydrate		300g	375g
Dietary Fiber		25g	30g

Calories per gram:
Fat 9 • Carbohydrate 4 • Protein 4

CONTAINS: Milk

Preheat the oven to 425° F. Place the squash on a baking pan lined with parchment paper and drizzle with about 2 tbsp. olive oil, salt, and pepper. Roast for 30 to 45 minutes until the squash is tender. Remove and allow the squash to cool. When ready to prepare, heat a medium saucepan with about 1 tbsp. olive oil over medium heat. Cook the shallots until soft, about 1 to 2 minutes. Add the squash and heat. Allow it to gently mash into smaller chunks as you cook it, about another 8 to 12 minutes. Add the pomegranate seeds, cream, and butter or Smart Balance. Remove from heat, season, and serve.

healthy bytes Pomegranate is rich in potassium and vitamin C and has three times the antioxidants of red wine or green tea. It aids in keeping fatty deposits down in arteries, therefore potentially reducing the risk of heart disease, stroke, Alzheimer's disease, and cancer.

SPANIKOPITA

I LOVE GREEK and Mediterranean food. The style is fresh food cooked lightly and simply. It is rich in vegetables, citrus, and seafood. This is a great example, using a light phyllo dough and spinach filling. Experiment with various fillings after you gain some comfort working with the phyllo. It is not difficult; just keep it moist. Don't fret if a sheet tears; just keep going.

1 tbsp. olive oil
20 oz. spinach leaves (2 bunches)
¼ tsp. nutmeg
2 tbsp. pine nuts
16 oz. feta
¼ c. onion, chopped
1 tbsp. fresh thyme
1 tbsp. fresh oregano, chopped
1 tbsp. fresh basil, chopped
3 garlic cloves, minced
1 lemon, juiced
1 tsp. lemon zest
1 tsp. smoked paprika
1 egg
1 tsp. salt
½ tsp. black pepper
1 box phyllo dough
Approximately 2 tbsp. manchego, finely grated
Approximately 1 tbsp. sesame seeds

Nutrition Facts

Serving Size 1 oz (28g)
Servings Per Container 20

Amount Per Serving	
Calories 70	Calories from Fat 45

	% Daily Value*
Total Fat 5g	8%
Saturated Fat 2.5g	12%
Trans Fat 0g	
Cholesterol 10mg	3%
Sodium 100mg	4%
Total Carbohydrate 4g	1%
Dietary Fiber 1g	2%
Sugars 0g	
Protein 2g	

Vitamin A 20%	•	Vitamin C 4%	
Calcium 4%	•	Iron 4%	

* Percent Daily Values are based on a 2,000 calorie diet. Your daily values may be higher or lower depending on your calorie needs.

		Calories	2,000	2,500
Total Fat	Less than		65g	80g
Sat Fat	Less than		20g	25g
Cholesterol	Less than		300mg	300mg
Sodium	Less than		2,400mg	2,400mg
Total Carbohydrate			300g	375g
Dietary Fiber			25g	30g

Calories per gram:
Fat 9 • Carbohydrate 4 • Protein 4

CONTAINS: Milk, Nuts

Preheat the oven to 425° F. Heat the olive oil over medium heat in a large saucepan. Add the spinach and the nutmeg, and cook until reduced and most of the liquid has evaporated. In a small pan, lightly toast the pine nuts. Remove from the heat, and allow to cool. Place the spinach in a sieve or colander, and press to remove as much moisture as possible. Mix the spinach, pine nuts, feta, onion, thyme, oregano, basil, garlic, lemon juice, lemon zest, paprika, and egg together, and season with salt and pepper. Cover the phyllo with a damp paper towel to keep it moist while you work with it. Layer 10 sheets of phyllo for the bottom on a sheet pan larger than the sheets. Spread the filling in the middle. Layer about 6 layers on top. Place grated manchego or other sheep's milk cheese and sesame seeds on top. Bake for about 20 minutes or until golden brown and crispy.

healthy bytes   Pine nuts are actually the seed of certain varieties of pine trees. They are found on the pine cones covered by a hard coat and can be eaten raw, toasted, roasted, or mashed. Pine nuts are nature's only source of pinoleic acid, which stimulates hormones and helps diminish your appetite. Pine nuts have one of the highest concentrations of oleic acid, which is a monounsaturated fat that aids the liver in eliminating triglycerides from your body and helps protect the heart. Pine nuts are also packed with 3 mg of iron per 1 ounce serving. Iron is a key component of hemoglobin, the oxygen-carrying pigment in blood that supplies energy. They are rich in magnesium, which helps alleviate muscle cramps, tension, and fatigue. Pine nuts contain a fair amount of fiber and are high in protein. There are some areas that harvest pine nuts for a coffee called piñon, which is rich and nutty tasting.

SPINACH DHAL

I AM EXCITED by Indian cuisine. There is a Northern and a Southern cuisine, not unlike here in the United States. I love both; the flavors are sweet, spicy, and deep, as there is generous spice usage. Using a lot of spice for flavor is a key component of Grassroots Gourmet cooking. By using spices to build flavor, we rely less on fat, salt, and sugar. I think that's one reason Indian cuisine is in general very healthful.

8 oz. lentils
2 c. water
2 c. vegetable nage or chicken stock (see recipes in chapter 19)
½ tsp. turmeric
1 tsp. freshly ground ginger
5 oz. baby spinach
½ c. fresh cilantro, chopped
1 tbsp. olive oil
3 garlic cloves, thinly sliced

2 tbsp. shallot, thinly sliced
1 tsp. ground cumin seed
2 tsp. mustard seed
1 tsp. curry powder
1 tsp. ground coriander seed
1 hot chili, thinly sliced
Salt and pepper
Naan

In a medium saucepan over medium heat, bring the lentils (after rinsing) to a boil with the water, nage or stock, turmeric, and ginger. Reduce the heat to a simmer for 20 minutes, until the lentils are tender. Add the spinach and cilantro, and cook for another 8 to 10 minutes. In a small pan, heat the oil and add the garlic, shallot, cumin seed, mustard seed, curry, coriander seed, and hot chili. Cook over high heat for 2 minutes to release the flavors. Add this to the lentils, stir, season with salt and pepper, and serve with warm naan.

healthy bytes Mustard seed is a source of allyl isothiocyanate, which is believed to play a role in tumor prevention. It belongs to the Brassica family, which also contains cabbage, broccoli, and kale as members. Mustard seed stands prominent in the ancient Christian faith and was often worn in a locket to signify that something so seemingly small and unimportant, when nurtured and nourished, will grow into something of great strength and power.

STOVETOP APPLESAUCE

"**PORK CHOPS** and applesauce," as the classic Peter Brady line goes. I love pork and apple. It is another American classic. Applesauce is also great with any number of meats, including a lot of game meats. Here is an easy way to make some fresh applesauce right on the stovetop and a great way to use some apples that may be starting to lose their crunch.

¼ c. orange juice
2 apples, cored, peeled, and sliced
⅓ c. natural organic sugar
1½ tbsp. cinnamon

Nutrition Facts		
Serving Size 4 oz (113g)		
Servings Per Container 2		
Amount Per Serving		
Calories 70	Calories from Fat 20	
		% Daily Value*
Total Fat 2.5g		4%
Saturated Fat 0g		0%
Trans Fat 0g		
Cholesterol 0mg		0%
Sodium 10mg		0%
Total Carbohydrate 9g		3%
Dietary Fiber 3g		11%
Sugars 2g		
Protein 4g		
Vitamin A 15%	•	Vitamin C 4%
Calcium 4%	•	Iron 10%

* Percent Daily Values are based on a 2,000 calorie diet. Your daily values may be higher or lower depending on your calorie needs.

	Calories	2,000	2,500
Total Fat	Less than	65g	80g
Sat Fat	Less than	20g	25g
Cholesterol	Less than	300mg	300mg
Sodium	Less than	2,400mg	2,400mg
Total Carbohydrate		300g	375g
Dietary Fiber		25g	30g

Calories per gram:
Fat 9 • Carbohydrate 4 • Protein 4

Combine all ingredients and simmer on the stove over medium heat until the apples are soft and the liquid has reduced, about 30 to 45 minutes. Apples are high in pectin and will naturally thicken.

healthy bytes Pectin is a soluble type of fiber found in apples, peaches, carrots, peas, and citrus fruits. It has the potential to relieve diarrhea and acts to help detoxify the gastrointestinal tract. It may also stimulate the immune system. It improves the body's handling of insulin by potentially reducing the rate of glucose uptake following consumption of certain types of carbohydrates. It may also help promote satiety as well as impact gallstone formation. Several studies have reported a significant decrease in serum cholesterol and low-density lipoprotein (LDL or bad) cholesterol and an increase or no change in high-density lipoprotein (HDL or good) cholesterol in people with a diet rich in pectin-containing fruits and vegetables.[6] Diets containing pectin incorporated into a food source seem to be better tolerated than those who consume supplements.

TEMPURA VEGETABLES

YOU CAN DO anything here. Tempura dip vegetables for a side or main course or use shrimp, squid, or soft-shell crabs. I've even seen whole lobster tails cooked this way. For the best results, I like to use bite-sized pieces of yellow squash, parboiled fingerling potatoes, carrots, zucchini, mushrooms, and broccoli. Remember, the key is to heat the oil, have everything cut beforehand, mix your batter, wait 5 minutes, and start frying. Do not add too much in the way of pieces to the oil, or the temperature will drop and you will just get greasy nastiness.

Oil for frying
Tempura batter (see recipe in chapter 19)
Asian dipping sauce (see recipe in chapter 19)
16 oz. fresh vegetables, cut into bite-sized pieces
Salt
Pepper

Nutrition Facts

Serving Size 2 oz (57g)
Servings Per Container 8

Amount Per Serving

Calories 50   Calories from Fat 0

	% Daily Value*
Total Fat 0g	0%
Saturated Fat 0g	0%
Trans Fat 0g	
Cholesterol 0mg	0%
Sodium 0mg	0%
Total Carbohydrate 14g	5%
Dietary Fiber 1g	4%
Sugars 12g	
Protein 0g	

Vitamin A 0%	•	Vitamin C 6%
Calcium 0%	•	Iron 0%

* Percent Daily Values are based on a 2,000 calorie diet. Your daily values may be higher or lower depending on your calorie needs.

	Calories	2,000	2,500
Total Fat	Less than	65g	80g
Sat Fat	Less than	20g	25g
Cholesterol	Less than	300mg	300mg
Sodium	Less than	2,400mg	2,400mg
Total Carbohydrate		300g	375g
Dietary Fiber		25g	30g

Calories per gram:
Fat 9 • Carbohydrate 4 • Protein 4

Nutrition Facts

Serving Size 38/41 lbs (420g)
Servings Per Container 1

Amount Per Serving

Calories 550   Calories from Fat 60

	% Daily Value*
Total Fat 6g	10%
Saturated Fat 1.5g	9%
Trans Fat 0g	
Cholesterol 210mg	71%
Sodium 75mg	3%
Total Carbohydrate 104g	35%
Dietary Fiber 3g	10%
Sugars 0g	
Protein 18g	

Vitamin A 4%	•	Vitamin C 0%
Calcium 6%	•	Iron 25%

* Percent Daily Values are based on a 2,000 calorie diet. Your daily values may be higher or lower depending on your calorie needs.

	Calories	2,000	2,500
Total Fat	Less than	65g	80g
Sat Fat	Less than	20g	25g
Cholesterol	Less than	300mg	300mg
Sodium	Less than	2,400mg	2,400mg
Total Carbohydrate		300g	375g
Dietary Fiber		25g	30g

Calories per gram:
Fat 9 • Carbohydrate 4 • Protein 4

CONTAINS: Eggs

Heat some oil in a Dutch oven or fryer to 375° F. Have your vegetables ready. Make the batter and allow to rest 5 minutes. Dip the vegetables in the batter, fry, season, and enjoy.

ZUCCHINI SLAW

THIS IS A crunchy, delicious, Asian-type slaw with some amazing seasoning from South Africa. It also has a touch of heat from the piri-piri. You can serve it as a side with anything. If you like a more traditional type, just substitute cabbage for the zucchini.

2 medium zucchini

2 carrots

2 tbsp. toasted sesame oil

¼ c. rice wine vinegar

½ tsp. Doc's South African five-spice blend (see recipe in chapter 19)

½ tsp. Doc's piri-piri sauce (see recipe in chapter 19)

2 tsp. honey

1 tbsp. soy sauce

½ c. mayo

Nutrition Facts		
Serving Size 4 oz (113g)		
Servings Per Container 6		
Amount Per Serving		
Calories 200	Calories from Fat 160	
		% Daily Value*
Total Fat 18g		28%
Saturated Fat 1.5g		8%
Trans Fat 0g		
Cholesterol 10mg		4%
Sodium 670mg		28%
Total Carbohydrate 9g		3%
Dietary Fiber 1g		5%
Sugars 8g		
Protein 1g		
Vitamin A 60%	•	Vitamin C 20%
Calcium 2%	•	Iron 2%

* Percent Daily Values are based on a 2,000 calorie diet. Your daily values may be higher or lower depending on your calorie needs.

	Calories	2,000	2,500
Total Fat	Less than	65g	80g
Sat Fat	Less than	20g	25g
Cholesterol	Less than	300mg	300mg
Sodium	Less than	2,400mg	2,400mg
Total Carbohydrate		300g	375g
Dietary Fiber		25g	30g

Calories per gram:
Fat 9 • Carbohydrate 4 • Protein 4

CONTAINS: Eggs, Soy

Using a mandolin or slicing finely, cut the zucchini and carrots into ⅛-inch strips. Combine the remaining ingredients in a bowl and mix. Toss enough of the dressing with zucchini and carrots to lightly coat them.

healthy bytes Carrots are high in carotenoids. Researchers believe that an increase in carotenoids is associated with a reduction in many cancers. Carrots are also high in lutein and zeaxanthin, carotenoids that protect eye health. Cooking carrots changes the nutritional content slightly and makes some of the nutrients more bioavailable. Eating carrots with a little good fat releases the carotenoids and vitamin A, both of which are fat-soluble nutrients. Carrot oil is believed to help reduce dryness and wrinkles in mature skin.

PARMESAN TRUFFLE FRIES

OKAY, OKAY. I know this one is not super healthy, but it is super delicious. And every now and then, if you have a celebratory reason or perhaps for no reason at all, break out the fry-o-later for this code delicious. The occasion should merit really good champagne because that is what this meal demands. The salty, crunchy, truffled potato with the cheese just begs for the yeasty acidity of the champagne, the perfect foil. This is so delicious that with the champagne I call them pomme frites.

> 2 Idaho potatoes (about 1 lb.), the bigger and longer the better, peeled and cut into ¼ to ½ inch fries
> Vegetable oil for frying (roughly 2 qts.)
> 2 tsp. salt
> Truffle oil
> ⅓ c. parmesan, finely ground

Nutrition Facts		
Serving Size 3 1/2 oz (99g)		
Servings Per Container 6		
Amount Per Serving		
Calories 150	Calories from Fat 80	
		% Daily Value*
Total Fat 9g		**13%**
Saturated Fat 3g		**16%**
Trans Fat 0g		
Cholesterol 10mg		**4%**
Sodium 1410mg		**59%**
Total Carbohydrate 12g		**4%**
Dietary Fiber 2g		**7%**
Sugars 0g		
Protein 7g		
Vitamin A 2%	•	Vitamin C 25%
Calcium 15%	•	Iron 4%

* Percent Daily Values are based on a 2,000 calorie diet. Your daily values may be higher or lower depending on your calorie needs.

	Calories	2,000	2,500
Total Fat	Less than	65g	80g
Sat Fat	Less than	20g	25g
Cholesterol	Less than	300mg	300mg
Sodium	Less than	2,400mg	2,400mg
Total Carbohydrate		300g	375g
Dietary Fiber		25g	30g

Calories per gram:
Fat 9 • Carbohydrate 4 • Protein 4

CONTAINS: Milk

Place the cut fries in ice water for at least 30 minutes. You will see the starch release into the water. Remove the fries and place in a fresh ice bath. Set the frying oil to 275 to 280° F. Dry off the potatoes prior to frying to reduce splatter. Place in small batches for 6 to 8 minutes until they turn semitranslucent white. Do not put too many fries in at once, or you drop the oil temperature, and they won't turn out properly. Remove from the heat, and let rest at least 30 minutes on a cooling rack set over a sheet pan to catch the oil so it drains away. When you are ready to serve, heat the oil to 375° F, and cook the fries, again in small batches, until golden brown. It should take around 3 minutes. Place on the rack, and after a few minutes, transfer to a bowl. Sprinkle with salt and truffle oil. It is important to do this while the fries are hot as this is when they will absorb the flavors. Toss in the cheese, and serve.

healthy bytes These make you feel good.

mains (recipes)

THIS IS the heart of the matter as far as mealtime goes. The mains discussed here are also known as the main course, main entrée, dinner course, main or large plates, and so on. Like with the firsts, the important considerations here are the portion size. This part of the meal should be arriving fifteen to twenty-five minutes after the appetizer. You can use the firsts to accompany the main to provide a meal with the traditional meat, starch, and vegetable that you find so often when dining out. You can also turn firsts into mains: A little larger serving of soup with some bread makes a meal. A salad with some fresh seafood also makes a delicious main. Vegetables that are not deep fried or drowned in butter and cream or cheese sauce are also welcome guests to any main. In fact, many of the weight loss programs that sell you prepared foods require generous portions of salad or vegetables that you buy and prepare yourself as part of their plan. Make the main the focus, accompany with a starch, and fill in the "sides" with unlimited vegetable-focused dishes. What you will have are restaurant quality meals every night to be enjoyed slowly with a glass or two of wine. Here is what we want to accomplish with this service:

- Serve this course fifteen to twenty-five minutes after you serve the first course.
- Either before or during, serve an eight-ounce glass of water to accompany.
- Limit wine to one to three glasses.
- Grassroots Gourmet–prepared vegetables are the "unlimited" side.

- If you are serving dessert, use smaller portions.
- As always, season with salt and pepper as you cook and at the end unless otherwise noted.

NORTH CAROLINA OVEN-BAKED BARBECUE CHICKEN TWO WAYS

I LIKE TO call this dish "a house divided." I spent some time working in North Carolina and still have great friends I visit there. People tend to lump "southern barbecue" into a narrow flavor profile. In truth, there are many different styles and flavor combinations. Just within the state of North Carolina, there is an ongoing debate regarding the merits of the eastern North Carolina mustard-based sauces versus the western tomato-and-vinegar–based preparations. Calling it a debate is putting it mildly. Know where you are and what to ask for, or you risk being labeled a "damn Yankee." We served this during one of our first community cooking demos. It was well received, but it was fairly equally divided as to which was preferred. The debate rages on.

4 skinless chicken breasts
Peach-mustard grilling sauce (see recipe in chapter 19)
Western North Carolina barbecue sauce (see recipe in chapter 19)

Nutrition Facts		
Serving Size 4 oz (113g)		
Servings Per Container 8		
Amount Per Serving		
Calories 300	Calories from Fat 140	
		% Daily Value*
Total Fat 16g		25%
Saturated Fat 5g		25%
Trans Fat 0g		
Cholesterol 105mg		36%
Sodium 200mg		8%
Total Carbohydrate 2g		1%
Dietary Fiber 0g		0%
Sugars 1g		
Protein 34g		
Vitamin A 4%	•	Vitamin C 2%
Calcium 2%	•	Iron 8%
* Percent Daily Values are based on a 2,000 calorie diet. Your daily values may be higher or lower depending on your calorie needs.		

	Calories	2,000	2,500
Total Fat	Less than	65g	80g
Sat Fat	Less than	20g	25g
Cholesterol	Less than	300mg	300mg
Sodium	Less than	2,400mg	2,400mg
Total Carbohydrate		300g	375g
Dietary Fiber		25g	30g

Calories per gram:
Fat 9 • Carbohydrate 4 • Protein 4

Preheat the oven to 425° F. Place the breasts in a resealable plastic bag, and gently pound until the breasts are about ½ inch thick. Making the breasts the same thickness by pounding tenderizes and also makes them cook at the same rate. Remove and place on a baking sheet. Cover two with the peach-mustard sauce and two with the barbecue sauce. Bake for approximately 25 minutes or until done using a meat thermometer or until the juices run clear. Rest the breasts for 5 minutes before serving.

healthy bytes Peaches originated in China, and the peach tree was considered the tree of life by the ancients. Peaches have to be picked ripe; they will not ripen much after picking, and one small bruise can ruin the whole peach. Peaches are low in calories, high in fiber, and contain some vitamin C and vitamin A. They also contain some beta-cryptoxanthin, which is believed to have anti-inflammatory and anticancer properties.

OVEN-ROASTED MUSHROOM-STUFFED QUAIL WITH BLUEBERRY CHIMICHURRI

THIS DISH can be adapted for Cornish hens and other small game birds. This is really delicious on a serving of warm white corn grits. Most of the quail come cleaned and deboned; if not, your butcher can do it for you.

3 c. mixed mushrooms, like shiitake, button, portabella, and oyster
4 oz. turkey sausage
¼ c. onion, finely chopped
1 tbsp. garlic, finely chopped
2 tbsp. olive oil
Salt
Pepper
½ c. white wine
½ c. breadcrumbs
¼ c. panko crumbs
8 quail, cleaned and boned, except for legs
1 tsp. parsley, finely chopped
Blueberry Chimichurri Sauce (see recipe in chapter 19)

Nutrition Facts		
Serving Size 9 oz (255g)		
Servings Per Container 8		
Amount Per Serving		
Calories 480	Calories from Fat 250	
		% Daily Value*
Total Fat 28g		**43%**
Saturated Fat 7g		**37%**
Trans Fat 0g		
Cholesterol 155mg		**52%**
Sodium 310mg		**13%**
Total Carbohydrate 10g		**3%**
Dietary Fiber 1g		**5%**
Sugars 2g		
Protein 47g		
Vitamin A 10%	•	Vitamin C 15%
Calcium 6%	•	Iron 45%

*Percent Daily Values are based on a 2,000 calorie diet. Your daily values may be higher or lower depending on your calorie needs.

		Calories	2,000	2,500
Total Fat	Less than		65g	80g
Sat Fat	Less than		20g	25g
Cholesterol	Less than		300mg	300mg
Sodium	Less than		2,400mg	2,400mg
Total Carbohydrate			300g	375g
Dietary Fiber			25g	30g

Calories per gram:
Fat 9 • Carbohydrate 4 • Protein 4

Preheat the oven to 375° F. Place the mushrooms, turkey sausage, onion, and garlic in a food processor, pulsing until you have a paste. Stop and scrape the sides as needed. In a medium saucepan over medium heat, add the olive oil and mushroom-sausage mixture. Season the mixture with salt and pepper. Stir for about 5 minutes, and then add white wine, stirring for another minute. Remove from heat, and add breadcrumbs and panko. Remove and allow the mixture to come to room temperature. Season each quail with salt and pepper. Using about ¼ c. of stuffing per bird, stuff each bird. Using a sharp knife, make a small slit at the tail end on the breast side on both sides of the bird. Place each leg through the slit on the opposite side so they cross. Bake the birds for approximately 20 minutes or until the skin is golden brown, basting intermittently with 1 tsp. of the chimichurri sauce. If you need to, place under the broiler for 1 to 2 minutes to crisp the skin. Rest the birds before serving. Serve with 1 tbsp. of the sauce ladled over the top of each bird.

healthy bytes Blueberries are brain food. They help you keep your brain young and working properly by helping to enhance memory and ward off inflammation and oxidative stress, which causes many diseases. Blueberries have enough healthy benefits to fill pages, but it is important to note that they fight the aging process, combat cardiovascular disease, and fight cancer cells. You can benefit from eating just a half cup of blueberries a day. Fresh or frozen, both are packed with healthy nutrients.

WOOD PLANK MEDITERRANEAN CHICKEN (OR SALMON)

This could just as easily be a salmon dish. I like to cook this on an oak grilling plank; the salmon variation is fantastic on a cedar grilling plank. In fact, for a fancy dinner party, you can make the Mediterranean marinade for both chicken and some salmon fillets and put both on the grill. This offers your guests a delicious choice of related but distinctly different flavor combinations. I recommend this with a bright New Zealand sauvignon blanc like Kim Crawford Marlborough.

Nutrition Facts		
Serving Size 4 3/5 oz (130g)		
Servings Per Container 8		
Amount Per Serving		
Calories 170	Calories from Fat 60	
		% Daily Value*
Total Fat 7g		11%
Saturated Fat 1g		6%
Trans Fat 0g		
Cholesterol 75mg		25%
Sodium 290mg		12%
Total Carbohydrate 0g		0%
Dietary Fiber 0g		0%
Sugars 0g		
Protein 25g		
Vitamin A 0%	•	Vitamin C 4%
Calcium 0%	•	Iron 2%

* Percent Daily Values are based on a 2,000 calorie diet. Your daily values may be higher or lower depending on your calorie needs.

		Calories	2,000	2,500
Total Fat	Less than		65g	80g
Sat Fat	Less than		20g	25g
Cholesterol	Less than		300mg	300mg
Sodium	Less than		2,400mg	2,400mg
Total Carbohydrate			300g	375g
Dietary Fiber			25g	30g

Calories per gram:
Fat 9 • Carbohydrate 4 • Protein 4

> Mediterranean marinade (see recipe in chapter 19)
> 4 skinless chicken breasts or 2 salmon fillets
> 4 oak (or cedar for the salmon) grilling planks (2 packages)
> Olive oil

For the chicken: Follow the directions for the marinade. Place the chicken breasts along with the marinade into a resealable plastic bag. Squeeze out the air, and set in a flat-bottomed container so the breasts rest covered in the marinade. Refrigerate for at least 4 hours, preferably overnight, remove, and allow to come up to room temperature. Follow the soaking directions for the wood grill planks. When ready, run a little olive oil on the planks so the chicken does not stick. Cook over medium heat on the grill (or in a 325° F oven) for about 25 minutes or until done by a meat thermometer (about 160° F—remember to allow for carryover) or the juices run clear. Allow the breasts to rest about 5 minutes. The nutritional information provided is for the chicken.

For the salmon: Follow the directions for the marinade. Place the salmon fillets along with the marinade in a resealable plastic bag. Squeeze out the air, and set in a flat-bottomed container so the fillets rest covered in the marinade. Refrigerate for at least 4 hours, preferably overnight, remove, and allow to come up to room temperature. Follow the soaking directions for the wood grill planks. When ready, run a little olive oil on the planks so the salmon does not stick. Cook over medium heat on the grill (or in a

325° F oven) for about 18 to 20 minutes, depending on the thickness of the fillets. When done, the flesh should separate easily, revealing a uniform color, and release easily from the skin. I use a fish spatula to get between the fillet and the skin; I don't like to serve fish with skin that is not crispy. Allow the fillets to rest for about 5 minutes.

healthy bytes Thyme contains thymol, a powerful antiseptic. Thymol is a wonderful anti-inflammatory agent. It has a long history as a digestive aid and helps to loosen chest and respiratory congestion. It is often used in over-the-counter natural vapor rubs and cough drops. The following is a historic remedy for coughs: steep 3 tbsp. of dry thyme in some boiling water, remove, and add 1 tbsp. of honey. This quiets the cough without the drug side effects and sugar.

SLOW-ROASTED DUCK WITH BLUEBERRY SAUCE

I LOVE DUCK. However, people need to realize duck is not chicken. It can dry out quickly and should be served when slightly pink, for example, when it is pan fried. Overcooked duck tastes like an old boot—the bottom of an old boot that's been in the lake for a year or two. When prepared correctly it is absolutely scrumptious, and the skinless breasts contain about half the saturated fat of a boneless, skinless chicken breast.

1 (approximately 4 lbs.) Muscovy duck (you can use Pekin duck if you can't find Muscovy)
Salt
Freshly ground pepper
½ tsp. onion powder
½ tsp. paprika
½ tsp. garlic powder
½ tsp. dried thyme
½ tsp. dried oregano
¼ tsp. cayenne
2 tbsp. fresh sage, finely chopped
2 tbsp. shallot, finely chopped, divided
1 medium bulb fresh ginger (7–9 oz.)
½ bulb garlic, roughly chopped
2 ribs celery, roughly chopped
2 carrots, roughly chopped
1 yellow onion, peeled and quartered
8 oz. fortified wine, like marsala

Nutrition Facts		
Serving Size 8 oz (227g)		
Servings Per Container 6		
Amount Per Serving		
Calories 370	Calories from Fat 160	
		% Daily Value*
Total Fat 19g		**28%**
Saturated Fat 5g		**27%**
Trans Fat 0g		
Cholesterol 165mg		**55%**
Sodium 620mg		**26%**
Total Carbohydrate 11g		**4%**
Dietary Fiber 2g		**7%**
Sugars 6g		
Protein 39g		
Vitamin A 2%	•	Vitamin C 8%
Calcium 6%	•	Iron 20%

* Percent Daily Values are based on a 2,000 calorie diet. Your daily values may be higher or lower depending on your calorie needs.

	Calories	2,000	2,500
Total Fat	Less than	65g	80g
Sat Fat	Less than	20g	25g
Cholesterol	Less than	300mg	300mg
Sodium	Less than	2,400mg	2,400mg
Total Carbohydrate		300g	375g
Dietary Fiber		25g	30g

Calories per gram:
Fat 9 • Carbohydrate 4 • Protein 4

1 c. dark chicken stock (see recipe in chapter 19)
⅓ c. champagne vinegar
2 tbsp. honey
1 bay leaf
1 sprig of fresh thyme
1 pt. fresh blueberries
2 oz. butter or Smart Balance substitute

Preheat the oven to 350° F. Remove any giblets from the cavity of the duck, wash it off, and pat dry. Season the entire duck with salt and pepper. In a small mixing bowl combine the onion powder, paprika, garlic powder, thyme, oregano, cayenne, sage, 2 tbsp. of the shallots, ½ of the ginger, and ½ of the garlic, peeled and finely grated. Season the entire duck, including the inside cavity, with the mixture. Stuff the cavity with the remaining garlic and ginger, celery, carrots, and onion. Place the duck on the rack of a roasting pan, and roast for about an hour. You may have to drain the pan intermittently as it fills with the fat that drips off. After an hour, turn the heat down to 300° F, and cook for another 1 to 1½ hours, emptying the pan of fat as needed. The duck is done when the skin is crispy and the leg bones easily pull away. Remove and drain off any remaining fat. Allow the duck to rest. While the duck is resting, place the roasting pan on the stovetop, and over high heat use ½ of the marsala to deglaze the bottom. Pour that into a medium saucepan. Add the stock, vinegar, honey, bay leaf, remaining marsala, and thyme. Bring to a boil stir, and reduce by ½ to ⅔ until it is thickened. Remove thyme and bay leaf. Run the sauce through a sieve, and return to the saucepan. Add the blueberries and reduce heat to a simmer, for about 5 minutes, or until the blueberries are soft and have started bursting. Remove from heat, continue stirring, and add the butter or Smart Balance. Remove the duck skin and carve. Drizzle 1 to 2 tsp. of the sauce over the duck meat.

healthy bytes Skinless duck breast has much less saturated fat than even some lean beef selections. It is a great source of both niacin and selenium, which is needed for good heart function. It also provides more iron per serving than chicken, turkey, Cornish game hens, and some cuts of beef. Many markets now carry frozen duck. Better yet, visit your local butcher, and see if he or she can get some fresh for you.

CHICKEN YAKITORI

YAKITORI IS a traditional Japanese kebab. You can still get this great street food all around Japan. There you can find not just chicken but also squid, fish, and other assorted meats cooked over a charcoal grill. Feel free to substitute other meats or seafood.

1 lb. chicken pieces
1 tsp. salt
½ tsp. freshly ground pepper
¼ c. mirin
¼ c. sake
3 tbsp. sesame oil
1½ tsp. fresh ginger, finely minced
1 tbsp. fresh lime juice
1 tsp. roasted garlic puree (see recipe in chapter 19)
16 bamboo skewers (or other kebab holder), soaked

Nutrition Facts		
Serving Size 4 oz (113g)		
Servings Per Container 4		
Amount Per Serving		
Calories 190	Calories from Fat 90	
		% Daily Value*
Total Fat 10g		15%
Saturated Fat 2g		9%
Trans Fat 0g		
Cholesterol 55mg		18%
Sodium 290mg		12%
Total Carbohydrate 13g		4%
Dietary Fiber 0g		0%
Sugars 7g		
Protein 13g		
Vitamin A 2%	•	Vitamin C 0%
Calcium 2%	•	Iron 4%

* Percent Daily Values are based on a 2,000 calorie diet. Your daily values may be higher or lower depending on your calorie needs.

	Calories	2,000	2,500
Total Fat	Less than	65g	80g
Sat Fat	Less than	20g	25g
Cholesterol	Less than	300mg	300mg
Sodium	Less than	2,400mg	2,400mg
Total Carbohydrate		300g	375g
Dietary Fiber		25g	30g

Calories per gram:
Fat 9 • Carbohydrate 4 • Protein 4

Season the chicken pieces with salt and pepper. Combine the mirin, sake, sesame oil, ginger, lime juice, and roasted garlic puree in a medium saucepan, and bring to a boil. Reduce to a simmer, and simmer for 5 to 10 minutes. Remove from the heat, and let cool to room temperature. While the sauce cools, soak the skewers in water. Cut the chicken pieces into fairly uniform, bite-sized chunks. Reserve ⅓ of the sauce. Place the chicken in the remaining sauce to marinate for several hours. Place about 1 oz. of chicken per skewer, and lay the skewers on a grill at medium heat. Cook for about 6 to 8 minutes per side until the pieces are done and no longer pink in the middle. The exact time will depend on the thickness of the pieces. Use the reserved sauce to apply the glaze to each piece as it cooks on the grill. The sauce can be made in advance and will keep for about 2 weeks in the refrigerator.

healthy bytes Ginger is best known as a remedy for upset stomach and nausea. In addition ginger has anti-inflammatory properties; it contains the antioxidant gingerol, which has been shown to inhibit the growth of cancer cells in some forms of colorectal cancer. It is thought that ginger contains antimicrobial and antiviral properties as well. Another benefit of ginger is the ability to improve circulation. While ginger has very few side effects, one should exercise caution if taking blood-thinning drugs, as there is a potential for interaction with high doses.

CRISPY PRESSED TOFU AND CRAB SALAD–STUFFED PORTOBELLO MUSHROOMS

LOOKING AT my recipe collection and reflecting on my personal experience, my familiarity with tofu always seems to be paired with some Asian flavors. Not a bad thing but a rather pedestrian approach. I always eat delicious tofu preparations when I visit the Orient, but how about something different? Tofu is extremely versatile and is a flavor chameleon. Rather bland in and of itself, it can add texture and acts to provide a canvas upon which to paint a dish's flavor profile. After a *long* day in the test kitchen, we emerged with an absolute winner. The tofu in this dish takes on a meat-like texture when prepared this way, which accentuates the natural meatiness of the portobello. It has a light surf-and-turf feel to it. If you want an all-veggie version, just double the amount of tofu you use and leave out the crab.

Nutrition Facts		
Serving Size 10 oz (283g)		
Servings Per Container 12		
Amount Per Serving		
Calories 230	Calories from Fat 100	
		% Daily Value*
Total Fat 12g		18%
Saturated Fat 3g		14%
Trans Fat 0g		
Cholesterol 20mg		7%
Sodium 410mg		17%
Total Carbohydrate 22g		7%
Dietary Fiber 3g		13%
Sugars 7g		
Protein 15g		
Vitamin A 6%	•	Vitamin C 130%
Calcium 20%	•	Iron 15%

* Percent Daily Values are based on a 2,000 calorie diet. Your daily values may be higher or lower depending on your calorie needs.

	Calories	2,000	2,500
Total Fat	Less than	65g	80g
Sat Fat	Less than	20g	25g
Cholesterol	Less than	300mg	300mg
Sodium	Less than	2,400mg	2,400mg
Total Carbohydrate		300g	375g
Dietary Fiber		25g	30g

Calories per gram:
Fat 9 • Carbohydrate 4 • Protein 4

CONTAINS: Milk, Nuts, Shellfish

Mediterranean marinade (see recipe in chapter 19)
4 tbsp. pine nuts, toasted
12 large portobello mushroom caps
1 14 oz. package extra-firm tofu
Oil
8 oz. crabmeat (backfin is fine)
½ c. red onion, finely chopped
2 celery stalks, finely chopped
½ c. water chestnuts (roughly 2½ oz. when drained), finely chopped
1 lemon, juiced
1 tbsp. fresh basil, chopped
Approximately 5 oz. plain Greek yogurt
½ tsp. Old Bay spice
1¼ tsp. smoked paprika
¼ tsp. onion powder
¼ tsp. garlic powder
¼ tsp. dried oregano
¼ tsp. dried thyme
¼ tsp. cayenne
1 tsp. salt
1 tsp. freshly cracked black pepper
4 oz. chèvre (preferably herbed)

Prepare the marinade and set aside. Toast the pine nuts and set aside. Clean the portobello caps, removing the stems and the dark gills from the underside. Remove the tofu block (do not substitute; if it is not extra firm, the tofu will crumble), and gently press between paper towels or dish towels to remove the water. Cut the extra-firm tofu block in half so you now have 2 blocks with half the original thickness but the original length and width. Now cut each of those blocks in half lengthwise so there are now 4 tofu blocks of equal proportions. Gently press again to remove as much water as possible. Set the tofu blocks in the marinade, and marinate for at least 1 hour and up to 12 hours. In a separate bowl, combine the crabmeat, red onion, celery, water chestnuts, lemon juice, basil, yogurt, Old Bay, paprika, onion powder, garlic powder, oregano, thyme, cayenne, salt, and pepper. When the tofu has finished marinating, remove and place on a hot sauté pan that has been lightly oiled over medium heat. Place another pan on top and weigh down (any canned goods work well here). The tofu will have absorbed the oil, so it should not stick, and therefore you only need very little oil in the pan. Cook 3 to 4 minutes or until a golden-brown skin forms on the tofu. Flip and repeat. Remove from the stove, and cube the tofu into bite-sized pieces. Mix with the crab salad and fill each mushroom cap. You can just reserve some of the salad if you do not want to place it all in the mushroom caps. Divide the chèvre among the stuffed caps, and place under the broiler for 3 to 4 minutes or until the chèvre has melted and starts to brown. Serve immediately.

healthy bytes Tofu is bean curd made by adding mineral salt and water to a soybean mash. The mineral salt makes the protein and fiber in the soy mash turn thick and smooth. Tofu is rich in calcium and is an inexpensive source of protein, making it a good vegetarian substitute for meat or dairy products. Plain tofu has almost no taste, but it readily absorbs the flavor of herbs and spices added when you prepare a meal. Tofu is a versatile food and an important part of East Asian cuisines. The special health benefits of tofu have been attributed to two major components: isoflavones and amino acids. Isoflavones are a special group of bioflavonoids found more highly concentrated in soy than in any other food.

CHICKEN POT PIE

THIS IS A classic winter comfort food. I like to make this in individual ramekins for portion control as well as convenience. You can freeze the pot pies and reheat later.

6 tbsp. olive oil
1 medium yellow onion, chopped (about 1 c.)
1 can sliced water chestnuts (8 oz.), chopped
Salt
Freshly ground pepper
4 tbsp. all-purpose flour
2 tbsp. masa corn flour
2 c. light chicken stock (see recipe in chapter 19)
6 oz. fat-free ricotta cheese
2 c. diced Yukon gold potatoes, blanched
1 c. diced carrots, blanched
1 c. frozen sweet peas, defrosted
2 tbsp. parsley, finely chopped
2 c. cooked chicken, shredded
1 savory basic pie crust (see recipe in chapter 19)

Nutrition Facts

Serving Size 7 oz (198g)
Servings Per Container 15

Amount Per Serving

Calories 380	Calories from Fat 200

	% Daily Value*
Total Fat 23g	35%
Saturated Fat 3g	16%
Trans Fat 0g	
Cholesterol 80mg	27%
Sodium 670mg	28%
Total Carbohydrate 24g	8%
Dietary Fiber 2g	7%
Sugars 3g	
Protein 21g	

Vitamin A 30%	•	Vitamin C 15%	
Calcium 8%	•	Iron 10%	

* Percent Daily Values are based on a 2,000 calorie diet. Your daily values may be higher or lower depending on your calorie needs.

	Calories	2,000	2,500
Total Fat	Less than	65g	80g
Sat Fat	Less than	20g	25g
Cholesterol	Less than	300mg	300mg
Sodium	Less than	2,400mg	2,400mg
Total Carbohydrate		300g	375g
Dietary Fiber		25g	30g

Calories per gram:
Fat 9 • Carbohydrate 4 • Protein 4

CONTAINS: Milk

Preheat the oven to 400° F. Lightly grease or use cooking spray on fifteen 7 oz. ramekins. In a large sauce pan, heat the olive oil. Add the onions and water chestnuts, and sauté for 2 minutes. Season this dish with salt and pepper as you build each flavor layer. Stir in both the all-purpose flour and corn masa flour, and cook for about 3 to 4 minutes. The mixture will take on the consistency of wallpaper paste. This is a blond roux. Add the chicken stock, and bring the liquid to a boil. Reduce to a simmer, and continue to cook for about 8 to 10 minutes or until the sauce starts to thicken. Stir in the ricotta cheese, and continue to cook for about 5 minutes until everything is thoroughly combined. Add the potatoes, carrots, peas, parsley, and chicken, mixing thoroughly. Divide the filling among the ramekins. Roll out the crust, and cut circles just slightly larger than the ramekins (you can trace around an inverted ramekin with a paring knife). Place the crust on top of the filling. Make sure you seal the pastry at the edges of the ramekins, and place them on a baking sheet. Place the sheet in the oven, and bake for 25 to 30 minutes or until the crust is golden brown. Remove from the oven, and cool for several minutes prior to serving.

healthy bytes Water chestnuts are not nuts at all. They are tubers that are grown in marshy areas in Asia. Nutritionally, water chestnuts are a good source of potassium and fiber. They are low in sodium, and fat is virtually nonexistent. Caloriewise, one cup of water chestnut slices contains about 130 calories. Water chestnuts are high in carbohydrates. They have a sweet crunch and are thought to sweeten the breath.

SAFFRON RISOTTO WITH MUSHROOMS, PEAS, AND PEARL ONIONS

I LOVE RISOTTO. This makes a great meal in itself or as a side or an appetizer in a smaller portion. This basic recipe yields a lovely, creamy risotto with a little *al dente* crunch in the rice, the way I think it should be; mushy risotto should just be illegal. To use the basic recipe, eliminate the saffron, mushrooms, and peas and replace the pearl onions with shallots (¼ c. finely chopped) and yellow onions (¼ c.). Once you have mastered the stirring, which produces the creaminess by slowly releasing the starches, then add ingredients to create your own variations.

Approximately 2¾ c. light chicken stock, divided
    (see recipe in chapter 19)
½ tsp. saffron threads
4½ tbsp. olive oil, divided
½ c. pearl onions, roughly chopped if they are on the large side
1 garlic clove, finely chopped
1 cup arborio rice
8 oz. shiitake mushrooms, chopped
½ c. sake or white wine
1 c. frozen spring garden peas or fresh English garden peas
2 tbsp. butter or Smart Balance substitute
¼ c. parmesan cheese, finely grated
1 tbsp. mascarpone cheese
Salt
White pepper

Nutrition Facts		
Serving Size 7 oz (198g)		
Servings Per Container 6		
Amount Per Serving		
Calories 300	Calories from Fat 120	
		% Daily Value*
Total Fat 14g		21%
Saturated Fat 3g		16%
Trans Fat 0g		
Cholesterol 10mg		3%
Sodium 460mg		19%
Total Carbohydrate 33g		11%
Dietary Fiber 2g		7%
Sugars 2g		
Protein 5g		
Vitamin A 8%	•	Vitamin C 10%
Calcium 6%	•	Iron 6%

* Percent Daily Values are based on a 2,000 calorie diet. Your daily values may be higher or lower depending on your calorie needs.

		Calories	2,000	2,500
Total Fat	Less than		65g	80g
Sat Fat	Less than		20g	25g
Cholesterol	Less than		300mg	300mg
Sodium	Less than		2,400mg	2,400mg
Total Carbohydrate			300g	375g
Dietary Fiber			25g	30g

Calories per gram:
Fat 9 • Carbohydrate 4 • Protein 4

CONTAINS: Fish, Milk

Warm 1 c. of chicken stock and dissolve the saffron threads in the stock. In a saucepan over medium heat, add 2½ tbsp. of olive oil. Add the onions and garlic, season, and cook for approximately 2 minutes. Add the rice, and cook another 1 to 2 minutes, stirring constantly. Add about ½ of the saffron broth, and cook, stirring frequently and allowing the liquid to reduce between additions. Add more saffron stock, and then plain chicken stock, warmed, as needed. Stir frequently over the next 18 to 20 minutes. Simultaneously in another pan, heat the remaining oil and cook the mushrooms over medium heat. Add the wine in small increments, letting it be absorbed by the mushrooms. Add the peas. Remove from heat. Add the butter or Smart Balance, parmesan cheese, and mascarpone cheese to the risotto. Add in the peas and mushrooms. Season with salt and white pepper. Serve immediately.

healthy bytes Saffron has been one of the most highly prized spices since antiquity. It has been sought after for its color, flavor, and medicinal properties. It is the dried stigma, or threads, of the flower of the crocus plant. The active components in saffron have many therapeutic applications in many traditional medicines, such as an antiseptic, antidepressant, antioxidant, and digestive aid. The α-crocin, a carotenoid compound that gives the spice its characteristic golden yellow color, has antioxidant, antidepressant, and anticancer properties.

FRENCH OMELET WITH TRUFFLE BUTTER AND BRIE

ALTHOUGH IT appears simple, mastering the omelet and properly cooking eggs in general demands culinary precision. If you want to test a chef, ask him or her to perfectly poach or fry an egg or better yet make an omelet. This measure of culinary ability is not just a Western standard. If you want to determine a sushi chef's ability, have them prepare *tamago*. This is a sweet, folded, custard-like egg preparation often served as a final sushi course or starter, again to demonstrate the chef's ability. You can grab a glass of wine and make this dish to restore the harmony of your universe. Or you can just enjoy its elegant simplicity: a simple omelet served with toast and wine. Everyone knows the recipe, but not everyone does it well. If you have any questions on how to perform the trifold French omelet, grab a pan, some bowls, and a few dozen eggs and practice.

3 eggs
1 tbsp. truffle butter
¼ tsp. salt
1 oz. brie cheese
Parsley

Nutrition Facts		
Serving Size 8 oz (227g)		
Servings Per Container 1		
Amount Per Serving		
Calories 480	Calories from Fat 340	
		% Daily Value*
Total Fat 38g		59%
Saturated Fat 18g		92%
Trans Fat 0g		
Cholesterol 830mg		277%
Sodium 1030mg		43%
Total Carbohydrate 2g		1%
Dietary Fiber 0g		0%
Sugars 0g		
Protein 29g		
Vitamin A 35%	•	Vitamin C 0%
Calcium 15%	•	Iron 15%

* Percent Daily Values are based on a 2,000 calorie diet. Your daily values may be higher or lower depending on your calorie needs.

	Calories	2,000	2,500
Total Fat	Less than	65g	80g
Sat Fat	Less than	20g	25g
Cholesterol	Less than	300mg	300mg
Sodium	Less than	2,400mg	2,400mg
Total Carbohydrate		300g	375g
Dietary Fiber		25g	30g

Calories per gram:
Fat 9 • Carbohydrate 4 • Protein 4

CONTAINS: Milk

Place the uncracked eggs in some warm water (warm, not hot—you're not cooking them yet), and allow them to warm for 5 minutes. Heat the truffle butter over medium heat in a nonstick pan. Mix the eggs and salt in a bowl. When the butter has stopped foaming, add the eggs, and stir for 5 to 15 seconds with a spatula. When the eggs start to set, stop stirring. Loosen the omelet around the edges, and pour any liquid toward the edges by tilting the pan. When there is no liquid flowing, cook an additional 10 to 15 seconds. Place any filling, in this case the cheese, in the middle. Tilt the edge of the pan furthest away from you up and flip ⅓ of the omelet back on itself. Tilt the same edge down and flip the back ⅓ of the omelet on itself. Plate, garnish with parsley, serve, and enjoy.

healthy bytes Eggs were previously much maligned. Currently enjoying a resurgence as part of a healthy, balanced diet, the incredible, edible egg is now often referred to as "nature's perfect food." They are cheap, easy to prepare in many ways, and one of the best sources of protein around. Egg yolks also contain nine essential amino acids and are loaded with vitamins and minerals that aid your eyes, brain, and heart. Egg yolks are also a great source of choline, a nutrient that is essential for cardiovascular and brain function as well as cell membrane health. The choline in the yolk is actually what helps to prevent the buildup of cholesterol and fat in the liver. Free-range eggs are higher in beneficial omega-3 fatty acids.

JENNY AND FORREST FETTUCCINE

"**ME AND JENNY** goes together like peas and carrots," so said the sage Forrest Gump. And this dish goes together like Bubba and shrimp. The dish is easy to prepare, does not take much time, and is incredibly delicious. Use the basic pasta recipe in chapter 19, which you can make ahead of time.

   Basic pasta (see recipe in chapter 19)
   Olive oil
   ⅓ c. carrot, sliced
   ⅔ c. peas
   1 tbsp. shallot, finely minced
   Salt
   Alfredo sauce (see recipe in chapter 19)
   Cheese, such as parmesan
   Parsley

Coat the basic pasta lightly with olive oil, wrap in plastic wrap, and let it rest in the refrigerator for at least an hour or

Nutrition Facts		
Serving Size 8 oz (227g)		
Servings Per Container 4		
Amount Per Serving		
Calories 520	Calories from Fat 80	
		% Daily Value*
Total Fat 10g		**15%**
Saturated Fat 2.5g		**13%**
Trans Fat 0g		
Cholesterol 5mg		**2%**
Sodium 570mg		**24%**
Total Carbohydrate 90g		**30%**
Dietary Fiber 4g		**17%**
Sugars 3g		
Protein 20g		
Vitamin A 50%	•	Vitamin C 6%
Calcium 10%	•	Iron 15%

* Percent Daily Values are based on a 2,000 calorie diet. Your daily values may be higher or lower depending on your calorie needs.

	Calories	2,000	2,500
Total Fat	Less than	65g	80g
Sat Fat	Less than	20g	25g
Cholesterol	Less than	300mg	300mg
Sodium	Less than	2,400mg	2,400mg
Total Carbohydrate		300g	375g
Dietary Fiber		25g	30g

Calories per gram:
Fat 9 • Carbohydrate 4 • Protein 4

CONTAINS: Milk

overnight. Allow the dough to come up to room temperature. Divide the dough into 4 even pieces. Roll the dough out thinly by hand, or run it through a pasta machine. Cut the noodles by hand, or run them through the cutter attachment on the pasta machine, and hang to dry. Heat some olive oil in a pan over medium heat, then add the carrots and peas with the shallot. When ready to serve, add the pasta noodles to a pan of boiling, salted water to which you have added a dash of olive oil. The pasta will cook very quickly, within a few minutes. Remove; drain; and toss with the peas, carrots, and shallots. Top with Alfredo sauce and some additional cheese, like parmesan, if desired, and garnish with parsley. Serve with some warm bread.

healthy bytes Peas are high in vitamin K, vitamin B_1, vitamin B_2, vitamin B_6, folic acid, and niacin. Peas are also rich in iron and vitamin C. Peas do, however, contain purines. Purines are commonly found to occur naturally in both plants and animals. In some individuals who are susceptible to purine-related problems, excessive intake of these substances can cause health problems. Gout and kidney stones are two of these conditions.

BUTTERNUT SQUASH RAVIOLI WITH SAGE BROWN BUTTER

A DELICIOUS classic and easy to make. Follow the basic pasta recipe in chapter 19; I use a Kitchen Aid stand mixer with dough hook and pasta roller accessories, but you can just as easily do it all by hand (I've done it that way, too). Let the pasta dough rest at least an hour in the refrigerator. It will keep wrapped for several days if you need to make it well ahead of time. Let it come up to room temperature, then work it through the rollers on your pasta machine to get sheets or roll out by hand.

Nutrition Facts		
Serving Size 8 oz (227g)		
Servings Per Container 6		
Amount Per Serving		
Calories 360	Calories from Fat 140	
		% Daily Value*
Total Fat 16g		24%
Saturated Fat 4.5g		22%
Trans Fat 0g		
Cholesterol 10mg		4%
Sodium 1010mg		42%
Total Carbohydrate 47g		16%
Dietary Fiber 5g		20%
Sugars 4g		
Protein 9g		
Vitamin A 140%	•	Vitamin C 20%
Calcium 4%	•	Iron 6%

* Percent Daily Values are based on a 2,000 calorie diet. Your daily values may be higher or lower depending on your calorie needs.

	Calories	2,000	2,500
Total Fat	Less than	65g	80g
Sat Fat	Less than	20g	25g
Cholesterol	Less than	300mg	300mg
Sodium	Less than	2,400mg	2,400mg
Total Carbohydrate		300g	375g
Dietary Fiber		25g	30g

Calories per gram:
Fat 9 • Carbohydrate 4 • Protein 4

1 (1–2 lb.) butternut squash, peeled, seeded, and roughly
    chopped
3 tbsp. olive oil
1 tsp. salt
½ tsp. freshly ground black pepper
Basic pasta (see recipe in chapter 19)
2 tbsp. butter
2 tsp. sage, finely chopped
2 tbsp. shallot, finely chopped

Preheat the oven to 425° degrees F. Place the squash on a baking pan lined with parchment paper and drizzle with olive oil, salt, and pepper. Roast for 30 to 45 minutes until the squash is tender. Remove and allow the squash to cool. While the squash cools, roll out the pasta into sheets. I put about 1 to 2 tsp. of squash in the middle of each ravioli piece and fold over, crimping the dough. Heat the butter in a pan with the shallots and sage until it starts to foam and gets a light brown color with a nutty aroma. Quickly add the ravioli (the butter can burn quickly once it turns). Season with salt and pepper, and serve immediately.

healthy bytes Olive oil is mainly made up of monounsaturated fat; the most important is oleic acid. It is a very heart-healthy ingredient thought to lower LDL (bad cholesterol) and raise HDL (good cholesterol). Olive oil is also high in phenols, which are antioxidants that combat the oxidative process that may cause some forms of cancer. Extra virgin olive oil is essentially the unprocessed first press of the oil. This has the best nutrient base and the most healthful properties.

CURRY SMOKED SALMON WITH BLOOD ORANGE CURRY SAUCE

IF YOU DO not have access to a smoker, you can season the salmon and broil it. The fish is done when the flesh flakes away from the skin and bone. This sauce is also incredible served over some lamb or other meat with a vegetable couscous.

Salmon fillet, approximately 3 lbs.
2 tsp. salt
1 tsp. freshly ground black pepper
1 tbsp. curry spice
Blood orange curry sauce (see recipe in chapter 19)

Prepare the fillet with salt, pepper, and curry spice. Have the smoker ready, or place under the broiler. The exact time will depend on the size and thickness of the fillet. Serve the fish over rice or couscous, and ladle the curry sauce on top.

healthy bytes Curry powder is actually a mixture of any number of spices. One main spice in most curry powders is turmeric. This is the spice that gives curry its yellow color and is also responsible,

Nutrition Facts		
Serving Size 8 oz (227g)		
Servings Per Container 8		
Amount Per Serving		
Calories 420	Calories from Fat 180	
		% Daily Value*
Total Fat 20g		**32%**
Saturated Fat 4.5g		23%
Trans Fat 0g		
Cholesterol 90mg		**31%**
Sodium 660mg		**27%**
Total Carbohydrate 28g		**9%**
Dietary Fiber 15g		59%
Sugars 2g		
Protein 37g		
Vitamin A 15%	•	Vitamin C 25%
Calcium 25%	•	Iron 80%

* Percent Daily Values are based on a 2,000 calorie diet. Your daily values may be higher or lower depending on your calorie needs.

	Calories	2,000	2,500
Total Fat	Less than	65g	80g
Sat Fat	Less than	20g	25g
Cholesterol	Less than	300mg	300mg
Sodium	Less than	2,400mg	2,400mg
Total Carbohydrate		300g	375g
Dietary Fiber		25g	30g

Calories per gram:
Fat 9 • Carbohydrate 4 • Protein 4

CONTAINS: Fish

at least in part, for some of the health benefits of curried dishes. A member of the ginger family, turmeric has long been associated with its healing properties. Used as a common antiseptic in India, turmeric is used regularly to treat damaged skin, such as cuts or burns. It's even being touted as a possible cure for Alzheimer's disease. Curry can also have coriander, cumin, and red pepper. All these ingredients have their own curative properties.

LAMB AND TURKEY GYROS

GYROS ARE a favorite sandwich of mine. I remember the first time I was ever in Athens, Greece. It was many years ago. I must have walked the whole city looking for a "traditional Athenian gyro" like the ones I had eaten at home. I finally got a sandwich when someone corrected my anglicized pronunciation: it's pronounced "yee-roh," not "hero" or "ji-roh." Replacing some of the ground lamb with leaner turkey makes it a healthier alternative without sacrificing the flavor, as the turkey will take on the essence of the lambs and herbs. If you want to make a souvlaki sandwich instead of the gyro, just top this with some feta cheese.

Nutrition Facts		
Serving Size 4 oz (113g)		
Servings Per Container 12		
Amount Per Serving		
Calories 190	Calories from Fat 120	
		% Daily Value*
Total Fat 13g		**20%**
Saturated Fat 5g		26%
Trans Fat 0g		
Cholesterol 65mg		**21%**
Sodium 790mg		**33%**
Total Carbohydrate 2g		**1%**
Dietary Fiber 0g		0%
Sugars 1g		
Protein 15g		
Vitamin A 0%	•	Vitamin C 2%
Calcium 2%	•	Iron 8%

* Percent Daily Values are based on a 2,000 calorie diet. Your daily values may be higher or lower depending on your calorie needs.

	Calories	2,000	2,500
Total Fat	Less than	65g	80g
Sat Fat	Less than	20g	25g
Cholesterol	Less than	300mg	300mg
Sodium	Less than	2,400mg	2,400mg
Total Carbohydrate		300g	375g
Dietary Fiber		25g	30g

Calories per gram:
Fat 9 • Carbohydrate 4 • Protein 4

½ c. yellow onion, chopped
1 tbsp. garlic, finely minced
1 lb. ground turkey
1 lb. ground lamb
1 tsp. salt
½ tsp. freshly ground black pepper
1 tbsp. marjoram, finely minced
½ tsp. rosemary (leaves only), finely diced
Pita bread
Lettuce, shredded (optional)
Tomato, shredded (optional)
Onion, shredded (optional)
Feta cheese (optional)
Tzatziki sauce (see recipe in chapter 19)

Preheat an oven to 325° F. Place the onion and garlic in a food processer and puree, stopping to scrape down the sides with a spatula as needed. Remove the mixture and place in a sieve over a sink or bowl. Use a spatula or the back of a wooden spoon to push the liquid out of the mixture. Once this is done, empty back into the food processor, and add the ground turkey, ground lamb, salt, pepper, marjoram, and rosemary. Pulse intermittently for 8 to 12 seconds, stopping as needed to scrape the sides. The meat mixture should now resemble a thick paste. Place the mixture in a loaf pan. Set the pan in a water bath, and bake about 1 to 1½ hours. Remove from the oven, remove the loaf from the pan, and allow to rest, loosely covered with foil, for 15 to 20 minutes. Cut the tops off some pita bread to make some pockets. To dress, place some loaf slices into the pita bread. Add desired toppings, such as lettuce, tomatoes, onions, and feta, and a generous serving of tzatziki. Fold and enjoy.

healthy bytes   Dill, as found in the tzatziki sauce, is often used in cooking to flavor fish, salads, dressings, and many other dishes. It has medicinal uses as a digestive aid. It also has antibacterial properties. It is believed to be an active cancer-fighting agent because it can neutralize some carcinogens. Dill is also a good source of calcium, iron, fiber, and magnesium.

FAJITAS

WE USE flank steak, which is the traditional beef cut used for fajitas, here, but you can make this with seafood, like shrimp, or poultry as well. It is delicious served on fresh corn tortillas with guacamole salad and salsa. (See chapter 17 for those recipes.)

Fajita marinade (see recipe in chapter 19)
Approximately 3 lbs. flank steak
1 sweet green pepper
1 sweet red pepper
1 sweet Vidalia onion
1 tsp. salt
½ tsp. freshly ground black pepper
2 tbsp. olive oil

Nutrition Facts		
Serving Size 3 oz (85g)		
Servings Per Container 16		
Amount Per Serving		
Calories 140	Calories from Fat 40	
		% Daily Value*
Total Fat 4.5g		7%
Saturated Fat 1.5g		8%
Trans Fat 0g		
Cholesterol 25mg		9%
Sodium 70mg		3%
Total Carbohydrate 0g		0%
Dietary Fiber 0g		0%
Sugars 0g		
Protein 24g		
Vitamin A 0%	•	Vitamin C 0%
Calcium 2%	•	Iron 10%

* Percent Daily Values are based on a 2,000 calorie diet. Your daily values may be higher or lower depending on your calorie needs.

		Calories	2,000	2,500
Total Fat	Less than		65g	80g
Sat Fat	Less than		20g	25g
Cholesterol	Less than		300mg	300mg
Sodium	Less than		2,400mg	2,400mg
Total Carbohydrate			300g	375g
Dietary Fiber			25g	30g

Calories per gram:
Fat 9 • Carbohydrate 4 • Protein 4

Mix the marinade and add the steak. Allow to marinate at least 8 hours, preferably overnight. Slice the vegetables thinly. Season the meat with salt and pepper, then place the fajita meat on the grill over medium-high heat until cooked to your liking. I like to cook it until it is medium rare. While the meat is cooking, heat the olive oil over medium-high heat in a sauté pan. Sauté the vegetables, seasoning with salt and pepper as needed, and set aside. Allow the meat to rest for 10 minutes once removed from the grill, then thinly slice the meat against the grain, add vegetables, and serve, on tortillas if desired.

healthy bytes Grapefruit contains pectin, a form of soluble fiber that has been shown in animal studies to slow down the progression of atherosclerosis. Grapefruit is also rich in vitamin C and lycopene, which helps to fight free radicals, thereby fighting cellular damage. Grapefruit juice is also thought to help reduce kidney stones by adjusting the urinary pH value and increasing citric acid excretion. This decreases the risk of forming calcium oxalate stones. Check with your health care provider about consuming grapefruit juice if you're taking prescription drugs. Certain drugs combined with grapefruit juice affect their bioavailabilty.

BASIC HUMMUS

THIS IS NOT a mistake. A meal of hummus, or several types of flavored hummus, along with baked pita chips and a vegetable tray can be a filling, satisfying, and scrumptious meal. When the weather is hot and you feel like you need a snack plus a little something extra, this can hit the spot. Once you have the basic recipe down, there is no limit to the variations to suit your taste. Try roasted garlic instead of the regular garlic. Add in roasted red peppers for some natural sweetness or chipotle peppers for spicy smokiness. My favorite is the basic, with two whole heads of roasted garlic, two chopped ancho chilis, and a tablespoon of adobo sauce. I like to put one head of garlic (along with the chilis and adobo) in the food processor and fold one head in with the herbs so you get chunks of sweet, roasted, garlicky goodness.

Nutrition Facts		
Serving Size 4 1/2 oz (128g)		
Servings Per Container 12		
Amount Per Serving		
Calories 350	Calories from Fat 180	
		% Daily Value*
Total Fat 21g		**32%**
Saturated Fat 3g		**14%**
Trans Fat 0g		
Cholesterol 0mg		**0%**
Sodium 25mg		**1%**
Total Carbohydrate 31g		**10%**
Dietary Fiber 4g		**15%**
Sugars 0g		
Protein 12g		
Vitamin A 2%	• Vitamin C 8%	
Calcium 15%	• Iron 20%	
* Percent Daily Values are based on a 2,000 calorie diet. Your daily values may be higher or lower depending on your calorie needs.		

	Calories	2,000	2,500
Total Fat	Less than	65g	80g
Sat Fat	Less than	20g	25g
Cholesterol	Less than	300mg	300mg
Sodium	Less than	2,400mg	2,400mg
Total Carbohydrate		300g	375g
Dietary Fiber		25g	30g

Calories per gram:
Fat 9 • Carbohydrate 4 • Protein 4

> 1 bag (16 oz.) of dried chick peas, reconstituted, or 2 cans (15.5 oz.), drained
> 1 c. chicken stock or vegetable nage (use if reconstituting dried chick peas; see recipes in chapter 19)
> 1½ c. water (use if reconstituting dried chick peas), divided
> 2 garlic cloves, roasted and chopped
> 1 tsp. salt
> 1 c. sesame tahini (about one 12 oz. can)
> 1 lemon, juiced
> ½ c. good-quality olive oil
> ¼ c. fresh flat-leaf parsley, finely chopped
> ¼ c. cilantro, finely chopped

Reconstitute the chick peas with 1 c. of the vegetable nage mixed with 1 c. of water. Add the garlic, salt, tahini, and lemon juice to a food processor, and puree along with the olive oil. Continue pureeing, slowly adding ½ c. of water until the desired consistency is achieved (I like it about a creamy-porridge consistency). Fold in the parsley and cilantro.

healthy bytes Sesame seeds have been used in food preparation as far back as 1600 B.C. They are an incredible source of copper, manganese, and tryptophan. They also contain significant amounts of calcium, magnesium, iron, phosphorus, zinc, fiber, and thiamin. Two unique compounds found in sesame are sesamin and sesamolin. These substances are known as lignans. Lignans have been shown to lower cholesterol and blood pressure, resulting in improved cardiovascular health. They may also act to increase vitamin E bioavailability. Sesamin has been found to protect the liver from oxidative damage. Sesame may be of value in treating rheumatoid arthritis, asthma, colon cancer, migraines, and osteoporosis.

PORCINI MUSHROOM AND ARTICHOKE HEART RAGOUT

THIS IS A deliciously hearty stew, and the earthy porcinis add a beef-like quality. It can be very hard to find fresh porcini mushrooms. Fortunately, they retain their flavor well when dried. By reconstituting in a dark chicken or beef stock, a whole additional flavor profile joins the dish. This is unbelievably satisfying served over some fresh fettuccine pasta.

2 oz. dried porcini mushrooms or other exotic mushrooms
½ c. dark chicken or beef stock (see recipe in chapter 19)
2 shallots, minced
4 tbsp. butter or Smart Balance substitute
2 garlic cloves, finely minced
1 tsp. fresh thyme, finely chopped
1 tsp. salt
½ tsp. freshly ground pepper
¾ c. light chicken stock (see recipe in chapter 19)
16 oz. artichoke hearts
1 tbsp. flat-leaf parsley, finely chopped
2 tbsp. fat-free ricotta cheese
½ oz. parmesan cheese strips

Nutrition Facts

Serving Size 6 oz (170g)
Servings Per Container 6

Amount Per Serving

Calories 130   Calories from Fat 50

	% Daily Value*
Total Fat 6g	10%
Saturated Fat 3.5g	18%
Trans Fat 0g	
Cholesterol 20mg	6%
Sodium 800mg	33%
Total Carbohydrate 16g	5%
Dietary Fiber 3g	13%
Sugars 2g	
Protein 6g	

Vitamin A 4%	•	Vitamin C 15%
Calcium 10%	•	Iron 8%

* Percent Daily Values are based on a 2,000 calorie diet. Your daily values may be higher or lower depending on your calorie needs.

	Calories	2,000	2,500
Total Fat	Less than	65g	80g
Sat Fat	Less than	20g	25g
Cholesterol	Less than	300mg	300mg
Sodium	Less than	2,400mg	2,400mg
Total Carbohydrate		300g	375g
Dietary Fiber		25g	30g

Calories per gram:
Fat 9 • Carbohydrate 4 • Protein 4

CONTAINS: Milk

Reconstitute the dried porcinis with hot dark chicken or beef stock. Once the mushrooms have rehydrated, pick them out, discarding any woody debris. Reserve the liquid by pouring the used stock through a fine sieve to catch any woody detritus. Using a medium-sized saucepan over medium heat, sauté the shallots in the butter or Smart Balance for 3 to 4 minutes. Add the garlic, thyme, salt, pepper, and mushrooms, and cook until any liquid has about evaporated. Add the reserved liquid, light chicken stock, artichoke hearts, parsley, and ricotta. Cook until the liquid is reduced by half. Season with salt and pepper. Make the parmesan strips by using a peeler to peel 2 to 3 strips of parmesan cheese, and place these on top of individual bowls of the ragout.

healthy bytes There are three types of mushrooms with the greatest health benefits: maitake, shiitake, and reishi. Mushrooms are a fungus; they scavenge on organic matter, which means they can absorb and eliminate toxins. The reishi mushroom is believed in Chinese medicine to be "elixir of immortality" due to the special chemical makeup of the mushroom.

VEGETARIAN CHILI

THIS IS A great meal for any season. Make it very vegetarian by using the vegetable nage. The wheat berry gives the chili a great texture. The unsweetened cocoa adds a deep smoky flavor and the corn masa leaves a gentle backdrop of corn flavor and thickens the chili at the same time. Substitute some earthy exotic mushrooms, like black poplar, porcini, portabella, or nameko, for an even heartier flavor. If you want to keep it mostly vegetarian but add in some meaty flavor, substitute beef or chicken stock for the vegetable nage. This dish also serves as a great base for any meat chili; just add whatever type of meat you like.

2 tbsp. olive oil
1 large yellow onion, chopped
1 large green bell pepper, chopped
2 tbsp. garlic, finely minced
1½ lbs. mushrooms, diced into chunks
1 tsp. dried oregano, Mexican if possible
1 tsp. dried basil
1 tsp. dried thyme
2 tbsp. chili powder

Nutrition Facts		
Serving Size 6 oz (170g)		
Servings Per Container 40		
Amount Per Serving		
Calories 470	Calories from Fat 320	
		% Daily Value*
Total Fat 36g		55%
Saturated Fat 5g		25%
Trans Fat 0g		
Cholesterol 0mg		0%
Sodium 270mg		11%
Total Carbohydrate 34g		11%
Dietary Fiber 2g		10%
Sugars 1g		
Protein 6g		
Vitamin A 15%	•	Vitamin C 15%
Calcium 8%	•	Iron 20%

* Percent Daily Values are based on a 2,000 calorie diet. Your daily values may be higher or lower depending on your calorie needs.

	Calories	2,000	2,500
Total Fat	Less than	65g	80g
Sat Fat	Less than	20g	25g
Cholesterol	Less than	300mg	300mg
Sodium	Less than	2,400mg	2,400mg
Total Carbohydrate		300g	375g
Dietary Fiber		25g	30g

Calories per gram:
Fat 9 • Carbohydrate 4 • Protein 4

2 tsp. fresh ground cumin
½ tsp. smoked paprika
½ tsp. dried oregano
½ tsp. dried thyme
½ tsp. onion powder
½ tsp. garlic powder
1 tsp. salt
½ tsp. freshly ground pepper
¼ tsp. cayenne
5 large tomatoes, peeled, seeded, and chopped (or 1 can diced tomatoes, 28 oz.)
1 tbsp. unsweetened cocoa
8 oz. dried black beans, soaked overnight and reconstituted
8 oz. dried kidney beans, soaked overnight and reconstituted
1 c. winter wheat berries, cooked
1 can (15 oz.) tomato sauce
1–2 chipotle peppers in adobo sauce, finely minced
4 c. water
1 c. vegetable nage (see recipe in chapter 19)
3 tbsp. corn flour masa
¼ c. fresh cilantro leaves, chopped
1 avocado, thinly sliced
Fat-free sour cream
Green onions, chopped

In a large heavy pot or Dutch oven, heat the oil over medium-high heat. Add the onion, green pepper, and garlic, cook, stirring occasionally until just translucent, about 3 minutes. Add mushrooms, and cook, stirring occasionally until vegetables start to brown, about another 5 minutes. Add the oregano, basil, thyme, chili powder, cumin, paprika, oregano, thyme, onion powder, garlic powder, salt, pepper, and cayenne, and cook about another 30 seconds. Add the tomatoes and their liquid, unsweetened cocoa, black and kidney beans, winter wheat berries, tomato sauce, chipotle peppers, water, and vegetable nage, combining well. Bring to a boil. Remove some of the broth, and in a separate bowl, mix in the masa flour to form a thin paste. Return to the pot, stirring as you add the paste back. Reduce the heat to medium-low and simmer, stirring occasionally, for about 1 to 2 hours. Check every 30 minutes or so, and if the chili becomes too thick, add additional vegetable nage or water. If you need additional spicy heat as you cook and taste, add some (in ½ tsp. increments) adobo sauce. Remove from the heat, and add the cilantro. Reseason if needed. Garnish in the bowl with thin slices of avocado around the edges, a dollop of sour cream in the middle, and green onions on the sour cream.

Wheat berries are produced by removing the husk of whole wheat grains. The bran, germ, and endosperm are left intact, making them exceptionally nutritious. They are rich in folic acid, protein, B-complex vitamins, and vitamin E. They are also a great source of fiber. In holistic regimens, wheat berries are viewed as a cleansing agent and are believed to have anti-aging capabilities. Diets rich in whole grains like wheat berries have been associated with less obesity, diabetes, and cardiovascular and periodontal disease.

SHABU-SHABU

THIS IS REALLY more of a technique of preparation than any one particular dish. I often have this dish at my friend's home when visiting Japan. On a cold night, eating this delicious, homey potluck-type meal prepared by his wife brings comfort just in its very remembrance. It is divine with nice, chilled sake, which is Japanese rice wine. This dish is traditionally prepared with a dashi, or Japanese fish stock prepared from bonito. I think it works delightfully well prepared with a slightly diluted light chicken stock mixed with some white wine. It is an excellent way to eat lean game meat without overcooking, not to mention an excuse to pull the fondue pot out of the attic.

Nutrition Facts		
Serving Size 8 oz (227g)		
Servings Per Container 4		
Amount Per Serving		
Calories 200	Calories from Fat 80	
		% Daily Value*
Total Fat 9g		14%
Saturated Fat 2g		9%
Trans Fat 0g		
Cholesterol 60mg		20%
Sodium 750mg		31%
Total Carbohydrate 6g		2%
Dietary Fiber 1g		3%
Sugars 2g		
Protein 25g		
Vitamin A 8%	•	Vitamin C 30%
Calcium 6%	•	Iron 20%

* Percent Daily Values are based on a 2,000 calorie diet. Your daily values may be higher or lower depending on your calorie needs.

		Calories	2,000	2,500
Total Fat	Less than		65g	80g
Sat Fat	Less than		20g	25g
Cholesterol	Less than		300mg	300mg
Sodium	Less than		2,400mg	2,400mg
Total Carbohydrate			300g	375g
Dietary Fiber			25g	30g

Calories per gram:
Fat 9 • Carbohydrate 4 • Protein 4

CONTAINS: Soy

1 c. white wine

2½ c. light chicken stock, divided (see recipe in chapter 19)

1¼ c. water, divided

¼ lb. Chinese or napa cabbage, shredded

8 ribs bok choy, white parts only, cut thin lengthwise

1 leek, white part only, thinly sliced

4 oz. mushrooms, preferably shiitake

4 portions (4 oz. each) bison steak or other lean game meat, cut extremely thin

¼ sake

2 tsp. sesame oil

3 tbsp. soy sauce

1 tsp. rice wine vinegar

Prepare a fondue pot for use or use a pot that can be heated (like a crockpot) and add the wine, allowing it to gently heat until it is warmed. In a saucepan on the stove, bring 2 c. stock plus 1 c. water to a boil. Remove from the heat, and add to the heated wine. Add the cabbage, bok choy, leek, and mushrooms to the pot. Meanwhile, for the dipping sauce, mix together ½ c. stock, ¼ c. water, sake, sesame oil, soy sauce, and rice wine vinegar. Place each serving of the meat, along with the dipping sauce, in front of each diner. Allow each diner to dip the meat into the heated vegetables and stock for 10 to 15 seconds to cook. Remove the meat (and some veggies), dip in the sauce, and repeat.

healthy bytes Bok choy is a member of the cabbage family and is sometimes referred to as Chinese white cabbage. It is a rich source of vitamins A, C, and K; beta-carotene; calcium; and fiber. It also contains potassium and vitamin B_6 and is believed to help aid digestion.

HERB-CRUSTED PORK CHOPS

PORK IS LEAN. This is something most people don't appreciate, and therefore it tends to be overcooked and arrive tough and dried out. It should be served when just slightly pink on the inside with clear running juices. If you're unsure, just use your meat thermometer. Remember to remove from the heat a few degrees shy of done to allow for carryover. I recommend serving this with the pan-simmered apples and napa cabbage from chapter 17.

Nutrition Facts		
Serving Size 5 oz (142g)		
Servings Per Container 4		
Amount Per Serving		
Calories 280	Calories from Fat 140	
		% Daily Value*
Total Fat 16g		24%
Saturated Fat 6g		29%
Trans Fat 0g		
Cholesterol 75mg		25%
Sodium 890mg		37%
Total Carbohydrate 6g		2%
Dietary Fiber 1g		3%
Sugars 0g		
Protein 29g		
Vitamin A 8%	•	Vitamin C 4%
Calcium 4%	•	Iron 8%

* Percent Daily Values are based on a 2,000 calorie diet. Your daily values may be higher or lower depending on your calorie needs.

	Calories	2,000	2,500
Total Fat	Less than	65g	80g
Sat Fat	Less than	20g	25g
Cholesterol	Less than	300mg	300mg
Sodium	Less than	2,400mg	2,400mg
Total Carbohydrate		300g	375g
Dietary Fiber		25g	30g

Calories per gram:
Fat 9 • Carbohydrate 4 • Protein 4

1 tsp. salt
½ tsp. freshly ground black pepper
4 boneless pork chops, 4–6 oz. each (about ½ in. in thickness)
2 tbsp. fresh basil, chopped
1 tbsp. fresh sage, finely chopped
1 tbsp. fresh flat-leaf parsley, finely chopped
2 tsp. fresh thyme, finely chopped
2 tsp. fresh marjoram, finely chopped
1 tsp. balsamic vinegar
1 tbsp. crushed corn flakes
1 tbsp. masa corn flour
2 tbsp. fresh breadcrumbs
2 tbsp. olive oil
1 tsp. salt
½ tsp. freshly ground black pepper
2 oz. butter or Smart Balance substitute

Preheat oven to 375° F. Salt and pepper both sides of the chops. Place the basil, sage, parsley, thyme, marjoram, vinegar, corn flakes, masa corn flour, and breadcrumbs into a bowl. Add enough olive oil to make a thick paste. Heat some olive oil in a pan over high heat until smoking. Season with salt and pepper, then sear the chops for about 10 to 15 seconds each side, just long enough to get a brown crust. Remove from heat. Get an oven proof baking dish just large enough to hold the chops side by side. Layer about ⅓ of the herb paste on the bottom. Place the chops into the baking dish and pack the remaining herb mixture on top. Divide the butter or Smart Balance on top of the chops. Finish in the oven for about 20 minutes.

healthy bytes Marjoram is one of the few herbs to have a city named after it. Marjoram, located in Sicily, is among the Mediterranean areas in which marjoram is a native inhabitant. Marjoram's flavor, unlike some other herbs, can intensify when dried. It yields a powerful oil, widely used in aromatherapy. It is used in the treatment of sore muscles, asthma, and headaches and as a digestive aid. It has also been used in the treatment of bronchitis, sinusitis, and sinus headaches. In holistic circles, it is considered a calming herb. Some of the flavonoids in marjoram have a tranquilizing effect and may also promote cardiovascular health and prevent the development of Alzheimer's disease. Marjoram is also considered a detoxifying herb in holistic regimens because it stimulates perspiration. This promotes detoxification through sweating.

PORK BARBECUE

YOU SIMPLY cannot be from the South and not have some barbecue recipe. Moderation is the key with meals like this, so enjoy the succulent, melt-in-your-mouth pork in long, drawn-out bites. The pork butt is actually from the shoulder and is my favorite barbecue cut.

> 1 pork butt, 6–8 lbs.
> Wild game brine (see recipe in chapter 19)
> Doc's barbecue spice rub (see recipe in chapter 19)
> Hickory or other wood for smoking

Place the pork butt in the wild game brine for 6 to 24 hours. Remove and pat dry. Apply the rub generously to the pork butt. The butt often has a cap of fat on top. If so, use a boning knife or other thin blade to cut the cap back about ¾ of the way so that there is a flap you can lift and see the surface of the meat. Place the rub directly on the meat, put the cap in place, and continue to cover all exposed surfaces. Set the

Nutrition Facts

Serving Size 4 oz (113g)
Servings Per Container 30

Amount Per Serving	
Calories 290	Calories from Fat 160

	% Daily Value*
Total Fat 18g	28%
Saturated Fat 7g	34%
Trans Fat 0g	
Cholesterol 105mg	35%
Sodium 360mg	15%
Total Carbohydrate 1g	0%
Dietary Fiber 0g	0%
Sugars 0g	
Protein 28g	

Vitamin A 6%		•	Vitamin C 0%
Calcium 4%		•	Iron 10%

* Percent Daily Values are based on a 2,000 calorie diet. Your daily values may be higher or lower depending on your calorie needs.

	Calories	2,000	2,500
Total Fat	Less than	65g	80g
Sat Fat	Less than	20g	25g
Cholesterol	Less than	300mg	300mg
Sodium	Less than	2,400mg	2,400mg
Total Carbohydrate		300g	375g
Dietary Fiber		25g	30g

Calories per gram:

Fat 9 • Carbohydrate 4 • Protein 4

smoker to about 210 to 215° F, using hickory wood (or any other flavor you prefer). Smoke for 8 to 12 hours at this temperature. Check frequently so you make sure you have continuous smoke. If you have a regular charcoal grill, use as a smoker by placing the coals on half of the coal area. When the coals are hot, add the wood. Place the butt over to the side with no direct heat. Use a thermometer to gauge and maintain appropriate heating if your grill doesn't have one. The meat is ready when it easily pulls away from the bone. When done, remove from smoker, loosely cover with foil, and allow it to rest for an hour or two.

healthy bytes Paprika is derived from paprika chili peppers. It contains capsicum, as all members of that family do. Paprika has antimicrobial properties and can act to reduce hypertension and improve circulation. It increases saliva production and aids in digestion. It is also rich in vitamin C, containing six to nine times as much as a similar weight of tomatoes. When peppers are processed commercially under high heat, much of the vitamin value can be lost; sun-dried peppers retain much more of the vitamin benefit.

GRILLED STEAK ITALIANO

BEEF, AND STEAK in particular, sometimes gets a bad rap. But a reasonable serving of good, lean beef should be part of a delicious and nutritious diet. One of the keys is to source your meat. I know my butcher, so I can get him to trim it for me. I also get organic, grass-fed, free-range beef. I make sure I get it from a reliable source. Great beef doesn't need a lot to make it a great meal. Grill it properly until rare to medium rare, allow it to rest, and serve with a side of your choice. And don't forget a glass of a big, bold red wine. The enjoyment is total self-satisfying mastication.

Approximately 1½ lbs. of steak, like rib eye, strip, T-bone,
    or porterhouse
Herbed olive oil (see recipe in chapter 19)
Salt
Freshly ground pepper

Nutrition Facts		
Serving Size 6 oz (170g)		
Servings Per Container 4		
Amount Per Serving		
Calories 340	Calories from Fat 130	
		% Daily Value*
Total Fat 14g		22%
Saturated Fat 4.5g		23%
Trans Fat 0g		
Cholesterol 130mg		43%
Sodium 640mg		27%
Total Carbohydrate 0g		0%
Dietary Fiber 0g		0%
Sugars 0g		
Protein 48g		
Vitamin A 0%	•	Vitamin C 0%
Calcium 2%	•	Iron 25%

* Percent Daily Values are based on a 2,000 calorie diet. Your daily values may be higher or lower depending on your calorie needs.

		Calories	2,000	2,500
Total Fat	Less than		65g	80g
Sat Fat	Less than		20g	25g
Cholesterol	Less than		300mg	300mg
Sodium	Less than		2,400mg	2,400mg
Total Carbohydrate			300g	375g
Dietary Fiber			25g	30g

Calories per gram:
Fat 9 • Carbohydrate 4 • Protein 4

Allow steak to sit at room temperature. Coat both sides with herbed olive oil, salt, and pepper. Grill to desired doneness. Allow to rest 5 minutes, then slice, serve, and smile.

Sage has been valued by many different cultures for more than two thousand years. In ayurvedic medicine it is considered a purifying herb. Sage contains thujone, which is an effective agent against salmonella and candida. In holistic use sage is considered a warming and strengthening herb and clears congestion, coughs, sore throats, and laryngitis. It is also considered a grounding herb and is used frequently for hot flashes in menopausal women.

GRILLED PORK LOIN MARGARITA

PORK LOIN is tender, and, contrary to what a lot of people think, generally extremely lean. You can buy center-cut pork loins ready to use or larger entire pork loins, which is what I like to do. Trim the ends and cut the center piece out (the size you want) for this preparation. Remember to watch the loin carefully on the grill; because it is lean, it can easily overcook. An instant-read thermometer is a good investment here.

1 pork loin, trimmed (approximately 3 lbs.)
Margarita marinade (see recipe in chapter 19)
Salt
Freshly ground pepper

Nutrition Facts		
Serving Size 4 1/2 oz (128g)		
Servings Per Container 12		
Amount Per Serving		
Calories 150	Calories from Fat 40	
		% Daily Value*
Total Fat 4.5g		**7%**
Saturated Fat 1.5g		**7%**
Trans Fat 0g		
Cholesterol 70mg		**23%**
Sodium 290mg		**12%**
Total Carbohydrate 1g		**0%**
Dietary Fiber 0g		**0%**
Sugars 0g		
Protein 26g		
Vitamin A 2%	•	Vitamin C 2%
Calcium 0%	•	Iron 6%

* Percent Daily Values are based on a 2,000 calorie diet. Your daily values may be higher or lower depending on your calorie needs.

	Calories	2,000	2,500
Total Fat	Less than	65g	80g
Sat Fat	Less than	20g	25g
Cholesterol	Less than	300mg	300mg
Sodium	Less than	2,400mg	2,400mg
Total Carbohydrate		300g	375g
Dietary Fiber		25g	30g

Calories per gram:
Fat 9 • Carbohydrate 4 • Protein 4

Place the pork loin and marinade in a resealable plastic bag, reserving some marinade for later. Place the bag in the refrigerator and marinate for about 4 hours. Place on the grill over medium-high heat. Turn several times over the next 15 to 25 minutes (depending on thickness). The loin is done when the meat thermometer reads about 140° F. Remove and let rest loosely covered with aluminum foil for about 5 minutes. Then pour in reserved marinade and let rest an additional 5 minutes. Slice, season with salt and freshly ground pepper, and serve.

Mint has long been enjoyed for its aroma and taste. It has also been long used for its health benefits, including soothing an upset stomach and aiding digestion. It has shown promise in helping to relieve the symptoms associated with irritable bowel syndrome. It has documented antifungal properties and has been used in the treatment of allergies and asthma. A specific component of mint, perillyl alcohol, has been shown to have activity in fighting cancers, such as lung, colon, and skin.

GROUND TURKEY SLOPPY JOSÉ

I LIKE TO use ground turkey, but you could also use lean, free-range, grass-fed beef or even ground bison. Because you add the sauce as soon as the meat is cooked, the turkey doesn't dry out. You can also grind you own meat, which is a very economical use of parts if you purchase the whole bird.

Olive oil
1 lb. ground turkey
1 medium onion, chopped
2 tsp. shallot, minced
1 tsp. garlic, minced
¼ tsp. dried oregano
¼ tsp. dried thyme
¼ tsp. onion powder
¼ tsp. garlic powder
¼ tsp. cayenne
¼ tsp. Chinese five-spice powder
¼ tsp. ancho chili pepper
½ tsp. salt
½ tsp. freshly ground pepper
½ c. green pepper, chopped
1 c. enchilada sauce (see recipe in chapter 19)

Nutrition Facts		
Serving Size 4 1/4 oz (120g)		
Servings Per Container 8		
Amount Per Serving		
Calories 120	Calories from Fat 50	
		% Daily Value*
Total Fat 6g		9%
Saturated Fat 1.5g		7%
Trans Fat 0g		
Cholesterol 45mg		15%
Sodium 260mg		11%
Total Carbohydrate 5g		2%
Dietary Fiber 1g		5%
Sugars 2g		
Protein 11g		
Vitamin A 10%	•	Vitamin C 20%
Calcium 2%	•	Iron 8%

* Percent Daily Values are based on a 2,000 calorie diet. Your daily values may be higher or lower depending on your calorie needs.

	Calories	2,000	2,500
Total Fat	Less than	65g	80g
Sat Fat	Less than	20g	25g
Cholesterol	Less than	300mg	300mg
Sodium	Less than	2,400mg	2,400mg
Total Carbohydrate		300g	375g
Dietary Fiber		25g	30g

Calories per gram:
Fat 9 • Carbohydrate 4 • Protein 4

Heat some olive oil in a medium saucepan. Brown the turkey, remove from the pan, drain any oil, and set aside. Add onions, shallots, and garlic to the pan. Cook over medium heat until translucent, about 3 to 5 minutes. Add the oregano, thyme, onion powder, garlic powder, cayenne, Chinese five-spice powder, ancho chili pepper, salt, and pepper, and cook another 30 seconds. Add green pepper, and cook 1 minute. Add sauce and the browned ground turkey, and simmer for 10 to 15 minutes. You can serve this with bread, on a roll, or in a bowl.

healthy bytes Star anise is found in Chinese five-spice powder. Star anise is actually the fruit of an evergreen plant, *Tillicum verum*. It contains anethole, which gives it a licorice flavor, and it is often used as a mouth freshener in the Orient. It can be applied externally for the treatment of many skin diseases. The fruit is helpful in digestion, colic, and eliminating discomfort due to intestinal gas. Star anise is also used in the prevention of headaches. It is a component in the process used to extract shikimic acid, which is used for making the antiviral medicine Tamiflu and for the prevention of avian influenza. In addition, it also has diuretic medicine properties.

BLACKENED REDFISH TACOS

TACOS ARE an easy fix and are delectable when served with some salsa and guacamole salad (see the recipes in chapter 17). If you cannot find redfish, any light, white-fleshed fish, like tilapia, will work. Make sure the pan is hot, and let the fish blacken, otherwise the fish may stick to the pan if you try to turn it too early.

2 redfish fillets, 6–8 oz. each
1 c. buttermilk
2 tbsp. Doc's blackening blend (see recipe in chapter 19)
½ tsp. cayenne pepper
Oil
½ c. lettuce, shredded
Corn tortillas (see recipe in chapter 17)
½ c. tomatoes, diced
Salsa (see recipe in chapter 17)
Guacamole salad (see recipe in chapter 17)

Nutrition Facts

Serving Size 6 oz (170g)
Servings Per Container 6

Amount Per Serving	
Calories 240	Calories from Fat 120

	% Daily Value*
Total Fat 14g	**21%**
Saturated Fat 3.5g	18%
Trans Fat 0g	
Cholesterol 55mg	**19%**
Sodium 85mg	**4%**
Total Carbohydrate 4g	**1%**
Dietary Fiber 0g	0%
Sugars 1g	
Protein 25g	

Vitamin A 10%	•	Vitamin C 15%
Calcium 4%	•	Iron 8%

* Percent Daily Values are based on a 2,000 calorie diet. Your daily values may be higher or lower depending on your calorie needs.

	Calories	2,000	2,500
Total Fat	Less than	65g	80g
Sat Fat	Less than	20g	25g
Cholesterol	Less than	300mg	300mg
Sodium	Less than	2,400mg	2,400mg
Total Carbohydrate		300g	375g
Dietary Fiber		25g	30g

Calories per gram:
Fat 9 • Carbohydrate 4 • Protein 4

CONTAINS: Fish

Soak the redfish fillets in the buttermilk for 30 minutes to 1 hour. Remove the fillets and pat dry. Season both sides with Doc's blackening blend and cayenne. Heat a cast-iron skillet with a little oil until smoking. Place the fillets on the skillet, cooking 2 to 4 minutes per side, depending on the thickness of the fillets. Remove the fillets, and place a ½ fillet on lettuce in a tortilla and dress with tomatoes, salsa, and guacamole salad.

healthy bytes Seafood is one of the healthiest foods around. Fish in general provide a large range of health benefits. White-fleshed fish are lower in fat than any other source of animal protein. They contain many beneficial vitamins and minerals and are a great source of iodine, iron, and choline. Fish is a food that is high in protein and low in calories. Most fish are naturally low in inflammatory omega-6 fats. Such fish as wild salmon are high in beneficial omega-3 fatty acids. More nutrients are retained in fish that is baked or broiled rather than processed and fried. It is not just brain food or heart food but also recommended for overall good health as well.

HERB-CRUSTED GROUPER

FRESH FISH is simply amazing, and I believe it is a lot more versatile than most people realize. A lot of people who don't like fish have had a bad experience, the likeliest of which is dried-out fish. It is very important not to overcook it, which results in tough meat with poor flavor. Properly cooked fish is tender, juicy, and just flakes away from the fillet when done. The herb crust acts to help the fillets retain moisture, so this recipe is a little more forgiving.

½ tsp. salt
½ tsp. freshly cracked black pepper
1 large grouper fillet, approximately 2 lbs.
2 tbsp. fresh basil, chopped
1 tbsp. cilantro, finely chopped
1 tbsp. flat-leaf parsley, finely chopped
2 tsp. thyme, finely chopped
1 tsp. dill, finely chopped
1 tbsp. crushed corn flakes
1 tbsp. masa corn flour
2 tbsp. fresh breadcrumbs
1 lemon, juiced
Approximately ¼ c. + 2 tbsp. olive oil, divided
2 oz. butter or Smart Balance substitute
5 oz. grape tomatoes

Nutrition Facts		
Serving Size 6 oz (170g)		
Servings Per Container 6		
Amount Per Serving		
Calories 240 Calories from Fat 120		
		% Daily Value*
Total Fat 14g		21%
Saturated Fat 3.5g		18%
Trans Fat 0g		
Cholesterol 55mg		19%
Sodium 85mg		4%
Total Carbohydrate 4g		1%
Dietary Fiber 0g		0%
Sugars 1g		
Protein 25g		
Vitamin A 10%	•	Vitamin C 15%
Calcium 4%	•	Iron 8%

* Percent Daily Values are based on a 2,000 calorie diet. Your daily values may be higher or lower depending on your calorie needs.

	Calories	2,000	2,500
Total Fat	Less than	65g	80g
Sat Fat	Less than	20g	25g
Cholesterol	Less than	300mg	300mg
Sodium	Less than	2,400mg	2,400mg
Total Carbohydrate		300g	375g
Dietary Fiber		25g	30g

Calories per gram:
Fat 9 • Carbohydrate 4 • Protein 4

CONTAINS: Fish

Preheat oven to 375° F. Salt and pepper the fillet. Place the basil, cilantro, parsley, thyme, dill, corn flakes, masa corn flour, and breadcrumbs in a bowl. Add the lemon juice and enough olive oil (approximately ¼ c.) to make a thick paste. Get an oven proof baking dish just large enough to hold the fillet. Place the fillet in the baking dish, skin side down, and pack the herb mixture on top. Put dabs of the butter or Smart Balance on top. Place the tomatoes around the sides, drizzle with remaining olive oil, and season with salt and pepper. Bake in the oven for about 20 minutes. Remove the fish by sliding the fish spatula between the fillet and the skin (I don't like serving fish with skin unless the skin is crispy). Slice the tomatoes, and place on top. This is great with noodles or lightly tossed pasta on the side.

Parsley is one of the most popular herbs in the world. It was known to the ancient Greeks as "rock celery" and is indeed a relative of celery. It is an extremely good source of vitamins K, C, and A and also contains folate and iron. Parsley contains myristicin, which has been shown to have antitumor activity. It is believed that this compound activates the enzyme glutathione S-transferase, which helps protect against oxidative damage. Other compounds, such as the flavonoid luteolin, have also shown antioxidant activity. Chewed after eating garlic, it can help remove any offensive odors, and its high levels of vitamin C may be protective against rheumatoid arthritis.

GRILLED SHELLFISH SALAD

HERE'S AN incredible summer recipe. If you are cooking at the beach, you can make the marinade ahead of time, get some fresh shellfish and veggies, and grill it on the beach. Enjoy this meal while watching the sun set over the ocean just refills the soul. And don't forget to refill your glass with a crisp white wine, like a viognier or chenin blanc, and you'll know what they're serving in heaven tonight!

4 large prawns (heads on if possible) or 8 large shrimp
4 large diver scallops or 8 large regular scallops
Shellfish marinade (see recipe in chapter 19)
1 Vidalia or other sweet onion, sliced
1 zucchini, sliced
1 red pepper
1 carrot, cut thinly
4 oz. fresh sugar snap peas
1 cucumber, peeled, seeded, and sliced
8 oz. of mixed greens
1 large tomato, sliced
1/3 c. Greek yogurt
1 lemon, juiced
1 lime, juiced
2 avocados (Haas)
4 anchovy fillets
4 tsp. cilantro, finely chopped
1/2 c. good-quality olive oil
2 tbsp. roasted garlic puree (see recipe in chapter 19)
1 tbsp. fresh basil, finely chopped
1 tbsp. hot sauce

Nutrition Facts

Serving Size 12 oz (340g)
Servings Per Container 8

Amount Per Serving

Calories 290   Calories from Fat 170

	% Daily Value*
Total Fat 19g	30%
Saturated Fat 2g	10%
Trans Fat 0g	
Cholesterol 35mg	11%
Sodium 250mg	11%
Total Carbohydrate 13g	4%
Dietary Fiber 7g	30%
Sugars 7g	
Protein 17g	

Vitamin A 60%	•	Vitamin C 70%	
Calcium 6%	•	Iron 10%	

* Percent Daily Values are based on a 2,000 calorie diet. Your daily values may be higher or lower depending on your calorie needs.

	Calories	2,000	2,500
Total Fat	Less than	65g	80g
Sat Fat	Less than	20g	25g
Cholesterol	Less than	300mg	300mg
Sodium	Less than	2,400mg	2,400mg
Total Carbohydrate		300g	375g
Dietary Fiber		25g	30g

Calories per gram:
Fat 9   •   Carbohydrate 4   •   Protein 4

CONTAINS: Fish, Shellfish

Place the prawns, diver scallops, and marinade in a resealable plastic bag, and refrigerate for 4 to 8 hours. Combine the yogurt, lemon juice, lime juice, avocados, anchovies, cilantro, olive oil, roasted garlic puree, basil, and hot sauce in a food processor and blend until smooth. Remove and refrigerate. When ready to grill, remove the prawns and scallops from the marinade. Start the vegetables (onion, zucchini, and red pepper) slightly ahead of the shellfish, as they will cook quickly. When grilling the pepper, allow the skin to burn and blister. Then remove the burned skin, and slice before serving. After the vegetables are done grilling, combine them with the carrot, peas, cucumber, mixed greens, and tomato in a large bowl, and toss with the dressing. Portion the plates, and divide the shellfish on top. A slice of grilled bread is an outstanding accompaniment.

healthy bytes Scallops are a rich source of tryptophan, vitamin B_{12}, phosphorus, magnesium, and potassium. They are an excellent source of low-fat protein. Like other seafood, they contain beneficial omega-3 polyunsaturated fatty acids, which promote cardiovascular health. Diets rich in foods like scallops can help prevent lethal and nonlethal heart dysrhythmias, reduce the risk of heart attack and stroke, and reduce hypertension.

CRABBY PATTIES

I LOVE CRAB cakes any time of year, but what I hate are crab cakes that are all bread and no crab. So these cakes have a minimum amount of binder like breadcrumbs. You will especially like biting into one and getting a mouthful of luscious, sweet lump crabmeat. It is important to fold the ingredients into the mix instead of vigorously mixing so you don't tear up the lumps of crabmeat. If you're doing that, you might as well buy the less-expensive backfin. I don't ever recommend claw for cakes. The combination of the seasoned cornflakes and panko make for an amazing, crunchy, golden-brown complement to this sweet patty party.

2 tbsp. olive oil
1 c. sweet onion, finely diced
½ c. water chestnuts, chopped
½ c. green pepper, diced
1 tbsp. garlic, finely chopped
Salt
Pepper
2 tbsp. green onion (green part only), chopped

Nutrition Facts

Serving Size 4 oz (113g)
Servings Per Container 12

Amount Per Serving

Calories 140   Calories from Fat 40

	% Daily Value*
Total Fat 4.5g	7%
Saturated Fat 1g	5%
Trans Fat 0g	
Cholesterol 70mg	24%
Sodium 300mg	12%
Total Carbohydrate 13g	4%
Dietary Fiber 1g	4%
Sugars 3g	
Protein 13g	

Vitamin A 2%	Vitamin C 15%
Calcium 8%	Iron 6%

* Percent Daily Values are based on a 2,000 calorie diet. Your daily values may be higher or lower depending on your calorie needs.

		Calories	2,000	2,500
Total Fat	Less than		65g	80g
Sat Fat	Less than		20g	25g
Cholesterol	Less than		300mg	300mg
Sodium	Less than		2,400mg	2,400mg
Total Carbohydrate			300g	375g
Dietary Fiber			25g	30g

Calories per gram:
Fat 9 • Carbohydrate 4 • Protein 4

CONTAINS: Milk, Shellfish

¼ c. parmesan cheese, finely grated
2 tbsp. fresh cilantro, finely chopped
1 tsp. dry mustard powder
2 tbsp. Dijon mustard
1 lemon, juiced
2 limes, juiced
½ c. Greek yogurt
1 egg
¾ c. seasoned breadcrumbs
¼ tsp. white pepper
Dash hot sauce
1 tsp. Worcestershire sauce
1 lb. fresh lump crabmeat (make sure you look for shells and bits)
¼ c. all-purpose flour combined with 1 tbsp. Emeril Creole spice
1 egg beaten with 1 tbsp. water
¼ c. panko + ¼ c. crushed cornflakes combined with 1 tbsp. Emeril Creole spice
Vegetable oil for frying
Crabby patty dressing (see recipe in chapter 19)

Over medium heat in a medium saucepan, heat the olive oil. Add the sweet onion, water chestnuts, green pepper, and garlic. Season with salt and pepper, and cook for about 5 minutes, or until the vegetables have sweated. Allow to cool to room temperature. Mix in the green onion, parmesan cheese, cilantro, mustard powder, Dijon mustard, lemon juice, lime juice, yogurt, egg, breadcrumbs, white pepper, hot sauce, and Worcestershire sauce. Fold in the crabmeat. Using a scale to weigh or a 4 oz. scoop, scoop out the patties into balls and lay out on wax paper. In a separate series of bowls, place a bowl of the seasoned flour followed by the egg and water followed by the seasoned panko and cornflakes. Flatten each ball into a patty shape, and dip into the flour, shaking off any excess. Then place into the egg, allowing excess to drip off. Finally place into the seasoned panko mixture to coat. Cook the patties in some vegetable oil in a medium pan over medium-high heat until golden brown and delicious on both sides. Serve the patties with a little dab of crabby patty dressing on top.

healthy bytes Crab is a great source of low-fat protein. Like other types of seafood, they are rich in omega-3s. It is a good source of vitamins A and C, thiamin, riboflavin, niacin, and pantothenic acid. Crab is also a great source of sodium, potassium, phosphorus, calcium, magnesium, iron, zinc, manganese, and selenium.

AVOCADO AND TOMATO SOUP

AVOCADOS CAN be a little tricky to work with. To keep them from turning brown after you remove them from the pit and skin, hit them with some mild acid, like lemon or lime juice. This keeps them green. By adding the avocado after the soup is cooked, we avoid trying to actually cook the avocado, and it retains its creaminess and fresh flavor.

<table>
<tr><td colspan="3">Nutrition Facts</td></tr>
<tr><td colspan="3">Serving Size 10 oz (283g)
Servings Per Container 12</td></tr>
<tr><td colspan="3">Amount Per Serving</td></tr>
<tr><td colspan="2">Calories 160</td><td>Calories from Fat 60</td></tr>
<tr><td colspan="3" align="right">% Daily Value*</td></tr>
<tr><td colspan="2">Total Fat 6g</td><td>10%</td></tr>
<tr><td colspan="2">Saturated Fat 0g</td><td>0%</td></tr>
<tr><td colspan="2">Trans Fat 0g</td><td></td></tr>
<tr><td colspan="2">Cholesterol 0mg</td><td>0%</td></tr>
<tr><td colspan="2">Sodium 180mg</td><td>7%</td></tr>
<tr><td colspan="2">Total Carbohydrate 25g</td><td>8%</td></tr>
<tr><td colspan="2">Dietary Fiber 8g</td><td>33%</td></tr>
<tr><td colspan="2">Sugars 12g</td><td></td></tr>
<tr><td colspan="3">Protein 7g</td></tr>
<tr><td>Vitamin A 60%</td><td colspan="2">• Vitamin C 50%</td></tr>
<tr><td>Calcium 8%</td><td colspan="2">• Iron 20%</td></tr>
</table>

* Percent Daily Values are based on a 2,000 calorie diet. Your daily values may be higher or lower depending on your calorie needs.

	Calories	2,000	2,500
Total Fat	Less than	65g	80g
Sat Fat	Less than	20g	25g
Cholesterol	Less than	300mg	300mg
Sodium	Less than	2,400mg	2,400mg
Total Carbohydrate		300g	375g
Dietary Fiber		25g	30g

Calories per gram:
Fat 9 • Carbohydrate 4 • Protein 4

Salt
Pepper
2 tbsp. olive oil
1 c. onion, chopped
½ c. celery, chopped
½ c. carrot, chopped
1 tbsp. garlic, chopped
1 tbsp. dried oregano
1 tbsp. dried thyme
6 oz. tomato paste
1 can (28 oz.) chopped tomatoes
2 c. vegetable nage (or chicken stock for a nonvegetarian version; see recipes in chapter 19)
1 c. water
1 c. white wine
1 tbsp. white wine vinegar
¼ c. fresh basil, chopped
1 bay leaf
2 avocados
Baguette cut into small rounds
Mozzarella cheese
Truffle oil for drizzle
Chives
Grape tomatoes

Throughout this recipe, do not forget to season with salt and pepper at each cooking stage. In a large, heavy-bottomed pot, heat the olive oil over medium heat, and add the onions, celery, and carrot. Sweat for about 2 to 3 minutes. Add the garlic, oregano, and thyme, and cook another minute. Add the tomato paste, and cook until the paste starts to turn a dark brick color (be careful not to burn). Add the chopped tomatoes, vegetable nage, water, wine, vinegar, basil, and bay leaf. Simmer for about an hour, or until the soup has reduced by about a third. Remove the bay leaf. Add the avocados, and with an immersion blender (or in small batches in a blender), blend the soup. Serve with the toasted baguette rounds topped with melted mozzarella and a drizzle of truffle oil. Split the grape tomatoes in half lengthwise, and with a paring knife, make a small *X* on the skin side. Place the chive into the *X* so it stands up, and place in soup. Serve hot.

healthy bytes Truffles are a type of tube mushroom known as ascomyzetes. Unique in flavor, truffles in cooking can be traced back to the Pharaoh Cheops, as these were among his most sought-after delicacies. Today they remain among the most expensive foodstuffs. If you enjoy their unique taste—they are not for everyone—an affordable way to experience it is through oil infused with truffle, or truffle oil. Although, like all mushrooms, they are almost entirely (approximately 73 percent) water, they do have a high content of proteins and minerals like potassium, calcium, and magnesium.

CHEDDAR CHEESE GRIT CAKES

I LOVE GRITS, the "Southern polenta." I prefer stone-ground, old-fashioned grits. The stone-ground contain the nutritious germ, and I find them much more flavorful and with a more pleasing texture than the bulk package usually found in the supermarket. I mail order mine, or I find locally produced grits that have outstanding taste and quality.

¼ tsp. salt
4 c. milk
1 c. stone-ground grits
8 oz. cheddar cheese, chopped

Nutrition Facts		
Serving Size 4 oz (113g)		
Servings Per Container 12		
Amount Per Serving		
Calories 170	Calories from Fat 80	
		% Daily Value*
Total Fat 9g		14%
Saturated Fat 6g		28%
Trans Fat 0g		
Cholesterol 30mg		9%
Sodium 200mg		8%
Total Carbohydrate 12g		4%
Dietary Fiber 0g		0%
Sugars 4g		
Protein 9g		
Vitamin A 10%	•	Vitamin C 0%
Calcium 25%	•	Iron 2%

* Percent Daily Values are based on a 2,000 calorie diet. Your daily values may be higher or lower depending on your calorie needs.

	Calories	2,000	2,500
Total Fat	Less than	65g	80g
Sat Fat	Less than	20g	25g
Cholesterol	Less than	300mg	300mg
Sodium	Less than	2,400mg	2,400mg
Total Carbohydrate		300g	375g
Dietary Fiber		25g	30g

Calories per gram:
Fat 9 • Carbohydrate 4 • Protein 4

CONTAINS: Milk

Add the salt to the milk in a medium saucepan over medium heat. Bring the milk to just under a boil, and add the grits. Reduce to a simmer. Stir constantly so the grits do not stick to the bottom of the pan and burn. Allow the mixture to thicken, about 20 to 30 minutes. Add the cheese and melt. Spread the grits over a half sheet pan covered with parchment paper. Allow to cool. Using a ring mold, press out circles. You can serve chilled or heated by serving as is or by placing on a hot griddle at 350° F, and allow a golden crust to form. Serve by heating one side only and flipping the noncrust side down on the serving platter.

Stone-ground grits are ground between stones that crush and grind the whole grain. This is done slowly and is accomplished without oxidizing the meal or destroying the nutrients with heat. In the more commercial, modern roller-milling method, there is heat, and parts are separated. In stone grinding nothing is separated or added to the natural grain. This process leaves the beneficial parts, like the germ, oil, and bran, intact. Whether it is meal, grits, or polenta is determined by setting the width of the stones and also the size of the screen the meal is sifted over after grinding.

OSSO BUCO

THIS IS A great-tasting dish but really depends on good technique to elevate it. The key is proper braising. The veal shank is a very tough but flavorful cut. It needs to be browned so it can develop that delicious brown coating, courtesy of the Maillard reaction. The Maillard reaction is a reaction between an amino acid and a reducing sugar. With some applied heat, this nonenzymatically browns the meat. This process results in that great crust and flavor. The meat then tenderizes in the liquid with a long, slow heat that breaks down the collagen, gelatin, and other components into a naturally thickened, delicious sauce and melt-in-your-mouth veal.

Nutrition Facts		
Serving Size 16 oz (454g)		
Servings Per Container 6		
Amount Per Serving		
Calories 250	Calories from Fat 90	
		% Daily Value*
Total Fat 10g		15%
Saturated Fat 2.5g		13%
Trans Fat 0g		
Cholesterol 80mg		26%
Sodium 360mg		15%
Total Carbohydrate 18g		6%
Dietary Fiber 2g		9%
Sugars 2g		
Protein 22g		
Vitamin A 90%	•	Vitamin C 70%
Calcium 4%	•	Iron 8%

* Percent Daily Values are based on a 2,000 calorie diet. Your daily values may be higher or lower depending on your calorie needs.

	Calories	2,000	2,500
Total Fat	Less than	65g	80g
Sat Fat	Less than	20g	25g
Cholesterol	Less than	300mg	300mg
Sodium	Less than	2,400mg	2,400mg
Total Carbohydrate		300g	375g
Dietary Fiber		25g	30g

Calories per gram:
Fat 9 • Carbohydrate 4 • Protein 4

2 c. all-purpose flour
1 tbsp. dried oregano
1 tbsp. dried thyme
1 tbsp. onion powder
1 tbsp. garlic powder
1 tbsp. paprika
1 tsp. cayenne pepper
1 tbsp. salt + more for seasoning
1 tsp. freshly cracked black pepper + more for seasoning
6 large veal shanks, roughly 2 in. thick
Butcher's twine
3 tbsp. unsalted butter + more as needed
3 tbsp. olive oil + more as needed
1½ c. white wine, divided
1 c. onion, finely chopped
½ c. carrots, finely chopped
½ c. celery, finely chopped

1 tbsp. garlic, minced

1 leek, finely chopped

3–4 c. chicken stock (light or dark; see recipes in chapter 19)

8 fresh plum tomatoes, seeded and chopped, or 1½ c. canned plum tomatoes, drained and chopped

6 fresh curly parsley sprigs

6 fresh thyme sprigs

2 bay leaves

Cheesecloth bag

2 tbsp. veal demi-glace

1 lemon, zested

½ c. fresh flat-leaf parsley, minced

Preheat the oven to 325° F. Heat a Dutch oven to moderately high heat on the stovetop. Make sure it is hot. Season the all-purpose flour with oregano, thyme, onion powder, garlic powder, paprika, cayenne pepper, 1 tbsp. salt, and 1 tsp. pepper. Pat the veal shanks dry. Tie them with butcher's twine (to hold the meat together after cooking), and then dredge them in the flour, shaking off the excess. Add the 3 tbsp. butter and 3 tbsp. oil over moderately high heat until the butter stops foaming, then add the veal shanks, and brown. Do not add all the shanks at once as this will drop the temperature. We are looking to form a browned crust, not cook the veal through. Add more butter and oil as necessary. After the meat has formed a crust, remove from the Dutch oven. Add ¾ c. of wine to the Dutch oven to release the brown bits on the bottom. Scrape all those bits loose with a wooden spoon. When almost all the wine has evaporated, add a little butter and olive oil. Then add the onion, carrots, celery, garlic, and leek until the vegetables are softened. Allow the vegetables to form a layer on the bottom. Then add back the veal shanks and any juices from the platter upon which they rested. Add the remaining wine and stock so it comes about ¾ the way up the shanks. Cover the top of the shanks with the tomatoes, and place the curly parsley, thyme, and bay leaves in the cheesecloth over the shanks. Salt and pepper to taste. Bring the liquid to a simmer over medium heat. Cover and place mixture in the oven for 2½ hours, or until the veal is tender. Remove the shanks and set aside. Strain the liquid, making sure to press the vegetables so all the juice is extracted, discard the vegetables, and reserve the juices. Return the shanks to the bottom of the Dutch oven. On the stovetop over high heat, add the juices. Add the demi-glace to the juices, and reduce by about half, until it is slightly thickened. Pour the sauce over the shanks and place back in the oven, top removed, for another 10 to 15 minutes. In a bowl, combine the lemon zest and parsley to make a gremolata. Remove the shanks, place on a serving platter, and remove the twine. Top with the gremolata.

Bay leaf is the leaf of the bay laurel (*Laurus nobilis*). It is also known as sweet bay, sweet laurel, laurel leaf, or bay laurel. Often removed prior to serving, bay leaves nonetheless can contribute flavors and nutrients as they cook along with the food. The leaves yield vitamins A and C and also contain significant amounts of iron and manganese as well as smaller amounts of calcium, potassium, and magnesium.

CACIO E PEPE

I KNOW *cacio e pepe* is a Roman pasta dish consisting of cheese, pepper, and pasta. There are many excellent recipes for it. This is a variation. Here we use spaghetti squash and zucchini instead of pasta, a little red pepper flake for heat, and some oven-roasted grape tomatoes for a little sweetness.

1 spaghetti squash, 2–3 lbs.
1 pt. grape tomatoes
½ tsp. salt
1 tsp. black pepper
1 tbsp. + 1 tsp. good-quality olive oil + more for roasting
1 tbsp. shallot, minced
1 tsp. garlic, minced
2 medium zucchini, cut julienne
4 oz. pecorino romano cheese, finely grated
2 tbsp. cream
1½ tsp. red pepper flakes
2 tbsp. flat-leaf parsley, finely chopped

Nutrition Facts		
Serving Size 12 oz (340g)		
Servings Per Container 6		
Amount Per Serving		
Calories 190	Calories from Fat 90	
		% Daily Value*
Total Fat 10g		16%
Saturated Fat 3.5g		19%
Trans Fat 0g		
Cholesterol 20mg		6%
Sodium 470mg		20%
Total Carbohydrate 18g		6%
Dietary Fiber 4g		16%
Sugars 7g		
Protein 9g		
Vitamin A 15%	•	Vitamin C 50%
Calcium 25%	•	Iron 6%
* Percent Daily Values are based on a 2,000 calorie diet. Your daily values may be higher or lower depending on your calorie needs.		

	Calories	2,000	2,500
Total Fat	Less than	65g	80g
Sat Fat	Less than	20g	25g
Cholesterol	Less than	300mg	300mg
Sodium	Less than	2,400mg	2,400mg
Total Carbohydrate		300g	375g
Dietary Fiber		25g	30g

Calories per gram:
Fat 9 • Carbohydrate 4 • Protein 4

Preheat the oven to 350° F. Split the spaghetti squash into quarters and place in a baking dish. Place the tomatoes in a separate baking dish, and season both with salt and pepper, and drizzle with olive oil for roasting. Place in the oven for 30 to 45 minutes; the squash is done when you can easily pass a knife through the rind into the soft flesh. Remove and cool. When cool enough to handle, scrape the inside of the squash to remove the flesh, which should come away in spaghetti-like strands. Heat 1 tbsp. of olive oil over medium heat in a saucepan. Add the shallot and garlic, and cook for 1 to 2 minutes. Add the spaghetti squash and zucchini, and cook for 3 to 5 minutes. Add the cheese, cream, and tomatoes, and cook another 1 to 2 minutes. Remove from heat, and toss with 1 tsp. of olive oil, red pepper flakes, salt, and pepper. Garnish with parsley, and serve with some bread.

Winter squash comes in many varieties, such as acorn, butternut, and spaghetti. Winter squash is higher than summer squash in carbohydrate content. Spaghetti squash specifically has almost no calories, at around 42 per cup. It contains fiber, potassium, and vitamin A. Squash in general has a high water content, which makes it bigger in volume, thus filling you up quicker for fewer calories.

SOUTH AFRICAN FIVE-SPICE MEATBALLS

WE USED THE Doc's South African five-spice blend and Doc's piri-piri sauce from chapter 19 to literally spice up a classic: meatballs and pasta. The panko gives the meatballs a satisfying crispness. For a more classic meatball, leave out the five-spice blend and piri-piri sauce. Either way, it's a delicious meal. I usually serve this with pasta made from the basic pasta recipe and sauce from the marinara sauce recipe, both also in chapter 19.

Nutrition Facts

Serving Size 1 1/2 oz (43g)
Servings Per Container 35

Amount Per Serving	
Calories 100	Calories from Fat 50

	% Daily Value*
Total Fat 6g	8%
Saturated Fat 2g	9%
Trans Fat 0g	
Cholesterol 25mg	9%
Sodium 210mg	9%
Total Carbohydrate 5g	2%
Dietary Fiber 0g	0%
Sugars 0g	
Protein 8g	

Vitamin A 2%	•	Vitamin C 0%
Calcium 4%	•	Iron 6%

* Percent Daily Values are based on a 2,000 calorie diet. Your daily values may be higher or lower depending on your calorie needs.

	Calories	2,000	2,500
Total Fat	Less than	65g	80g
Sat Fat	Less than	20g	25g
Cholesterol	Less than	300mg	300mg
Sodium	Less than	2,400mg	2,400mg
Total Carbohydrate		300g	375g
Dietary Fiber		25g	30g

Calories per gram:
Fat 9 • Carbohydrate 4 • Protein 4

CONTAINS: Milk

- 1 lbs. ground pork, 80/20
- 1½ lbs. ground beef
- 2 tbsp. olive oil + more for frying
- 2 tbsp. breadcrumbs
- 1½ tsp. dried basil
- 1½ tsp. dried oregano
- 1½ tsp. dried thyme
- 1½ tsp. sweet paprika
- 1 tsp. hot paprika
- ½ tsp. garlic powder
- ½ tsp. onion powder
- ½ tsp. cayenne pepper
- 1 tsp. fresh garlic, minced
- 1 tsp. anchovy paste
- 1 egg
- 1 tbsp. tomato paste
- 1 tbsp. Doc's South African five-spice blend (see recipe in chapter 19)
- 3 tbsp. parmesan cheese, grated
- 2 tbsp. shallots
- 1 tsp. prepared mustard
- 1 tsp. salt
- 1 tsp. freshly ground pepper
- 1 tsp. piri-piri sauce (or more for more heat; see recipe in chapter 19)
- 2 c. panko breadcrumbs

chapter eighteen

Preheat the oven to 350° F. Combine the ground pork, ground beef, 2 tbsp. of olive oil, 2 tbsp. of breadcrumbs, basil, oregano, thyme, sweet paprika, hot paprika, garlic powder, onion powder, cayenne pepper, garlic, anchovy paste, egg, tomato paste, five-spice blend, parmesan cheese, shallots, mustard, salt, pepper, and piri-piri sauce, and mix by hand in a bowl. Using a scale or 1-oz. scoop, measure out 1 to 2 oz. meatballs and form by rolling in the palm of your hand. Roll the formed meatballs in the 2 c. of panko. Brown the meatballs in a saucepan in the olive oil. Finish by cooking on a baking sheet in the oven for 15 to 20 minutes.

healthy bytes Anchovies, like most fish, are high in heart-friendly polyunsaturated fatty acids like omega-3s, which can lower cholesterol levels and reduce the risk of heart disease. Anchovies are also a good source of vitamins E and D, calcium, and selenium. Anchovies, unlike larger fish, contain less-heavy metal, such as mercury, lead, cadmium, and arsenic. In general they contain fewer toxins due to their smaller size and shorter lifespan.

GRILLED SHRIMP-STUFFED CALAMARI WITH POBLANO SAUCE

JUST LIKE with fish, a lot of people do not like squid or other mollusks because their experience with them has been tainted by overcooking. Overcooked, they taste like little pieces of leather. Cooked right, they are tender, succulent, and flavorful. The shrimp here are partially cooked and added to the stuffing. This assures that as the calamari quickly cook, the shrimp will be done and not raw. The trick here is to not fully cook the shrimp ahead nor overcook the calamari tubes; they only need a minute or so on each side. You can have the tubes stuffed ahead of time and just grill them when ready to serve, so this is also a great dinner-party-menu item.

2 tbsp. olive oil + more for cooking
8 oz. shrimp
¼ c. onion, finely minced
1 tbsp. garlic, finely chopped
2 tbsp. parsley, finely minced
1 tbsp. thyme, finely chopped
¼ c. parmesan cheese, finely grated
2 tbsp. breadcrumbs
Salt

Nutrition Facts		
Serving Size 4 1/2 oz (128g)		
Servings Per Container 6		
Amount Per Serving		
Calories 210	Calories from Fat 100	
		% Daily Value*
Total Fat 11g		**17%**
Saturated Fat 3g		**15%**
Trans Fat 0g		
Cholesterol 200mg		**66%**
Sodium 280mg		**12%**
Total Carbohydrate 5g		**2%**
Dietary Fiber 0g		**0%**
Sugars 1g		
Protein 20g		
Vitamin A 6%	•	Vitamin C 25%
Calcium 15%	•	Iron 10%

* Percent Daily Values are based on a 2,000 calorie diet. Your daily values may be higher or lower depending on your calorie needs.

	Calories	2,000	2,500
Total Fat	Less than	65g	80g
Sat Fat	Less than	20g	25g
Cholesterol	Less than	300mg	300mg
Sodium	Less than	2,400mg	2,400mg
Total Carbohydrate		300g	375g
Dietary Fiber		25g	30g

Calories per gram:
Fat 9 • Carbohydrate 4 • Protein 4

CONTAINS: Milk, Shellfish

Pepper
½–¾ lb. calamari tubes
Poblano sauce (see recipe in chapter 19)

Heat a pan with a drizzle of olive oil on medium-high heat. Place the shrimp in the pan, and partially cook, stirring occasionally. Remove from heat just as they're turning pink, about 2 minutes, depending on the size of the shrimp, and finely chop. Mix the shrimp with the onion, garlic, parsley, thyme, parmesan cheese, and breadcrumbs. Season with salt and pepper. Stuff each calamari tube full, lightly oil the tubes with olive oil, and season with salt and pepper. Place on a hot grill for about 30 seconds to 1 minute each side, just enough to ensure the stuffing is cooked (the shrimp bits should turn pink) and the calamari tubes get a nice char from the grill. Remove the calamari from the grill, place on a bed of poblano sauce, and serve.

healthy bytes Squid, often referred to as calamari, are a great source of omega-3s that are often associated with fatty fish like salmon. Although squid can be high in cholesterol, a study performed in mice found that a diet of shrimp, squid, and octopus actually lowered overall cholesterol.[1] Mollusks, such as squid, are also great sources of such minerals as zinc, selenium, and iron. The level of iron in mollusks is similar to that found in red meat.

JAPANESE NOODLES

WHEN I VISIT Japan, this is my basic staple. We may splurge at the sushi or sashimi bar a night or two, but this is the bulk of our diet. It is much more in keeping with what the native population eats. If you want to be very traditional, you can also serve this with a fish stock called dashi made from dried bonito, which is a type of fish and is related to the tuna. If you need a quick meal, just add the chopped veggies in raw form to the broth. If you like it a little heartier, you can add a few slices of thinly sliced pork (it cooks in the broth) or seafood. If you are all by yourself you can slurp the broth at the end. In Japan, slurping indicates a delicious dish.

3 c. vegetable nage (or light chicken stock; see recipes in chapter 19)
Somen, ramen, or other Japanese noodles (3 oz. per person, 1 bundle)

Nutrition Facts

Serving Size 5 5/67 lbs (2302g)
Servings Per Container 1

Amount Per Serving	
Calories 2740 Calories from Fat 360	

	% Daily Value*
Total Fat 41g	**62%**
Saturated Fat 6g	**28%**
Trans Fat 0g	
Cholesterol 40mg	**13%**
Sodium 8530mg	**355%**
Total Carbohydrate 467g	**156%**
Dietary Fiber 37g	**149%**
Sugars 22g	
Protein 129g	

Vitamin A 610%	•	Vitamin C 160%
Calcium 100%	•	Iron 110%

* Percent Daily Values are based on a 2,000 calorie diet. Your daily values may be higher or lower depending on your calorie needs.

		Calories	2,000	2,500
Total Fat	Less than		65g	80g
Sat Fat	Less than		20g	25g
Cholesterol	Less than		300mg	300mg
Sodium	Less than		2,400mg	2,400mg
Total Carbohydrate			300g	375g
Dietary Fiber			25g	30g

Calories per gram:
Fat 9 • Carbohydrate 4 • Protein 4

CONTAINS: Eggs

Tempura vegetables (see recipes in chapters 17 and 19)
Tofu, cut into bite-sized chunks
A few drops of toasted sesame oil
Soy sauce
Cilantro or green onion, chopped
Hot sauce (like sriracha)

Heat the nage up to a boil, and add the noodles. Reduce to a simmer, and cook like any other dried pasta to desired consistency. Pour noodles and broth into a bowl. Add tempura vegetables, and top with toasted sesame oil, tofu, soy sauce, cilantro or green onion, and hot sauce.

healthy bytes Stock contains minerals like calcium, magnesium, phosphorus, silicon, sulfur, and trace elements. It also contains chondroitin and glucosamine, which are good for joints. Fish stock provides iodine, which is necessary for proper thyroid functioning.

SMOKED AFRICAN SPICE–RUBBED PORK LOIN AND ZUCCHINI SLAW

YOU CAN USE this technique and flavoring on any meat you want to smoke. It is equally delicious on poultry or game meat. The zucchini slaw side has an Asian flavoring, so it adds a nice changeup to the palate.

1 pork loin, center cut, approximately 3–4 lbs.
5 garlic cloves, crushed
2 oz. Doc's barbecue spice rub (see recipe in chapter 19)
1 oz. Doc's South African five-spice blend (see recipe in chapter 19)
Zucchini slaw (see recipe in chapter 17)

Cut slits in the pork loin fat cap. Rub the loin with crushed garlic, and then place the garlic in slits. Combine the barbecue spice rub and five-spice blend together, and then coat the loin. Allow to rest refrigerated for several hours to overnight. Smoke for 3 to 4 hours, depending on the size of the loin. When done the meat should pull away easily. If there is any question, check the internal temperature with a meat thermometer, looking for an internal center temperature of 140° F. Serve with the zucchini slaw.

Nutrition Facts		
Serving Size 4 oz (113g)		
Servings Per Container 6		
Amount Per Serving		
Calories 140	Calories from Fat 25	
		% Daily Value*
Total Fat 3g		5%
Saturated Fat 0.5g		4%
Trans Fat 0g		
Cholesterol 50mg		17%
Sodium 390mg		16%
Total Carbohydrate 4g		1%
Dietary Fiber 1g		5%
Sugars 1g		
Protein 22g		
Vitamin A 10%	•	Vitamin C 2%
Calcium 4%	•	Iron 10%

* Percent Daily Values are based on a 2,000 calorie diet. Your daily values may be higher or lower depending on your calorie needs.

	Calories	2,000	2,500
Total Fat	Less than	65g	80g
Sat Fat	Less than	20g	25g
Cholesterol	Less than	300mg	300mg
Sodium	Less than	2,400mg	2,400mg
Total Carbohydrate		300g	375g
Dietary Fiber		25g	30g

Calories per gram:
Fat 9 • Carbohydrate 4 • Protein 4

Anise seed was used for health benefits as far back as the ancient Greeks. It can help to reduce bloating, flatulence, colic, and intestinal cramping. It has antispasmodic properties and can also relieve menstrual cramps. Anise seed is reputed to be able to stimulate the pancreas. Additionally it functions as an expectorant. Anise seed is reportedly useful as a sleep aid.

SOUTH AFRICAN–SPICED ROAST PORK STEW

ONE OF THE truly amazing things about South Africa was the diversity of cultures. The area, especially around Capetown, is a real melting pot. There are influences from Asia, India, Portugal, the Netherlands, France, Germany, and England, to name just a few. I had some very interesting dishes that combined Asian/Indian flavors with some "native" South African touches. Here is a roast pork stew that comforts me by taking me back to my visits there and provides great memories of places, people, and friends.

Nutrition Facts		
Serving Size 12 oz (340g)		
Servings Per Container 12		
Amount Per Serving		
Calories 360	Calories from Fat 100	
		% Daily Value*
Total Fat 12g		**18%**
Saturated Fat 2.5g		**14%**
Trans Fat 0g		
Cholesterol 85mg		**29%**
Sodium 610mg		**25%**
Total Carbohydrate 32g		**11%**
Dietary Fiber 12g		**49%**
Sugars 5g		
Protein 39g		
Vitamin A 60%	•	Vitamin C 30%
Calcium 15%	•	Iron 60%

*Percent Daily Values are based on a 2,000 calorie diet. Your daily values may be higher or lower depending on your calorie needs.

	Calories	2,000	2,500
Total Fat	Less than	65g	80g
Sat Fat	Less than	20g	25g
Cholesterol	Less than	300mg	300mg
Sodium	Less than	2,400mg	2,400mg
Total Carbohydrate		300g	375g
Dietary Fiber		25g	30g

Calories per gram:
Fat 9 • Carbohydrate 4 • Protein 4

4–5 lbs. trimmed pork (I use the end cuts of the loin)
1 tbsp. anchovy paste
2 garlic cloves, minced
1 tbsp. tomato paste
2–3 tbsp. olive oil
1½ c. carrots, cut into 1 in. chunks
1½ c. onion, thinly sliced
1 tbsp. Doc's South African five-spice blend
    (see recipe in chapter 19)
1 tbsp. garam masala
1 tsp. hot paprika
1 tsp. sweet paprika
1 tsp. turmeric
¼ c. all-purpose flour
2 c. white wine
2 c. chicken stock (see recipe in chapter 19)
2 bay leaves
2 sprigs fresh thyme
2 sprigs fresh cilantro

1 lb. potatoes, cut into 1 in. cubes
1 packet unflavored gelatin
1 c. frozen peas
½ c. pearl onions
Salt
Freshly ground pepper

Preheat the oven to 300° F. Cut the pork into roughly 1 in. bits, and set aside. Combine the anchovy paste, garlic, and tomato paste in a small bowl, and set aside. Using a Dutch oven or other heavy-bottomed oven proof pot, heat the oil until smoking over medium high heat. Brown and remove the pork in batches. Add back the meat, carrots, and sliced onions to the Dutch oven, and cook over medium heat until the onions have softened, around 1 to 2 minutes. Add the garlic, anchovy paste, and tomato paste mixture as well as the five-spice blend, garam masala, hot paprika, sweet paprika, and turmeric, and cook another 30 seconds. Add the flour, coating the components, and cook another 30 seconds. Add the wine, increase the heat to high, and cook for about 2 minutes, or until the liquid has slightly thickened. Add the chicken stock, bay leaves, thyme, and cilantro, and bring to a simmer. Transfer to the oven, and cook for 90 minutes. Add the potatoes, and cook for another 45 minutes. While this is cooking, bloom 1 packet of unflavored gelatin in a separate bowl by adding a little cold water to it. After the potatoes have cooked for 45 minutes, remove from the oven, and place over medium heat on the stovetop. Add the peas and pearl onions, and cook for about 10 to 15 minutes. Increase the heat to high, add the gelatin, and stir until dissolved, about 3 to 5 minutes. Remove from heat, season with salt and pepper, and serve.

healthy bytes Turmeric was first used as a dye in India more than 2,500 years ago. Since that time it has revealed itself to be a powerful anti-inflammatory and cancer-fighting compound. The active complex in turmeric is curcumin. Turmeric has antibacterial properties and is regarded as a natural liver-detoxifying agent. It may be helpful in preventing Alzheimer's disease, depression, and multiple sclerosis. It is a cyclooxygenase-2 (a type of enzyme involved in inflammation) inhibitor, thus it is beneficial in arthritis and other inflammatory conditions. It may also aid in weight loss by increasing fat metabolism.

SMOKED SPICED LEG OF LAMB

I LIKE TO serve this with oven-roasted rosemary potatoes (see recipe in chapter 17) and a rosemary red wine reduction sauce (see recipe in chapter 19). This makes a lot of lamb, but the smoked lamb can be used as a delicious first with some fresh fruits, vegetables, and cheese. If you are having guests over, this is a great recipe because everything but smoking the lamb and putting potatoes in the oven can be done ahead of time. The smell of the smoker is so tempting, your guests will follow you out to check on it and likely will stay there until the lamb comes off.

1 semiboneless leg of lamb, 4–6 lbs.
Doc's barbecue spice rub (see recipe in chapter 19)
½ c. yellow onion, chopped
1 tbsp. fresh garlic, chopped
1 tbsp. Doc's piri-piri sauce (optional for a little heat; see recipe in chapter 19)
1 tbsp. fresh ginger, chopped
2 tbsp. Doc's South African five-spice blend (see recipe in chapter 19)
½ tsp. onion powder
½ tsp. garlic powder
1½ tsp. smoked paprika, divided
½ tsp. dried oregano
½ tsp. dried thyme
¼ tsp. cayenne pepper
1 tsp. kosher salt
1 tsp. freshly ground black pepper
¼ tsp. allspice
¼ tsp. ground cloves
¼ tsp. cardamom
1 lemon, juiced
½ c. olive oil
Butcher's twine
Rosemary red wine reduction sauce (see recipe in chapter 19)
Fresh rosemary sprigs

Nutrition Facts		
Serving Size 4 oz (113g)		
Servings Per Container 24		
Amount Per Serving		
Calories 280	Calories from Fat 160	
		% Daily Value*
Total Fat 19g		**28%**
Saturated Fat 7g		**37%**
Trans Fat 0g		
Cholesterol 90mg		**31%**
Sodium 260mg		**11%**
Total Carbohydrate 2g		**1%**
Dietary Fiber 0g		**0%**
Sugars 0g		
Protein 25g		
Vitamin A 2%	•	Vitamin C 4%
Calcium 2%	•	Iron 10%

* Percent Daily Values are based on a 2,000 calorie diet. Your daily values may be higher or lower depending on your calorie needs.

	Calories	2,000	2,500
Total Fat	Less than	65g	80g
Sat Fat	Less than	20g	25g
Cholesterol	Less than	300mg	300mg
Sodium	Less than	2,400mg	2,400mg
Total Carbohydrate		300g	375g
Dietary Fiber		25g	30g

Calories per gram:
Fat 9 • Carbohydrate 4 • Protein 4

Place the leg of lamb fat side down, and split the leg to the bone. Leaving the bone attached at the midpoint, butterfly the leg. In a food processor, combine the barbecue spice rub, yellow onion, garlic, piri-piri sauce, ginger, five-spice blend, onion powder, garlic powder, smoked paprika, oregano, thyme, cayenne pepper, kosher salt, pepper, allspice, cloves, cardamom, lemon juice, and olive oil. Apply the paste to the leg of lamb, both inside and out. Reassemble the leg to its original shape, keeping the bone intact, and secure with butcher's twine. Place in a plastic bag, and allow to rest in a refrigerator overnight.

Prepare your smoker according to directions. Place the lamb in the smoker, and cook until done (about 3 to 5 hours, depending on the size); an instant-read thermometer should read about 145° F in the middle. Remove and allow to rest.

To serve, thinly slice the leg of lamb. Surround with a side, such as oven-roasted rosemary potatoes (see recipe in chapter 17), and drizzle with some rosemary red wine reduction sauce. Garnish with fresh rosemary sprigs.

healthy bytes Cardamom is actually the dried, unripened fruit of a perennial member of the ginger family. The pods contain this aromatic seed. Often used as a breath freshener, a bowl of seeds can often be found in Indian restaurants. Cardamom stimulates bile flow, for liver health and fat metabolism. It is also a wonderful aid for digestive issues; it eases stomach cramps, cuts mucus, and is a great remedy to relieve flatulence. Real cardamom is expensive, and only *Elettaria cardamomum* (botanical name) is the real deal.

SWEET AND SAVORY CURRY-SPICED EGGPLANT

I WAITED A long time to make this dish, mostly because I've despised eggplant. My mom was mostly a great cook but not when it came to eggplant. What I recall of eating eggplant was a bitter, slimy, gooey experience, which I imagine sucking a snail through a straw would be like. I've avoided eating or cooking it like the plague for years, but I've seen the prep methods and read the recipes and reviews. With newfound knowledge and technique, I faced my old foe. I drew the last bit of inspiration from some Indian dishes, and I set forth. The key for me was in the preparation of the eggplant. Eggplant contains a lot of water, and if not prepared correctly prior to frying, it can become the aforementioned ball of goo. I experimented with cuts of varying thickness, and with this preparation it is important that the slices be between ½ to ¾ inch thick, as this size reduces substantially with the preparation process. It results in an almost meaty texture with a pleasant squash-like taste. I assume this is what eggplant is supposed to be like. It was, I daresay, delicious. I never thought I would be saying this, but I look forward to having eggplant again. I served this with two curries, essentially the same spicy curry, with one made slightly sweet with orange juice and one savory by using spicy tomato juice. It was fantastic, and you can use this for any other main, such as chicken or fish. I serve this over Chinese emperor black rice in two small servings. Ladle the curry over each grouping of eggplant and rice.

1 eggplant, sliced into ½ to ¾ inch pieces
Approximately 2 tbsp. salt
2 tbsp. butter or Smart Balance substitute, divided
1 c. onion, finely chopped, divided
2 tsp. fresh ginger, grated and divided
4 tsp. garlic, minced and divided
8 tsp. curry spice
2 tbsp. lime juice
2 jalapeños or other hot chili, finely chopped (leave the seed and
    membrane if you want extra heat) and divided
1 c. vegetable nage or chicken stock, divided (see recipes in
    chapter 19)
1 c. coconut milk, divided
½ c. orange juice
½ c. spicy tomato juice
12 oz. plain yogurt, divided
1 c. cilantro, chopped and divided
1 tsp. salt
½ tsp. white pepper
Seasoned flour for dusting
2 eggs, well beaten
½ c. seasoned breadcrumbs mixed with ½ c. panko
Olive oil for frying

Nutrition Facts		
Serving Size 4 oz (113g)		
Servings Per Container 8		
Amount Per Serving		
Calories 170	Calories from Fat 50	
		% Daily Value*
Total Fat 6g		9%
Saturated Fat 4g		20%
Trans Fat 0g		
Cholesterol 15mg		6%
Sodium 210mg		9%
Total Carbohydrate 25g		8%
Dietary Fiber 2g		7%
Sugars 2g		
Protein 5g		
Vitamin A 4%	•	Vitamin C 10%
Calcium 2%	•	Iron 10%

* Percent Daily Values are based on a 2,000 calorie diet. Your daily values may be higher or lower depending on your calorie needs.

	Calories	2,000	2,500
Total Fat	Less than	65g	80g
Sat Fat	Less than	20g	25g
Cholesterol	Less than	300mg	300mg
Sodium	Less than	2,400mg	2,400mg
Total Carbohydrate		300g	375g
Dietary Fiber		25g	30g

Calories per gram:
Fat 9 • Carbohydrate 4 • Protein 4

To prepare the eggplant, clean the skin (or remove if you like), and slice. Place absorbent towels on a cookie sheet or baking pan large enough to accommodate the slices in a single layer. Sprinkle salt liberally on the towels, and place the slices on the salt. Sprinkle the tops liberally with salt, and cover with absorbent towels. Allow the slices to sit for approximately 1 hour; the salt will draw out moisture, and you may need to replace the towels. Remove the salt from the pan and eggplant, and replace the towels. Moisture will continue to wick away from the vegetable over the next several hours.

To prepare the curries, get two medium saucepans. In each saucepan, place half of the butter or Smart Balance and onions. Cook over medium heat until the onions are translucent. Add half of the ginger, garlic, and curry spice to each saucepan, and cook for another minute. Add half of the lime juice, jalapeños, nage, and coconut milk to each saucepan. To one pot add orange juice, and to the other the tomato juice. Bring to a boil, and then reduce to a simmer for about 30 minutes until the liquid is reduced by about half. Remove from heat, and cool slightly. Prepare two bowls, each with half of the yogurt and cilantro. Strain each mixture into one of the prepared bowls and mix, and season with salt and white pepper. For the eggplant, set up a three-step breading station: a bowl with seasoned flour, a bowl with beaten eggs, and a bowl with breadcrumbs and panko (I use homemade breadcrumbs from stale sourdough baguette mixed with spices). Dredge the eggplant in flour, and shake off the excess. Dip the eggplant in egg, and shake off the excess. Place the eggplant in breadcrumbs, and shake off the excess. Place in medium saucepan with olive oil heated to medium high. Cook until golden brown and delicious on both sides. Ladle the curry yogurt sauce over the eggplant, and serve.

healthy bytes Eggplant is a member of the nightshade family, along with tomatoes, sweet peppers, and potatoes. Eggplants contain fiber, potassium, manganese, copper, thiamin, pyridoxine, magnesium, tryptophan, and niacin. Eggplant also contains phenols, such as caffeic acid and chlorogenic acid. Benefits attributed to chlorogenic acid include cancer-fighting properties, antimicrobial and antiviral abilities, and the lowering of LDL ("bad") cholesterol. Eggplant also contains flavonoids like nasunin. Nasunin is an anthocyanin found in eggplant skin and is a potent antioxidant and free-radical scavenger that has been shown to protect cell membranes from damage.

TEA-SMOKED SALMON

THIS IS A really uniquely delicious dish. The tea smoke is delicate, and you can use it with any variety of fish. It works well for shellfish, like scallops, as well. Try different types of teas for different flavors.

 1 tbsp. Szechuan peppers
 2 tbsp. green tea leaves
 1 star anise pod, whole
 ½ c. rice wine vinegar
 ½ c. water
 3 tbsp. ponzu sauce
 ½ lime, juiced
 1 salmon fillet, approximately 3 lbs.
 Ceylon tea, approximately 3–6 oz.
 Cherry wood or other fruitwood chips, approximately 6–12 oz.

Combine the pepper, green tea, and star anise in a small saucepan and lightly toast. Combine in a bowl with the rice wine vinegar, water, ponzu sauce, and lime juice. Marinate the salmon in the mixture overnight. Prepare the smoker, and mix the chips with the ceylon tea in a 2:1 ratio. Smoke the salmon until it flakes easily. The exact time will depend on the thickness and size of the fillet.

healthy bytes Green tea contains polyphenols and catechins. The catechin epigallocatechin gallate (EGCG) is a particularly powerful antioxidant. EGCG is twice as powerful as resveratrol, thought to be the active antioxidant in red wine. Green tea has been used as medicine in the Orient for more than four thousand years. It is reputed to be an aid in fighting cancer, treating rheumatoid arthritis, reducing LDL ("bad") cholesterol, and improving immune function. Green tea may help increase metabolism and thus may be helpful to those looking to lose weight.

Nutrition Facts		
Serving Size 4 oz (113g)		
Servings Per Container 12		
Amount Per Serving		
Calories 170	Calories from Fat 70	
		% Daily Value*
Total Fat 8g		12%
Saturated Fat 1.5g		7%
Trans Fat 0g		
Cholesterol 55mg		19%
Sodium 480mg		20%
Total Carbohydrate 3g		1%
Dietary Fiber 0g		0%
Sugars 3g		
Protein 20g		
Vitamin A 4%	• Vitamin C 0%	
Calcium 0%	• Iron 2%	

* Percent Daily Values are based on a 2,000 calorie diet. Your daily values may be higher or lower depending on your calorie needs.

	Calories	2,000	2,500
Total Fat	Less than	65g	80g
Sat Fat	Less than	20g	25g
Cholesterol	Less than	300mg	300mg
Sodium	Less than	2,400mg	2,400mg
Total Carbohydrate		300g	375g
Dietary Fiber		25g	30g

Calories per gram:
Fat 9 • Carbohydrate 4 • Protein 4

CONTAINS: Fish, Soy

VEGGIE POT PIES

Vegetarian does not have to be boring. Very often a vegetarian offering consists of some grilled veggies, maybe mixed with some pasta. Here's a great dish that is hearty, filling, and delicious. You can place any fish or meat chunks in this, and it becomes another delicious variation.

- 1 block extra-firm tofu, sliced into ¼ in. chunks
- 1 sprig fresh rosemary
- 3–5 sprigs fresh thyme
- 2 sprigs fresh sage
- 1 c. + 2 tbsp. onion, diced and divided
- 1 tbsp. + 2 tsp. garlic, minced and divided
- ¼ c. mirin (sweet rice wine)
- ¼ c. rice wine vinegar
- 3 tbsp. soy sauce
- 5 tbsp. butter or Smart Balance substitute
- ½ c. celery, sliced
- 1 portobello mushroom, chopped
- 1 tsp. salt

½ tsp. freshly ground black pepper

5 tbsp. all-purpose flour

3 c. vegetable nage or chicken stock (for nonvegetarian versions, see recipes in chapter 19)

¼ c. cream

1½ lbs. fingerling potatoes, diced and blanched

1 c. carrots, diced and blanched

1 c. sweet peas

1½ tsp. poultry seasoning

¼ tsp. cayenne pepper

2 tbsp. flat-leaf parsley, finely chopped

1 savory basic pie crust (see recipe in chapter 19)

1 egg beaten with 1 tsp. water

Nutrition Facts

Serving Size 7 oz. (198g)
Servings Per Container 12

Amount Per Serving

Calories 280   Calories from Fat 150

	% Daily Value*
Total Fat 17g	**26%**
Saturated Fat 3.5g	18%
Trans Fat 0g	
Cholesterol 15mg	**6%**
Sodium 320mg	**13%**
Total Carbohydrate 24g	**8%**
Dietary Fiber 2g	10%
Sugars 3g	
Protein 8g	

Vitamin A 35%	•	Vitamin C 25%
Calcium 8%	•	Iron 10%

* Percent Daily Values are based on a 2,000 calorie diet. Your daily values may be higher or lower depending on your calorie needs.

	Calories	2,000	2,500
Total Fat	Less than	65g	80g
Sat Fat	Less than	20g	25g
Cholesterol	Less than	300mg	300mg
Sodium	Less than	2,400mg	2,400mg
Total Carbohydrate		300g	375g
Dietary Fiber		25g	30g

Calories per gram:
Fat 9 • Carbohydrate 4 • Protein 4

CONTAINS: Milk

Place the cut tofu into a container with the sprig of rosemary, sprigs of thyme, sprigs of sage, 2 tbsp. onion, 1 tbsp. garlic, mirin, rice wine vinegar, and soy sauce. Marinate overnight. Place in an oven preheated to 400° F, and bake about 15 minutes. Flip the pieces over, and cook another 15 minutes. The pieces should have dried out somewhat and obtained a meat-like texture. Leave oven on, and set aside.

Place the butter or Smart Balance in a large saucepan over medium heat. Cook 1 c. onions until translucent, about 3 to 5 minutes. Add 2 tsp. garlic and celery, and cook another 2 minutes. Add the mushroom, and season with salt and pepper. Add the flour to form a blond roux. Add the seasoned tofu and nage, bring up to a boil, and then reduce to a simmer. Cook until the liquid starts to thicken, approximately 5 minutes. Add the cream, potatoes, carrots, peas, poultry seasoning, cayenne pepper, and parsley, and cook for another 5 minutes.

Meanwhile, roll out the pie crust. Divide the vegetable mixture into twelve 7-oz. ramekins, and cover each ramekin with a piece of pastry. Brush the beaten egg and water on the pastry, and bake at 400° F for 20 to 25 minutes. You can freeze the extra pies and reheat as you need them.

healthy bytes Garlic has antibiotic properties and in holistic circles is used as a blood-cleansing agent. The allicin found in garlic increases the enzymatic activity of atalase and glutathione found in human cells. These enzymes perform an antioxidant function. The antibacterial properties of garlic are well known; it has about 1 percent of the antibacterial effect of penicillin. Garlic has also been shown to help reduce blood pressure and reduce LDL ("bad") cholesterol. Eating parsley after eating garlic can help remove an offending garlic odor.

PIPERADE

A **PIPERADE** is a Basque dish, which, according to *La Rousse Gastronomique*, is a "rich stew of tomatoes and sweet (bell) peppers, sometimes seasoned with onion and garlic, cooked in olive oil or goose fat and then mixed with beaten eggs and lightly scrambled."[2] This version will include some poached eggs instead. In dishes where there are subtle tomato flavors and the tomato is a highlight, I like to prepare a tomato *concassé*. This removes the skin and seeds. The olive oil taste comes through this dish, so use one with good quality.

Nutrition Facts		
Serving Size 12 oz (340g)		
Servings Per Container 2		
Amount Per Serving		
Calories 300	Calories from Fat 190	
		% Daily Value*
Total Fat 22g		33%
Saturated Fat 4g		21%
Trans Fat 0g		
Cholesterol 305mg		102%
Sodium 110mg		5%
Total Carbohydrate 16g		5%
Dietary Fiber 3g		12%
Sugars 2g		
Protein 12g		
Vitamin A 0%	•	Vitamin C 140%
Calcium 8%	•	Iron 10%

* Percent Daily Values are based on a 2,000 calorie diet. Your daily values may be higher or lower depending on your calorie needs.

	Calories	2,000	2,500
Total Fat	Less than	65g	80g
Sat Fat	Less than	20g	25g
Cholesterol	Less than	300mg	300mg
Sodium	Less than	2,400mg	2,400mg
Total Carbohydrate		300g	375g
Dietary Fiber		25g	30g

Calories per gram:
Fat 9 • Carbohydrate 4 • Protein 4

½ lb. tomatoes (roughly 2 medium tomatoes)
4 oz. sweet peppers (with the red tomatoes, I prefer green, yellow, or orange peppers)
2 tbsp. good-quality olive oil
¼ c. onion, finely chopped
2 tbsp. garlic, minced
1 tsp. fresh thyme, chopped
1 tsp. fresh seasoned breadcrumbs
2 eggs, poached

To prepare the tomato *concassé*, use a paring knife to mark an *X* on the bottom of the tomato, just deep enough to penetrate the skin. Blanch the tomatoes in boiling water for 20 to 30 seconds. Quickly refresh in an ice bath. Using the paring knife again, cut out the core, and peel the tomato. Cut the tomato in half. Squeeze the juice and seeds into a bowl. Chop the tomato flesh. Pour the juice through a fine mesh strainer and reserve. Roast the peppers, and then place in a plastic bag for several minutes. This will make them easier to peel and remove the skins. Remove the seeds and inner membrane, and julienne. Heat a medium pan over medium heat with some olive oil. Add the chopped onions and garlic, and cook until the onions become translucent. Add the roasted peppers and thyme, and cook until any liquid has evaporated. Add tomatoes, breadcrumbs, and reserved juice. Cook approximately 5 minutes, until the liquid has evaporated. Top with the poached egg, and serve.

healthy bytes Sweet peppers are not spicy because they lack capsaicin. All peppers begin as the green variety and as they mature become more colorful. Red peppers are usually the sweetest. Also, the thinner the skin, the more "peppery" the taste, while the thicker-skinned varieties tend to be sweeter. Peppers are low in calories and are great sources of vitamins A and C and potassium.

WEEKI WACHEE SHRIMP

INSPIRATION CAN occur anywhere. This dish was inspired by the lovely mermaids at Weeki Wachee Springs in Florida. I spent a Labor Day weekend in northern Florida near the bountiful Gulf of Mexico. As I was driving back home, I saw a sign for Weeki Wachee. Weeki Wachee? After a bit it came to me—the mermaids on some Travel Channel show. Now the possibility of viewing live mermaids was an experience I couldn't pass up. It had rained the day before, but now the sky was blue with not too much humidity. I arrived a bit before show time, and I hit the jackpot; it was mermaid calendar signing day. I purchased a calendar and dutifully stood in line as the shapely mermaids smiled and signed. How could you not be inspired? And on the menu was delicious, fresh tail—shrimp tail, of course!

Nutrition Facts	
Serving Size 1 1/2 oz (43g)	
Servings Per Container 24	
Amount Per Serving	
Calories 50	Calories from Fat 30
	% Daily Value*
Total Fat 3.5g	**5%**
Saturated Fat 0g	**0%**
Trans Fat 0g	
Cholesterol 30mg	**10%**
Sodium 140mg	**6%**
Total Carbohydrate 1g	**0%**
Dietary Fiber 0g	**0%**
Sugars 0g	
Protein 5g	
Vitamin A 8% • Vitamin C 6%	
Calcium 2% • Iron 4%	

* Percent Daily Values are based on a 2,000 calorie diet. Your daily values may be higher or lower depending on your calorie needs.

	Calories	2,000	2,500
Total Fat	Less than	65g	80g
Sat Fat	Less than	20g	25g
Cholesterol	Less than	300mg	300mg
Sodium	Less than	2,400mg	2,400mg
Total Carbohydrate		300g	375g
Dietary Fiber		25g	30g

Calories per gram:
Fat 9 • Carbohydrate 4 • Protein 4

CONTAINS: Nuts, Shellfish

4 garlic cloves, minced

4 oz. fresh parmesan cheese, grated

Approximately ¾ oz. pine nuts

Approximately 1½–2 oz. fresh basil

Approximately ⅓ c. good-quality olive oil

1 lb. fresh shrimp, at least 21–25 count size

⅓ c. mead (may substitute with white wine mixed with 1 tsp. honey)

2–3 sprigs oregano

2–3 sprigs thyme

1 bay leaf

1 tbsp. herbes de Provence

2 tsp. hot paprika

2 tsp. sweet paprika

1 fresh hot pepper, split lengthwise

1 tsp. salt

1 c. water

6 pieces Parma prosciutto, sliced paper thin

Preheat the broiler on high. Combine the garlic, cheese, pine nuts, basil, and olive oil to make a thick pesto paste using a mortar and pestle or in a food processor; set aside. Clean and devein the shrimp. Combine the mead, oregano, thyme, bay leaf, herbes de Provence, hot paprika, sweet paprika, hot pepper, salt, and water in a saucepan. Bring the liquid to a simmer. Add the shrimp, and poach for 2 minutes. They should be slightly underdone, just starting to turn pink. Remove from the heat, and place the shrimp in an ice bath to stop the shrimp from cooking. Lay out the prosciutto slices, and cut each into 4 sections so you now have about 24 pieces. Smear 1 side of the prosciutto with the pesto. Wrap the shrimps with a piece of prosciutto with the pesto side facing the shrimp. Arrange under the broiler, and broil for 1 to 2 minutes. The prosciutto should get just a little crisp to it. Remove and serve.

healthy bytes Honey was an important medicine from ancient times through the Middle Ages. It is used to treat respiratory, throat, and gastrointestinal ailments. Honey contains the simple sugar glucose, which is easily absorbed by the body and thus is a quick source of energy. It contains antimicrobial and antioxidant properties. It was often used externally to treat skin conditions as well. The particular properties of a honey can vary depending on where and from what it is produced.

stocks, sauces, and more tasty bits

"Beware of the person who can't be bothered by details."

—WILLIAM FEATHER (1889–1981)

I WOULD ADD especially beware of any chef who can't be bothered by the details. As the ocean is made up of individual drops of water, so a meal is nothing more than all its individual components. It is only as good as the weakest ingredient or preparation. If you work your butt off to cook an excellent protein, you can ruin the entire production with a poor sauce or side. The difference between being merely good and great lies completely in the execution of the details. Stock is where attention to detail starts. It is the base. One of the giants of cooking, Auguste Escoffier, remarked:

Indeed, stock is everything in cooking. . . . Without it nothing can be done. If one's stock is good, what remains of the work is easy; if on the other hand, it is bad, or merely mediocre, it is quite hopeless to expect anything approaching a satisfactory result. The cook mindful of success, therefore will naturally direct his attention to the faultless preparation of his stock.[1]

I would add that you need this type of focus when preparing the sides and any sauces, breads, and so on. It is easy to become focused on your main objective: the star of the dish. But a great meal is a team sport. This chapter contains nuggets of detail wisdom. Here are some basics, like how to easily make bread dough, sauces, and, importantly, stocks. Here you will also find scattered about a few dessert recipe ideas when you need that extra punch. Mastering these features is a critical step to becoming a Grassroots Gourmet. Explore this chapter, and pull from it as often as you need to consistently bring your "A" game to the kitchen.

BLOOD ORANGE CURRY SAUCE

THE BLOOD orange gives a brilliant color and a sweetness to blend with the heat. This is great with some chicken and served with naan bread or over rice. You can also simmer vegetables in the sauce for an exotic-tasting first or main, depending on portion size. Don't panic if your sauce turns out too hot because of the pepper. Simply use that as a base. Add about four tablespoons of the too-hot curry to an additional six ounces of plain yogurt and three tablespoons of coconut milk, adjusting to your taste.

1 tbsp. butter or Smart Balance substitute
½ c. onion, minced
2 tsp. garlic, minced
1 tsp. fresh ginger, grated
4 tsp. curry powder
1 jalapeño, finely chopped (leave the seed and membrane in if you want extra heat)
½ c. vegetable nage or light chicken stock (see recipes in this chapter)
½ c. blood orange juice (or regular orange juice if you cannot get blood oranges)
½ c. coconut milk
1 tsp. lime juice
½ c. cilantro
6 oz. plain yogurt
Salt
White pepper

Nutrition Facts		
Serving Size 1 oz (28g)		
Servings Per Container 24		
Amount Per Serving		
Calories 25	Calories from Fat 15	
		% Daily Value*
Total Fat 1.5g		2%
Saturated Fat 1g		6%
Trans Fat 0g		
Cholesterol 0mg		0%
Sodium 55mg		2%
Total Carbohydrate 2g		1%
Dietary Fiber 0g		0%
Sugars 1g		
Protein 1g		
Vitamin A 0%	•	Vitamin C 10%
Calcium 2%	•	Iron 2%

* Percent Daily Values are based on a 2,000 calorie diet. Your daily values may be higher or lower depending on your calorie needs.		
	Calories	2,000	2,500

		Calories	2,000	2,500
Total Fat	Less than	65g	80g
Sat Fat	Less than	20g	25g
Cholesterol	Less than	300mg	300mg
Sodium	Less than	2,400mg	2,400mg
Total Carbohydrate		300g	375g
Dietary Fiber		25g	30g

Calories per gram:
Fat 9 • Carbohydrate 4 • Protein 4

In a medium saucepan, melt the butter or Smart Balance, and cook the onions until translucent. Add the garlic, ginger, curry powder, jalapeño, vegetable nage or chicken stock, orange juice, coconut milk, and lime juice. Bring to a boil, and then reduce to a simmer for about 30 minutes, or until reduced by half. Strain the mixture, cool, and add the cilantro and yogurt. Season with salt and white pepper to taste.

FRESH FRUIT AND YOGURT PARFAIT

I THINK OF this as a summer seasonal treat. It actually makes for a great breakfast or brunch item as well. I think it tastes best when you can get whatever fresh fruits are in season; in spring and summer in Georgia, the peaches are available. For an added treat, when you have fruit like peaches, grill them with a touch of brown sugar and cinnamon. Then put them in the parfait with some fresh berries.

Approximately 16 oz. assorted fresh fruit
¼ c. + 2 tbsp. sugar, Splenda, or other sweetener, divided
Liqueur, such as Cointreau (optional)
Approximately 6 oz. vanilla yogurt
1 tsp. cinnamon
1 tsp. unsweetened cocoa

Place the fruit in a bowl with ¼ c. of sweetener, and let macerate for about 30 minutes. You can also soak in a liqueur, such as Cointreau, if desired. Divide the fruit into 4 glasses, alternating layers with the yogurt. Combine the remaining sweetener, cinnamon, and cocoa in a small bowl. Dust this on top of the parfait through a sieve, and serve.

Nutrition Facts

Serving Size 4 oz (113g)
Servings Per Container 6

Amount Per Serving

Calories 70 — Calories from Fat 0

	% Daily Value*
Total Fat 0g	0%
Saturated Fat 0g	0%
Trans Fat 0g	
Cholesterol 0mg	0%
Sodium 15mg	1%
Total Carbohydrate 18g	6%
Dietary Fiber 1g	5%
Sugars 17g	
Protein 2g	

Vitamin A 6%	•	Vitamin C 10%
Calcium 4%	•	Iron 2%

* Percent Daily Values are based on a 2,000 calorie diet. Your daily values may be higher or lower depending on your calorie needs.

	Calories	2,000	2,500
Total Fat	Less than	65g	80g
Sat Fat	Less than	20g	25g
Cholesterol	Less than	300mg	300mg
Sodium	Less than	2,400mg	2,400mg
Total Carbohydrate		300g	375g
Dietary Fiber		25g	30g

Calories per gram:
Fat 9 • Carbohydrate 4 • Protein 4

CONTAINS: Milk

FRESH PEACH AND BLUEBERRY
TARTLET WITH BLACKBERRY COULIS

THIS IS A companion dessert to the parfait. When the fresh peaches and blueberries are available, this makes an elegant and satisfying dessert or brunch snack. The healthier but equally delicious "deconstructed" version is included as well, and that is what is used for the nutritional analysis.

1 box puff pastry shells (6 shells; for "deconstructed" version use ½ c. granola)
2 fresh ripe peaches, chopped
4 tbsp. natural sugar, divided
2 tsp. cinnamon (or 1 stick fresh ground)
1 tsp. allspice
1 lemon, juiced
¼ tsp. lemon zest
1 pt. blackberries
½ pt. blueberries
6 oz. vanilla yogurt

Nutrition Facts	
Serving Size 5 oz (142g)	
Servings Per Container 8	
Amount Per Serving	
Calories 90	Calories from Fat 10
	% Daily Value*
Total Fat 1g	1%
Saturated Fat 0g	0%
Trans Fat 0g	
Cholesterol 0mg	0%
Sodium 25mg	1%
Total Carbohydrate 18g	6%
Dietary Fiber 4g	17%
Sugars 12g	
Protein 3g	
Vitamin A 6% • Vitamin C 25%	
Calcium 6% • Iron 4%	

* Percent Daily Values are based on a 2,000 calorie diet. Your daily values may be higher or lower depending on your calorie needs.

	Calories	2,000	2,500
Total Fat	Less than	65g	80g
Sat Fat	Less than	20g	25g
Cholesterol	Less than	300mg	300mg
Sodium	Less than	2,400mg	2,400mg
Total Carbohydrate		300g	375g
Dietary Fiber		25g	30g

Calories per gram:
Fat 9 • Carbohydrate 4 • Protein 4

CONTAINS: Milk

Follow directions for puff pastry shells. After the shells bake, I like to remove any extra layers in the interior of the shell; this maneuver cuts down on some of the fat from the puff pastry shells. (For the "deconstructed" version, don't use the puff pastry shells.) Place the fresh chopped peaches in a bowl; you can leave the skins on if you prefer. Heat 3 tbsp. of sugar with the cinnamon and allspice in a saucepan over medium heat until the sugar starts to dissolve, about 3 to 5 minutes. Add the lemon juice and zest and peaches, and let cook over medium heat until sauce thickens slightly, about 10 minutes. While the peaches cook, make the coulis. Place the blackberries and 1 tbsp. of sugar in a blender, and puree. Run the liquid through a sieve, discarding the remaining pulp. When the peaches are done, remove from heat, and allow to cool to room temperature. Remove the pastry shell tops, and fill the pastry shells with the peach mixture, adding the blueberries either in layers or all together, depending on your preference. For the "deconstructed" version, mix the granola with the peaches and blueberries, and divide the fruit and granola mix among 6 large ring molds. Top with 1 tsp. of yogurt, and drizzle the coulis over the top and sides. Replace the top, and serve.

TZATZIKI

THIS IS AN incredibly versatile topping sumptuous on fresh-grilled bread or instead of mayonnaise on a sandwich. This version is head and shoulders above the pathetic white goop draped on top of poor gyro pretenders. This is another "basic." I like the dill in the basic, but if you are a traditionalist, feel free to leave it out. I like the white pepper because I think freshly ground black pepper leaves unattractive black specks everywhere, but the choice is yours. Once you are comfortable, feel free to experiment. The smashed avocado version follows at the end. That on a fresh-grilled slice of baguette with a fresh tomato is a complete meal.

Nutrition Facts		
Serving Size 2 oz (57g)		
Servings Per Container 10		
Amount Per Serving		
Calories 25	Calories from Fat 0	
		% Daily Value*
Total Fat 0g		0%
Saturated Fat 0g		0%
Trans Fat 0g		
Cholesterol 0mg		0%
Sodium 260mg		11%
Total Carbohydrate 3g		1%
Dietary Fiber 0g		0%
Sugars 2g		
Protein 3g		
Vitamin A 0%	•	Vitamin C 2%
Calcium 0%	•	Iron 0%

* Percent Daily Values are based on a 2,000 calorie diet. Your daily values may be higher or lower depending on your calorie needs.

	Calories	2,000	2,500
Total Fat	Less than	65g	80g
Sat Fat	Less than	20g	25g
Cholesterol	Less than	300mg	300mg
Sodium	Less than	2,400mg	2,400mg
Total Carbohydrate		300g	375g
Dietary Fiber		25g	30g

Calories per gram:
Fat 9 • Carbohydrate 4 • Protein 4

1 cucumber
½ shallot (about 1 tbsp.)
1 container (10.6 oz.) Greek yogurt
½ lemon, juiced
⅛ tsp. cayenne
1 tsp. honey
1 garlic clove, chopped
2 sprigs fresh dill
Salt
White pepper

Peel the cucumber and split lengthwise into equal halves. Using a teaspoon, scoop out the seeds. Rough chop the cucumber, and place in a food processor, pulsing until it is a fine puree. Place the mixture in a sieve over the sink or bowl. Using a spatula or a wooden spoon, push the mixture against the sieve to force out the excess water. Transfer the remaining pulp to a separate bowl. Combine the shallot, yogurt, lemon juice, cayenne, honey, and garlic in the food processor, and puree. Rough chop the dill, and combine all ingredients. Season with salt and white pepper to taste. For the smashed avocado version, add 1 roughly chopped avocado to the food processor when processing the yogurt mixture. Then add approximately ⅛ c. of fresh cilantro, finely chopped, instead of adding the dill.

GOUGÈRES

THESE ARE basically savory cheese puffs made from a pâte à choux. This a savory variation of the basic method and ingredients used to create éclair and cream puff shells. They provide an automatic portion control given their small size. These are a favorite of mine when stuffed with fresh crisp lettuce; chopped garden tomatoes; a few pieces of crispy bacon, lardon style; and a bit of Greek yogurt on top (see the recipe for open-faced gougère mini-BLTs in chapter 17), all served with a bowl of roasted corn and tomato soup (see recipe in chapter 17). Truly a code delicious! Once made, the dough can be frozen or the shells made ahead of time and reheated at 400° F for about four to five minutes. Variations and stuffings abound—enjoy!

Nutrition Facts		
Serving Size 1 1/5 oz (34g)		
Servings Per Container 24		

Amount Per Serving		
Calories 150	Calories from Fat 130	
		% Daily Value*
Total Fat 15g		23%
Saturated Fat 5g		25%
Trans Fat 0g		
Cholesterol 15mg		6%
Sodium 20mg		1%
Total Carbohydrate 2g		1%
Dietary Fiber 0g		0%
Sugars 0g		
Protein 1g		

Vitamin A 4%	•	Vitamin C 2%
Calcium 2%	•	Iron 0%

* Percent Daily Values are based on a 2,000 calorie diet. Your daily values may be higher or lower depending on your calorie needs.

		Calories	2,000	2,500
Total Fat	Less than		65g	80g
Sat Fat	Less than		20g	25g
Cholesterol	Less than		300mg	300mg
Sodium	Less than		2,400mg	2,400mg
Total Carbohydrate			300g	375g
Dietary Fiber			25g	30g

Calories per gram:
Fat 9 • Carbohydrate 4 • Protein 4

CONTAINS: Milk

5 tbsp. unsalted butter
¼ tsp. salt + optional additional salt
¼ tsp. cayenne
¼ tsp. cumin
8 oz. water
4.5 oz (roughly 1 c.) all-purpose flour, sifted
¼ tsp. baking powder
3 eggs
⅓ c. Gruyère cheese, finely grated
⅓ c. parmesan cheese, finely grated
Milk (optional)
Additional cheese (optional)

Preheat the oven to 425° F. Place parchment paper on a baking sheet. In a 2 qt. saucepan over medium heat, melt butter slowly with salt, cayenne pepper, and ground cumin. When the butter is melted, add the water, and rapidly bring to a boil. Remove from heat, and add sifted flour and baking powder all at once. Combine with a wooden spoon. Mixing continuously, but not too vigorously (or the fat may separate out), place back on the heat for about a minute until the paste pulls away from the pan smoothly, leaving only a thin film. Transfer to a bowl, and allow to cool. The dough is done when it takes on a shiny gloss. Using the wooden spoon, or a paddle if using a mixing bowl, add the eggs one at a time. Add the Gruyère and parmesan cheeses, and combine. Transfer to a piping bag with a #6 tip (or use a resealable plastic bag with a hole cut in a bottom corner), and pipe approximately 1 in. rounds onto the baking sheet. You may top the pastry with a little milk, additional cheese, or salt as you desire. Bake for 10 minutes. Reduce the heat to 375° F for another 10 minutes. Continue to reduce the heat every few minutes (3- to 5-minute intervals) until 200° F is reached or the puffs turn golden brown, whichever occurs first. Do not open the oven too frequently while cooking; the puff is a steam-dependent process. Remove from the heat; the puffs should be dry. Pierce the top with a paring knife to let any steam escape (if it doesn't, the insides will get soggy). Allow to cool and cut the tops.

BLUEBERRY CHIMICHURRI SAUCE

THIS IS AN amazing variation of a chimichurri sauce. For a basic just omit the blueberries. These blueberries in the chimichurri work with any game meat, duck, goose, quail, and Cornish hens. Vary the additions, and create your own.

⅓ c. fresh blueberries
2 tbsp. water
1 c. extra-virgin olive oil
⅔ c. sherry wine vinegar
2 tbsp. lemon juice
⅓ c. fresh flat-leaf parsley, finely chopped
¼ c. fresh oregano, finely chopped
¼ c. fresh basil, finely chopped
1 garlic clove, peeled and chopped
2 tbsp. shallots, minced
1 fresh poblano pepper, coarsely chopped with the seeds left in
1 fresh serrano chili, coarsely chopped with the seeds removed
    (or left in for extra heat)
¼ tsp. freshly cracked black pepper
½ tsp. kosher salt
1 bay leaf

Nutrition Facts		
Serving Size 1 oz (28g)		
Servings Per Container 21		
Amount Per Serving		
Calories 80	Calories from Fat 70	
		% Daily Value*
Total Fat 8g		12%
Saturated Fat 1g		6%
Trans Fat 0g		
Cholesterol 0mg		0%
Sodium 55mg		2%
Total Carbohydrate 1g		0%
Dietary Fiber 0g		0%
Sugars 0g		
Protein 0g		
Vitamin A 2%	•	Vitamin C 15%
Calcium 0%	•	Iron 2%

* Percent Daily Values are based on a 2,000 calorie diet. Your daily values may be higher or lower depending on your calorie needs.

	Calories	2,000	2,500
Total Fat	Less than	65g	80g
Sat Fat	Less than	20g	25g
Cholesterol	Less than	300mg	300mg
Sodium	Less than	2,400mg	2,400mg
Total Carbohydrate		300g	375g
Dietary Fiber		25g	30g

Calories per gram:
Fat 9 • Carbohydrate 4 • Protein 4

Heat the blueberries and water in a small saucepan until the blueberries just begin to burst. Remove from the heat, and set aside to cool. Place the olive oil, sherry vinegar, lemon juice, parsley, basil, oregano, garlic, shallots, poblano pepper, and serrano chili in a food processor. Pulse until well blended, but do not puree. Season the mixture with the pepper and salt. Add the bay leaf and blueberries. Transfer the sauce to a nonreactive bowl, and cover with plastic wrap for at least 2 hours. Remove the bay leaf prior to serving. The sauce will keep in the refrigerator container for several days.

PEACH-MUSTARD GRILLING SAUCE

THIS IS A yummy changeup for the summer grill. This works great on chicken or pork and adds a sweet-and-sour flavor with a hint of spice. You can substitute mango for the peach for a grilling sauce with tropical overtones.

3 tbsp. butter or Smart Balance substitute
2 tbsp. onion, minced
2 garlic cloves, minced
3 tbsp. peach syrup
½ c. whole-grain mustard
¼ c. Dijon mustard
¾ c. fresh peaches, chopped
½ tsp. salt

Nutrition Facts		
Serving Size 1 oz (28g)		
Servings Per Container 16		
Amount Per Serving		
Calories 45	Calories from Fat 30	
		% Daily Value*
Total Fat 3g		5%
Saturated Fat 1.5g		7%
Trans Fat 0g		
Cholesterol 5mg		2%
Sodium 290mg		12%
Total Carbohydrate 3g		1%
Dietary Fiber 1g		2%
Sugars 2g		
Protein 1g		
Vitamin A 2%	•	Vitamin C 2%
Calcium 2%	•	Iron 2%

* Percent Daily Values are based on a 2,000 calorie diet. Your daily values may be higher or lower depending on your calorie needs.

	Calories	2,000	2,500
Total Fat	Less than	65g	80g
Sat Fat	Less than	20g	25g
Cholesterol	Less than	300mg	300mg
Sodium	Less than	2,400mg	2,400mg
Total Carbohydrate		300g	375g
Dietary Fiber		25g	30g

Calories per gram:
Fat 9 • Carbohydrate 4 • Protein 4

Place the butter or Smart Balance and onions in a saucepan over medium heat, and cook until onions are translucent, approximately 4 minutes. Add the rest of the ingredients, and bring to a boil. Reduce heat, and simmer 15 to 20 minutes. Remove from heat, and combine in a blender (in small batches), or use an immersion blender.

WESTERN NORTH CAROLINA BARBECUE SAUCE

THIS IS A more traditional barbecue and grilling sauce with flavors inspired by the mountainous regions of western North Carolina. This is a great and versatile basic recipe. I like it a little spicy, so this basic version has a little spice. Try the basic first. If you like it hotter, add more cayenne; if you like it a little sweeter, add more honey. If you like a little more tang in the taste, then add a touch more cider vinegar. You can really craft this one to your own preferences. Just remember to master the basic before experimenting with variations.

1½ c. onion, minced
4 tbsp. butter or Smart Balance substitute
4 garlic cloves, minced
½ tsp. dried oregano
½ tsp. dried thyme
2½ tsp. smoked paprika
½ tsp. onion powder
½ tsp. garlic powder

2 tsp. dry mustard
1 tsp. cayenne
2 tsp. Doc's barbecue spice rub (see recipe in this chapter)
½ tsp. black pepper
6 oz. tomato paste
1½ c. water
¾ c. cider vinegar
2 tbsp. honey

Place the onions and butter or Smart Balance in a saucepan over medium heat, and cook until onions are translucent, approximately 4 minutes. Add garlic, oregano, thyme, smoked paprika, onion powder, garlic powder, dry mustard, cayenne, Doc's barbecue spice rub, pepper, and tomato paste, and cook, stirring constantly, until the tomato paste turns brick in color, about 5 minutes. Add the water, vinegar, and honey, and bring to a boil, then reduce to a simmer, stirring frequently until reduced by about a third. Remove from heat, and cool. Use an immersion blender or place in batches into a blender to puree everything together.

Nutrition Facts		
Serving Size 1 oz (28g)		
Servings Per Container 40		
Amount Per Serving		
Calories 20	Calories from Fat 10	
		% Daily Value*
Total Fat 1g		2%
Saturated Fat 0g		0%
Trans Fat 0g		
Cholesterol 0mg		0%
Sodium 40mg		2%
Total Carbohydrate 3g		1%
Dietary Fiber 0g		0%
Sugars 2g		
Protein 0g		
Vitamin A 4%	•	Vitamin C 2%
Calcium 0%	•	Iron 2%

* Percent Daily Values are based on a 2,000 calorie diet. Your daily values may be higher or lower depending on your calorie needs.

	Calories	2,000	2,500
Total Fat	Less than	65g	80g
Sat Fat	Less than	20g	25g
Cholesterol	Less than	300mg	300mg
Sodium	Less than	2,400mg	2,400mg
Total Carbohydrate		300g	375g
Dietary Fiber		25g	30g

Calories per gram:
Fat 9 • Carbohydrate 4 • Protein 4

CONTAINS: Fish

MEDITERRANEAN MARINADE

THIS IS A delightful marinade that is equally at home for chicken or flavorful fish like salmon. The marinade can also be reduced in a hot pan and drizzled over the protein for a fantastic pan sauce. Remember, don't use any wine in cooking that you would not drink.

½ c. olive oil
1 sprig each fresh rosemary, oregano, thyme, basil
1 tbsp. red onion, chopped
1 garlic clove, crushed
1 lemon, juiced
1 tsp. hot sauce
1 c. white wine
2 tsp. salt
1 tsp. freshly ground black pepper

Combine all ingredients, and whisk together. Marinade may be stored several days in the refrigerator.

Nutrition Facts		
Serving Size 1 oz (28g)		
Servings Per Container 16		
Amount Per Serving		
Calories 80	Calories from Fat 70	
		% Daily Value*
Total Fat 8g		12%
Saturated Fat 1g		5%
Trans Fat 0g		
Cholesterol 0mg		0%
Sodium 320mg		13%
Total Carbohydrate 1g		0%
Dietary Fiber 0g		0%
Sugars 0g		
Protein 0g		
Vitamin A 0%	•	Vitamin C 2%
Calcium 0%	•	Iron 0%

* Percent Daily Values are based on a 2,000 calorie diet. Your daily values may be higher or lower depending on your calorie needs.

	Calories	2,000	2,500
Total Fat	Less than	65g	80g
Sat Fat	Less than	20g	25g
Cholesterol	Less than	300mg	300mg
Sodium	Less than	2,400mg	2,400mg
Total Carbohydrate		300g	375g
Dietary Fiber		25g	30g

Calories per gram:
Fat 9 • Carbohydrate 4 • Protein 4

SHELLFISH MARINADE

THIS IS A grand flavor booster to shellfish. I particularly like it with crabs, prawns, shrimp, squid, and scallops, but you can use it with any shellfish. It's fantastic to mix this up at the beach, marinate your catch, and grill on the sand.

4 lemons, juiced
½ tsp. lemon zest
¼ tsp. fresh ginger, grated
1 dried red chili, chopped (you can add another if you like for a
  little extra zing)
1 garlic clove, smashed and chopped
¼ c. peach (or apple) cider
1 scallion or green onion, chopped
⅓ c. olive oil
1 tsp. sesame oil
1 tsp. salt
½ tsp. pepper

Nutrition Facts		
Serving Size 1 oz (28g)		
Servings Per Container 12		
Amount Per Serving		
Calories 60	Calories from Fat 50	
		% Daily Value*
Total Fat 6g		9%
Saturated Fat 1g		4%
Trans Fat 0g		
Cholesterol 0mg		0%
Sodium 210mg		9%
Total Carbohydrate 2g		1%
Dietary Fiber 0g		0%
Sugars 1g		
Protein 0g		
Vitamin A 2%	•	Vitamin C 20%
Calcium 0%	•	Iron 0%

* Percent Daily Values are based on a 2,000 calorie diet. Your daily values may be higher or lower depending on your calorie needs.

	Calories	2,000	2,500
Total Fat	Less than	65g	80g
Sat Fat	Less than	20g	25g
Cholesterol	Less than	300mg	300mg
Sodium	Less than	2,400mg	2,400mg
Total Carbohydrate		300g	375g
Dietary Fiber		25g	30g

Calories per gram:
  Fat 9 • Carbohydrate 4 • Protein 4

Combine all ingredients, and whisk together. Marinade may be stored several days in the refrigerator.

BRINES

SO WHAT IS the difference between brine and a marinade? The key difference is the salt. The main focus of brine is to add moisture, and the simplest brine is salt and water. Flavor components can be added, but the purpose is to add moisture. The purpose of a marinade is to add flavor, but it can add moisture to the product as well. Clearly there can be a gray zone. Regardless of what you label this, I use it with wild game and pork, too, because the meat is so lean that it can easily dry out. That is especially true when smoking or cooking long and slow, which is how I like to cook some game meats. Those methods allow the finished result to be tender and juicy and don't add additional fats as happens in recipes recommending wrapping in bacon during the cooking process.

Wild Game Brine

3 c. pickling salt
1 c. brown sugar
4–5 qts. water
1 orange, quartered
1 lemon, quartered
4 sprigs thyme
2 sprigs rosemary
¼ c. garlic, smashed
1 jalapeño, sliced (keep the membrane and seeds intact if you like it hotter)
1 onion, quartered
3 ribs celery, roughly chopped
3 carrots, roughly chopped
⅓ c. apple cider vinegar
1 can Guinness beer

Add the salt and brown sugar to the water; bring to a boil to dissolve. As the mixture cools, add all the other ingredients. Allow to come to room temperature, and then add the game meat. Make sure the liquid is room temperature before adding any meat. It is important you do not cook or poach the meat. Brine the meat for 6 to 24 hours.

Poultry Brine

3 c. pickling salt
1 c. brown sugar
4–5 qts. water
1 orange, quartered
1 lemon, quartered
4 sprigs thyme
2 sprigs rosemary
¼ c. poultry seasoning
1 jalapeño, sliced (keep the membrane and seeds intact if you like it hotter)
1 onion, quartered
3 ribs celery, roughly chopped
3 carrots, roughly chopped
⅓ c. apple cider vinegar

Add the salt and brown sugar to the water; bring to a boil to dissolve. As the mixture cools, add all the other ingredients. Allow to come to room temperature, and then add the game meat. Brine for 8 to 48 hours.

STOCKS

WHAT'S THE difference between broth and stock? A stock is made with bones. Therefore, there really is no such thing as a vegetable stock. Anthony Bourdain writes that the difference between a lot of delicious restaurant food and mediocre home-cooked food is the stock. He's right. I think when a recipe calls for stock, there is no substitute for stock from scratch. You don't need a lot of different stocks. A light and dark chicken stock will work with about everything. There really is no reason not to have some on hand. It is made in bulk and freezes well. You'll use it up before it has a chance to go bad. A word of caution: Once you go homemade stock, there is no going back.

Light Chicken Stock

   3 chicken carcasses (fryer size)
   3 onions, peeled and quartered
   4 large garlic cloves, smashed and roughly chopped
   4 large carrots, peeled and cut in large chunks
   6 celery stalks, cut in large chunks (leaves attached)
   1 leek, chopped (optional)
   2 bay leaves
   3–5 sprigs thyme
   3–5 sprigs oregano
   3–5 sprigs parsley
   4–6 qts. water
   1 tbsp. whole black peppercorns

Place all ingredients together in a large stockpot. Make sure the water level covers the chicken. Bring to a simmer for 4 to 6 hours. Do not let it boil. Pour the liquid through a mesh strainer. Place in containers, let cool, and put in the refrigerator for several days, or freeze for a few months.

Dark Chicken (and Meat) Stock

   1–2 tbsp. vegetable oil
   3 chicken carcasses (fryer size), roughly chopped
   2 onions, peeled and quartered
   2 large garlic cloves, smashed and roughly chopped
   2 large carrots, peeled and cut in large chunks
   3 celery stalks, cut in large chunks (leaves attached)

1 leek, chopped (optional)
1 bay leaf
3–5 sprigs thyme
3–5 sprigs oregano
3–5 sprigs parsley
1½ qts. water
1 tbsp. whole black peppercorns

Preheat the oven to 450° F. Place a large roasting pan on the stovetop over high heat, and add the oil. After about a minute, add the chopped chicken carcasses. Stir, and then place in the oven. Roast for about 45 minutes. Then add the onions, garlic, carrots, celery, leek, bay leaf, thyme, oregano, and parsley, and roast for another 20 minutes. Add the water and peppercorns, and stir, loosening the brown bits. Roast for an additional 15 to 20 minutes, and then remove and let cool. Strain the liquid, and be sure to press the liquid out from all the solids. Place in containers, let cool, and put in the refrigerator for several days, or freeze for a few months. For a meat (beef or lamb) stock, use about 2 lbs. of meat bones instead of the chicken carcasses.

Fish and Shellfish Stock

2 lbs. fish bones or crustacean shells
1–2 tbsp. olive oil
2 onions, peeled and chopped
2 large garlic cloves, smashed and roughly chopped
2 large carrots, peeled and chopped
3 celery stalks, chopped (leaves attached)
1 leek, chopped (optional)
1 bay leaf
3–5 sprigs thyme
3–5 sprigs parsley
1½ qts. water

Quickly sweat the fish bones or crustacean shells in the olive oil over medium heat for several minutes. This step is optional but helps release additional flavor. Add everything to the water in a large stockpot and simmer (do not boil, or the stock will cloud) for 45 minutes. Strain the liquid, and be sure to press the liquid out from all the solids. Place in containers, let cool, and put in the refrigerator for several days, or freeze for a few months.

Fish Fumet

A fish fumet is much more strongly flavored than a fish stock. It is used when you need or desire a stronger flavor. Soups are a good example.

    2 lbs. fish bones or crustacean shells
    1–2 tbsp. olive oil
    ½ onion, peeled and chopped
    3–5 sprigs thyme
    3–5 sprigs parsley
    1½ qts. fish stock (see recipe in this chapter)
    1 c. white wine
    ½ lemon, juiced then sliced

Sweat the bones or shells in the olive oil over medium heat for several minutes. Add all the ingredients to a large stockpot, including the lemon juice and lemon slices as well. If you have leftover mushroom trimmings, they can be added to the fumet. Simmer (do not boil, or the stock will cloud) for 45 minutes. Strain the liquid, and be sure to press the liquid out from all the solids. Place in containers, let cool, and put in the refrigerator for several days, or freeze for a few months.

Vegetable Nage

I love having this base around. It supplies a light, delicate backdrop of flavor. A nage is an aromatic court bouillon. A court bouillon is a flavored liquid, usually water with wine or vinegar. You can use this to poach fish or other things; I use it as I would a vegetable "stock." If you are planning to do any vegetarian cooking, you absolutely need this preparation. Although the flavors are subtle, they give you a canvas. Without it, if you just used water for the soups or other instances when you use this, the meal will be bland. There are a number of dishes and vegetable sides that can be converted to completely vegetarian dishes by simply using this, in equal amounts, for a light chicken stock. If you're cooking for vegetarians, remember the stock counts!

    6 onions, quartered
    12 carrots, roughly chopped
    2 lemons, quartered
    4 celery stalks, roughly chopped
    1 tsp. white peppercorns
    1 tsp. pink peppercorns

2 bay leaves
8 star anise pods
4 qts. water
2 c. white wine
2–3 sprigs tarragon
2–3 sprigs basil
2–3 sprigs cilantro
2–3 sprigs thyme
2–3 sprigs parsley

Bring the first 8 ingredients to a boil in the water. If your tap has any off flavors, use bottled water, as the nage has very subtle flavor characteristics. Reduce to a simmer, and continue for about 15 minutes more. Remove from heat, and allow to cool to room temperature. Add the wine, and then strain the entire mixture. The resulting liquid should be clear. Add the herbs, refrigerate for 24 hours, and then strain again. Place in containers, let cool, and put in the refrigerator for several days, or freeze for a few months.

ROASTED GARLIC PUREE

THIS IS A great item to have around. It will keep in the refrigerator, and you can pull it out to add to a dish, or just smear on some bread or toast and you have easy and tasty garlic bread. You can also simply roast the heads of garlic at 225° F covered in aluminum foil, olive oil, salt, and pepper for about 45 minutes and extract the paste.

2 heads of garlic, paper and skins removed and roughly chopped
1 tbsp. olive oil
1 oz. butter or Smart Balance substitute
⅓ c. cider vinegar
¾ c. water

Sauté the garlic in the olive oil and butter or Smart Balance in a pan over medium heat. Once the garlic is golden brown, add the cider vinegar and water. Reduce the mixture until the liquid is almost gone. Place in a food processor and puree.

Nutrition Facts		
Serving Size 1 oz (28g)		
Servings Per Container 2		
Amount Per Serving		
Calories 30	Calories from Fat 25	
		% Daily Value*
Total Fat 2.5g		4%
Saturated Fat 1.5g		6%
Trans Fat 0g		
Cholesterol 5mg		2%
Sodium 0mg		0%
Total Carbohydrate 2g		1%
Dietary Fiber 0g		0%
Sugars 0g		
Protein 0g		
Vitamin A 2%	•	Vitamin C 2%
Calcium 2%	•	Iron 0%

* Percent Daily Values are based on a 2,000 calorie diet. Your daily values may be higher or lower depending on your calorie needs.

	Calories	2,000	2,500
Total Fat	Less than	65g	80g
Sat Fat	Less than	20g	25g
Cholesterol	Less than	300mg	300mg
Sodium	Less than	2,400mg	2,400mg
Total Carbohydrate		300g	375g
Dietary Fiber		25g	30g

Calories per gram:
Fat 9 • Carbohydrate 4 • Protein 4

HERBED OLIVE OIL

THIS IS REALLY useful to coat meats before grilling to add a subtle, herbed flavor. It is also nice for using in vinaigrettes. Make sure to use fresh herbs.

2 c. olive oil
2 tbsp. each of rosemary, sage, thyme, basil, and oregano, roughly chopped

Place all the ingredients in a saucepan with the oil. Bring to a medium heat, and then reduce the heat and simmer for 30 to 45 minutes. Strain the oil, and place in an airtight container. Use as needed.

MARINARA SAUCE

THIS IS A really simple sauce and made fresh will keep for several days in the refrigerator, if you don't eat it all up before then. Making it fresh also avoids the extra sugars, preservatives, and refined and processed foods in the store versions. If you can, get Italian San Marzano tomatoes. These are grown from the region near Mount Vesuvius, and the volcanic soil gives them a unique flavor profile.

Nutrition Facts	
Serving Size 4 oz (113g)	
Servings Per Container 16	

Amount Per Serving	
Calories 50	Calories from Fat 15

	% Daily Value*
Total Fat 2g	3%
Saturated Fat 0g	0%
Trans Fat 0g	
Cholesterol 10mg	3%
Sodium 250mg	10%
Total Carbohydrate 9g	3%
Dietary Fiber 2g	8%
Sugars 3g	
Protein 2g	

Vitamin A 20%	•	Vitamin C 15%
Calcium 2%	•	Iron 8%

* Percent Daily Values are based on a 2,000 calorie diet. Your daily values may be higher or lower depending on your calorie needs.

	Calories	2,000	2,500
Total Fat	Less than	65g	80g
Sat Fat	Less than	20g	25g
Cholesterol	Less than	300mg	300mg
Sodium	Less than	2,400mg	2,400mg
Total Carbohydrate		300g	375g
Dietary Fiber		25g	30g

Calories per gram:
Fat 9 • Carbohydrate 4 • Protein 4

2 tbsp. olive oil
½ c. yellow onion, chopped
1 garlic clove, finely chopped
¼ c. carrots, chopped
¼ c. celery, chopped
1 tsp. each of thyme, basil, and oregano, roughly chopped
¼ tsp. sage, finely chopped
1 tbsp. anchovy paste
2 tbsp. tomato paste
½ c. red wine
1 can (28 oz.) tomato puree
1 can (28 oz.) diced tomatoes
1 bay leaf
2 tbsp. fresh flat-leaf parsley, finely chopped

Heat the olive oil over medium-high heat. Add the onions and garlic, and cook for about 5 minutes until the onions are translucent. Add the carrots and celery. Sauté another 5 to

10 minutes until the vegetables are soft. Add the thyme, basil, oregano, and sage. Stir for another minute. Add the anchovy paste and tomato paste. Stir for one more minute. Add the wine, and let it sit for about 3 minutes. Add the tomato puree, diced tomatoes, bay leaf, and parsley. Reduce heat and simmer for about an hour, or until the sauce reduces and thickens. Remove bay leaf. Blend in small batches in a blender, or use an immersion blender so the sauce has a thick, even consistency.

MARGARITA MARINADE

THIS IS A delicious marinade for pork or chicken. Reserve some marinade when you make this before you place the meat into the marinade. Then, when it comes off the grill, place the meat in a bowl with some marinade and loosely cover with foil to rest. It'll grab some extra flavor this way.

2 tbsp. olive oil
3 limes, juiced
2 tbsp. light brown sugar
1 c. tequila
2 tsp. Dijon mustard
1 dried hot pepper, crushed
¼ tsp. freshly ground allspice
¼ tsp. dried oregano
¼ tsp. dried thyme
¼ tsp. onion powder
¼ tsp. garlic powder
¼ tsp. cayenne pepper
½ tsp. paprika
2 tbsp. fresh cilantro, chopped
1 tsp. fresh mint, chopped

Combine all ingredients in a bowl, and mix thoroughly.

Nutrition Facts		
Serving Size 1 oz (28g)		
Servings Per Container 18		
Amount Per Serving		
Calories 40	Calories from Fat 15	
		% Daily Value*
Total Fat 2g		3%
Saturated Fat 0g		0%
Trans Fat 0g		
Cholesterol 0mg		0%
Sodium 45mg		2%
Total Carbohydrate 4g		1%
Dietary Fiber 0g		0%
Sugars 1g		
Protein 0g		
Vitamin A 4%	•	Vitamin C 10%
Calcium 0%	•	Iron 2%

* Percent Daily Values are based on a 2,000 calorie diet. Your daily values may be higher or lower depending on your calorie needs.

	Calories	2,000	2,500
Total Fat	Less than	65g	80g
Sat Fat	Less than	20g	25g
Cholesterol	Less than	300mg	300mg
Sodium	Less than	2,400mg	2,400mg
Total Carbohydrate		300g	375g
Dietary Fiber		25g	30g

Calories per gram:
Fat 9 • Carbohydrate 4 • Protein 4

SAVORY BASIC PIE CRUST

THIS IS A basic pie crust recipe. Like all pie crusts, you must resist the temptation to overwork the dough, or it will be too tough.

    3¼ c. (approximately 14.5 oz.) all-purpose flour
    1 tsp. salt
    1 c. cold, solid vegetable shortening (Crisco), cut in small cubes
    ½ c. butter, cut in small cubes
    4–5 tbsp. ice water

Nutrition Facts		
Serving Size 13 1/2 oz (383g)		
Servings Per Container 2		
Amount Per Serving		
Calories 2020 Calories from Fat 1290		
		% Daily Value*
Total Fat 146g		**225%**
Saturated Fat 0.5g		3%
Trans Fat 0g		
Cholesterol 0mg		**0%**
Sodium 1170mg		**49%**
Total Carbohydrate 149g		**50%**
Dietary Fiber 1g		3%
Sugars 2g		
Protein 22g		
Vitamin A 0%	•	Vitamin C 0%
Calcium 4%	•	Iron 50%

* Percent Daily Values are based on a 2,000 calorie diet. Your daily values may be higher or lower depending on your calorie needs.

	Calories	2,000	2,500
Total Fat	Less than	65g	80g
Sat Fat	Less than	20g	25g
Cholesterol	Less than	300mg	300mg
Sodium	Less than	2,400mg	2,400mg
Total Carbohydrate		300g	375g
Dietary Fiber		25g	30g

Calories per gram:
Fat 9 • Carbohydrate 4 • Protein 4

In a large mixing bowl, combine the flour and salt. Add the shortening to the flour mixture. You do not need to worry about overworking the dough until you add the water. Work the shortening in with your hands until it resembles coarse bread crumbs. Add the butter, likewise working it in. Add the water, 1 tbsp. at a time, working it in with your hands. The dough should just adhere together. The exact amount of water will vary by flour, relative humidity, and so on. Add only as much as water as you need to the dough. Wrap it in plastic wrap and refrigerate for at least 30 minutes; overnight is better. Remove the dough from the refrigerator, and place it on a lightly floured surface. Cut the dough in two, rewrap the unused half in plastic wrap, and place in the refrigerator. For each crust roll the dough out on the floured surface until it is about ⅛ in. thick. The shape depends on what the application is for; the most common shape is round.

ENCHILADA SAUCE

THIS IS A tasty sauce with a lot of uses. The peppers are mild, so it has good flavor without overwhelming heat, but you can always "Doc" it up. The canned sauces cannot compare.

    2 tbsp. olive oil
    ½ c. yellow onion, chopped
    1 tsp. garlic, finely chopped
    1¼ tsp. dried oregano
    1 tsp. cumin

¼ tsp. dried thyme

¼ tsp. cayenne pepper

¼ tsp. onion powder

¼ tsp. garlic powder

½ tsp. paprika

3 dried California (usually Anaheim) peppers, chopped

1 can (28 oz.) chopped tomatoes

1 tbsp. corn masa flour

1 c. light or dark chicken stock (see recipes in this chapter)

Heat the olive oil over medium-high heat. Add onions and garlic. Cook for about 5 minutes, until the onions are translucent. Add the oregano, cumin, thyme, cayenne, onion powder, garlic powder, paprika, and peppers. Cook for another minute. Add the tomatoes, masa flour, and chicken stock, and bring to a boil. Reduce heat, and simmer for about an hour, or until the sauce reduces and thickens. Blend in small batches in a blender, or use an immersion blender so the sauce has a thick, even consistency.

BAKED PITA CHIPS

THIS IS A super-easy way to get some chips for hummus or other dipping sauces without the added fat of deep-fried chips. They will keep for several days in a plastic bag. You can use tortillas for tortilla chips prepared the same way. For tortilla chips, I like to sprinkle the chips with a little fresh lime juice when they come out of the oven. A great way to do that is to put the juice in a misting bottle and mist the chips. It's the same way I like to apply the olive oil.

As many pita rounds as you like (each round makes 8 chips; 4 chips per tortilla)
Olive oil
Salt

Preheat the oven to 450° F. Line a baking sheet with aluminum foil. Cut the pitas into quarters, and then take each triangle and break it in half at the base. Lay the triangles on the baking sheet. Mist with olive oil, and sprinkle with salt. Cook for 3 to 5 minutes, or until desired degree of crispness is achieved. Remove and cool.

Nutrition Facts

Serving Size 2 oz (57g)
Servings Per Container 22

Amount Per Serving

Calories 35	Calories from Fat 15

	% Daily Value*
Total Fat 1.5g	2%
Saturated Fat 0g	0%
Trans Fat 0g	
Cholesterol 0mg	0%
Sodium 70mg	3%
Total Carbohydrate 5g	2%
Dietary Fiber 1g	5%
Sugars 0g	
Protein 1g	

Vitamin A 15%	•	Vitamin C 6%
Calcium 2%	•	Iron 6%

* Percent Daily Values are based on a 2,000 calorie diet. Your daily values may be higher or lower depending on your calorie needs.

	Calories	2,000	2,500
Total Fat	Less than	65g	80g
Sat Fat	Less than	20g	25g
Cholesterol	Less than	300mg	300mg
Sodium	Less than	2,400mg	2,400mg
Total Carbohydrate		300g	375g
Dietary Fiber		25g	30g

Calories per gram:
Fat 9 • Carbohydrate 4 • Protein 4

FAJITA MARINADE

THIS IS A great marinade for flank steak, a perfect cut to throw on the grill and serve with tortillas, guacamole, salsa, grilled onions and peppers, and fresh veggie toppings for outstanding fajitas. The marinade will also work for chicken and shrimp as well. Marinate the steak at least 4 hours if using flank or other tougher cuts.

> 4 oz. olive oil
> 2 garlic cloves, smashed
> ½ tsp. dried oregano
> ½ tsp. dried thyme
> ½ tsp. cayenne
> ½ tsp. garlic powder
> ½ tsp. paprika
> 1 tbsp. + ½ tsp. onion powder
> 1 tbsp. chili powder
> 2 tsp. ground cumin
> 1 bay leaf
> Approximately 4 oz. of juice consisting of the juice of 1 grapefruit, 1 lemon, and 1 lime
> 3 tbsp. apple cider vinegar
> ½ tsp. salt
> ½ tsp. freshly ground black pepper

Nutrition Facts		
Serving Size 1 oz (28g)		
Servings Per Container 8		
Amount Per Serving		
Calories 90	Calories from Fat 80	
		% Daily Value*
Total Fat 9g		**14%**
Saturated Fat 1g		**6%**
Trans Fat 0g		
Cholesterol 0mg		**0%**
Sodium 200mg		**8%**
Total Carbohydrate 3g		**1%**
Dietary Fiber 1g		**2%**
Sugars 0g		
Protein 0g		
Vitamin A 6%	•	Vitamin C 10%
Calcium 2%	•	Iron 4%

* Percent Daily Values are based on a 2,000 calorie diet. Your daily values may be higher or lower depending on your calorie needs.

	Calories	2,000	2,500
Total Fat	Less than	65g	80g
Sat Fat	Less than	20g	25g
Cholesterol	Less than	300mg	300mg
Sodium	Less than	2,400mg	2,400mg
Total Carbohydrate		300g	375g
Dietary Fiber		25g	30g

Calories per gram:
Fat 9 • Carbohydrate 4 • Protein 4

Combine all ingredients and mix together well.

OLIVE OIL HOLLANDAISE

MY TRADITIONAL basic hollandaise is very easy, very good, and decadent. It has a stick of butter, the juice of two lemons, and 3 egg yolks. I have cooked the culinary school–version with vinegar reduction and so on. This version replaces the butter with olive oil, but it is still a very rich sauce. Use it sparingly, and enjoy. It is great for Sunday brunch and eggs Benedict; a little over some broccoli or other vegetables are delicious as well.

> ½ c. of olive oil (not extra-virgin olive oil)
> 3 egg yolks
> 2 lemons, juiced
> Salt
> White pepper

The key to making this sauce is to properly temper the egg yolks and form a liaison. A liaison is a mixture of egg yolks and usually a fat, such as heavy cream. This combination gently thickens a preparation. Tempering is a process where the temperature at which the egg yolks coagulate is raised by adding a hot liquid to the yolks in small amounts. Egg yolks normally coagulate between 149 and 158° F. By gently whisking in the heated oil, that coagulation point is raised to 180 to 185° F. That way the sauce can be made safely (over 140° F) and not curdle (under 185° F). Use a thermometer the first few times you do this. Heat the olive oil over medium-low heat. Do not allow the oil to get too hot, or you will make scrambled eggs. Meanwhile, mix the egg yolks and lemon juice. Slowly add ⅓ of the heated oil to the egg and lemon juice mixture while whisking. Add the rest of the oil. Whisk the egg, juice, and oil mixture in a bowl heated over some boiling water. This allows you to control the temperature by removing the bowl or placing it over the pot. The sauce should turn pale yellow and be light and frothy. Season with salt and white pepper.

PICKLED BEETS

I AM NOT a beet guy. I never really cared for them. We all like some foods more than others, and there are those we just care for less. One of the great things about cooking for others is that sometimes you end up cooking things you normally wouldn't if it were just for yourself. I've probably had beets about twelve times in twelve different ways, none of which I particularly enjoyed. But a menu called for some pickled beets. Consequently I got my basic quick-pickling recipe, changed the vinegar types, and added a dash of heat. I used some sweeter baby beets. A rule of cooking is that you must taste what you serve; therefore I had to eat the beet. Delicious! It just goes to show that, with an open mind and the right preparation, we can enjoy what we once disregarded; like the little ugly duckling this has grown up beautifully. So visit some ugly ducklings from your past, and see if you can give them a total makeover. This is a basic pickling recipe and can be used for any number of vegetables.

    1 c. apple cider vinegar
    ½ c. rice wine vinegar
    2 tbsp. pickling spice
    2 tbsp. sugar
    1 tbsp. salt
    1 cayenne or similar pepper, split lengthwise
    8 baby beets (approximately 1 lb.), cooked and peeled

Place the apple cider vinegar, rice wine vinegar, pickling spice, sugar, salt, and cayenne in a medium saucepan. Bring to a boil to dissolve the salt and sugar. Remove from heat, and bring to room temperature. Place the beets in sealable container (you may slice or place in whole) and cover with pickling liquid. Refrigerate overnight.

APPLE PIE GRANITA

THIS IS A great light dessert when you just need a little something to put that final *fini* with an exclamation point. A granita is also nice as a midcourse palate cleanser or even as part of an amuse-bouche. The granita here is another "basic," so you can substitute other juices and flavors, even alcoholic beverages, like margaritas. Just remember that alcohol lowers the freezing point, so too much alcohol, and you just get a really cold drink—not necessarily a negative.

Nutrition Facts		
Serving Size 1 1/2 oz (43g)		
Servings Per Container 24		
Amount Per Serving		
Calories 30	Calories from Fat 0	
		% Daily Value*
Total Fat 0g		0%
Saturated Fat 0g		0%
Trans Fat 0g		
Cholesterol 0mg		0%
Sodium 5mg		0%
Total Carbohydrate 7g		2%
Dietary Fiber 0g		0%
Sugars 6g		
Protein 0g		
Vitamin A 0%	•	Vitamin C 20%
Calcium 2%	•	Iron 0%

* Percent Daily Values are based on a 2,000 calorie diet. Your daily values may be higher or lower depending on your calorie needs.

	Calories	2,000	2,500
Total Fat	Less than	65g	80g
Sat Fat	Less than	20g	25g
Cholesterol	Less than	300mg	300mg
Sodium	Less than	2,400mg	2,400mg
Total Carbohydrate		300g	375g
Dietary Fiber		25g	30g

Calories per gram:
Fat 9 • Carbohydrate 4 • Protein 4

CONTAINS: Milk

⅓ c. sugar or Splenda/Truvia (use proper sweetness conversion)
3 c. apple juice
1 lime, juiced
2 tbsp. apple pie spice (see recipe in this chapter)
6–8 oz. vanilla yogurt

Combine sugar, apple juice, lime juice, and apple pie spice in a blender, and mix thoroughly. Pour into a saucepan, bring to a simmer (do not boil), and allow to cool gently back to room temperature. Filter through fine sieve lined with cheesecloth.
Pour the mixture into a 9 or 10 in. metal baking pan. Freeze the mixture, checking every hour or so to smash out lumps or chunks if they form. It should be fully frozen in 4 to 5 hours. To serve, place a tablespoon of yogurt on the bottom of a martini or other cocktail glass. Shave thin layers of the granita, and place on top. Serve immediately.

APPLE PIE SPICE

I love spice combinations that evoke complete experiences. Knowing how to make these spice combinations allows you to have them around anytime you need them. You can also vary to suit your palate. Need a little more cinnamon? Add it. Less cardamom, reduce. These spice combinations are simply bases from which you vary as you need. They also save you money from having to buy the premixed, often stale, spices from the mega-marts.

    4 tbsp. ground cinnamon
    2 tbsp. ground nutmeg
    1 tbsp. ground allspice
    1 tbsp. ground cardamom

Combine all ingredients in an airtight container, mix well, and store. This will keep for several months.

Nutrition Facts

Serving Size 1 oz (28g)
Servings Per Container 8

Amount Per Serving	
Calories 90	Calories from Fat 80

	% Daily Value*
Total Fat 9g	14%
Saturated Fat 1g	6%
Trans Fat 0g	
Cholesterol 0mg	0%
Sodium 200mg	8%
Total Carbohydrate 3g	1%
Dietary Fiber 1g	2%
Sugars 0g	
Protein 0g	

Vitamin A 6%	•	Vitamin C 10%
Calcium 2%	•	Iron 4%

* Percent Daily Values are based on a 2,000 calorie diet. Your daily values may be higher or lower depending on your calorie needs.

	Calories	2,000	2,500
Total Fat	Less than	65g	80g
Sat Fat	Less than	20g	25g
Cholesterol	Less than	300mg	300mg
Sodium	Less than	2,400mg	2,400mg
Total Carbohydrate		300g	375g
Dietary Fiber		25g	30g

Calories per gram:
Fat 9 • Carbohydrate 4 • Protein 4

CRABBY PATTY DRESSING

This is not only scrumptious on crabby patties but also great on any seafood. If you have shrimp, calamari, or any other shellfish, it is perfect to offer this as well as the more traditional cocktail-based sauce. I also love this on some fresh grilled fish between two slices of some homemade bread. It is easy, delicious, and nutritious as a main.

    1 tbsp. red onion
    1 c. Greek yogurt
    1 lemon, juiced
    1 tbsp. garlic, finely minced
    1 tbsp. parsley, finely minced
    2 tsp. capers
    2 tsp. kosher dill pickle, finely chopped
    2 tsp. pickle juice
    ½ tsp. cayenne
    1 tbsp. Old Bay seasoning

Nutrition Facts

Serving Size 2 oz (57g)
Servings Per Container 45

Amount Per Serving	
Calories 15	Calories from Fat 0

	% Daily Value*
Total Fat 0g	0%
Saturated Fat 0g	0%
Trans Fat 0g	
Cholesterol 0mg	0%
Sodium 55mg	2%
Total Carbohydrate 4g	1%
Dietary Fiber 0g	0%
Sugars 2g	
Protein 1g	

Vitamin A 0%	•	Vitamin C 35%
Calcium 0%	•	Iron 0%

* Percent Daily Values are based on a 2,000 calorie diet. Your daily values may be higher or lower depending on your calorie needs.

	Calories	2,000	2,500
Total Fat	Less than	65g	80g
Sat Fat	Less than	20g	25g
Cholesterol	Less than	300mg	300mg
Sodium	Less than	2,400mg	2,400mg
Total Carbohydrate		300g	375g
Dietary Fiber		25g	30g

Calories per gram:
Fat 9 • Carbohydrate 4 • Protein 4

Place the red onion in ice water for 15 minutes to remove some of the stronger, bitter flavors of the raw red onion. Remove the onion, chop, and place with all the other ingredients in a bowl. Mix thoroughly.

DOC'S BARBECUE SPICE RUB

THERE ARE as many spice rubs for Southern barbecue as there are people who eat it. This is a very basic barbecue spice rub to get you started. Continue to experiment with flavors you like and degrees of spice, and add to this "starter" kit. This barbecue rub is delicious on any meat. As a basic it allows you to spice or sweeten it up as you like; think of it as a blank canvas. I like to multiply the quantities and keep a large batch on hand. It stores well.

Nutrition Facts		
Serving Size 5 g		
Servings Per Container 9		
Amount Per Serving		
Calories 20	Calories from Fat 5	
		% Daily Value*
Total Fat 0.5g		1%
Saturated Fat 0g		0%
Trans Fat 0g		
Cholesterol 0mg		0%
Sodium 170mg		7%
Total Carbohydrate 3g		1%
Dietary Fiber 1g		4%
Sugars 1g		
Protein 1g		
Vitamin A 15%	• Vitamin C 2%	
Calcium 2%	• Iron 4%	

* Percent Daily Values are based on a 2,000 calorie diet. Your daily values may be higher or lower depending on your calorie needs.

	Calories	2,000	2,500
Total Fat	Less than	65g	80g
Sat Fat	Less than	20g	25g
Cholesterol	Less than	300mg	300mg
Sodium	Less than	2,400mg	2,400mg
Total Carbohydrate		300g	375g
Dietary Fiber		25g	30g

Calories per gram:
Fat 9 • Carbohydrate 4 • Protein 4

1 tsp. cumin seed
1 tsp. fennel seed
1 tsp. coriander seed
½ tsp. dried oregano
½ tsp. dried thyme
3 tsp. smoked paprika
½ tsp. onion powder
½ tsp. garlic powder
1½ tsp. cayenne pepper
2 tsp. dark brown sugar
1 tsp. dried ground chipotle chili pepper

Toast the cumin, fennel, and coriander seeds. Grind them together in a spice grinder or food processor. Combine with all the other ingredients, and mix well.

DOC'S SOUTH AFRICAN FIVE-SPICE BLEND

I WAS QUITE familiar with Chinese five-spice powder, but I had not heard of this combination until I visited South Africa. My thanks go out to Chef Tabitha at Ezard House in Camps Bay. She not only prepared some amazing local dishes, both beautiful to see and delicious to taste, but also let me into her kitchen. I am also indebted to her for turning me on to this amazing blend. I don't know how I got on without it. If you ever head toward Cape Town, I suggest you visit Chef Tabitha at the Ezard House, where I recommend you stay as well.

Nutrition Facts		
Serving Size 1 Tbs (6g)		
Servings Per Container 30		
Amount Per Serving		
Calories 25	Calories from Fat 10	
		% Daily Value*
Total Fat 1g		2%
Saturated Fat 0g		0%
Trans Fat 0g		
Cholesterol 0mg		0%
Sodium 0mg		0%
Total Carbohydrate 3g		1%
Dietary Fiber 2g		7%
Sugars 0g		
Protein 1g		
Vitamin A 0%	•	Vitamin C 0%
Calcium 4%	•	Iron 6%

* Percent Daily Values are based on a 2,000 calorie diet. Your daily values may be higher or lower depending on your calorie needs.

	Calories	2,000	2,500
Total Fat	Less than	65g	80g
Sat Fat	Less than	20g	25g
Cholesterol	Less than	300mg	300mg
Sodium	Less than	2,400mg	2,400mg
Total Carbohydrate		300g	375g
Dietary Fiber		25g	30g

Calories per gram:
Fat 9 • Carbohydrate 4 • Protein 4

1 oz. cinnamon
2 oz. cumin seed
1 oz. anise seed
2 oz. coriander seed
1 oz. ginger powder

Combine all ingredients, and blend in a spice blender. Store in an airtight container.

DOC'S BLACKENING BLEND

2 tsp. paprika
4 tsp. dried thyme
2 tsp. onion powder
2 tsp. garlic powder
1 tsp. sugar
2 tsp. salt
2 tsp. black pepper
1 tsp. Doc's chili powder (see recipe in this chapter)
1 tsp. dried oregano
1 tsp. dried basil
¾ tsp. ground cumin
½ tsp. ground ginger
½ tsp. ground coriander

Combine all ingredients, and mix well.

DOC'S CHILI POWDER

2 oz. chipotle or pasilla chilis, stems and seeds removed
2 oz. ancho chilis, stems and seeds removed
2 oz. California chilis, stems and seeds removed

Place all the chilis in a food processor or spice mill, and grind until the consistency is that of a fine powder. Using a medium sieve, run the powder through to remove any large parts that remain.

DOC'S PIRI-PIRI SAUCE

I HAD NEVER had this before going to South Africa. From what I can decipher, it seems to be Portuguese in origin, at least that's what my friends of Portuguese descent in South Africa told me. I love the heat, but unlike some sauces that just go for the burn, this has an amazing flavor. There were any number of variations of the sauce, and this is my take, which combines my favorite flavors from the different varieties I tasted. An amazing dish that I had a number of times was cooked chicken livers with some piri-piri and served with crackers or bread. I recommend you try it as a first.

Nutrition Facts		
Serving Size 1 Tbs (15g)		
Servings Per Container 100		
Amount Per Serving		
Calories 20	Calories from Fat 5	
		% Daily Value*
Total Fat 1g		1%
Saturated Fat 0g		0%
Trans Fat 0g		
Cholesterol 0mg		0%
Sodium 10mg		1%
Total Carbohydrate 3g		1%
Dietary Fiber 0g		0%
Sugars 0g		
Protein 1g		
Vitamin A 2%	•	Vitamin C 20%
Calcium 2%	•	Iron 2%

* Percent Daily Values are based on a 2,000 calorie diet. Your daily values may be higher or lower depending on your calorie needs.

	Calories	2,000	2,500
Total Fat	Less than	65g	80g
Sat Fat	Less than	20g	25g
Cholesterol	Less than	300mg	300mg
Sodium	Less than	2,400mg	2,400mg
Total Carbohydrate		300g	375g
Dietary Fiber		25g	30g

Calories per gram:
Fat 9 • Carbohydrate 4 • Protein 4

1 c. olive oil
20–25 hot red chilis (make sure they are red to get the right color)
2 jalapeños, roasted
1 poblano, roasted
1 red bell pepper, roasted
¼ c. cider vinegar
¼ c. lemon juice
3 tbsp. (about 5 cloves) garlic, chopped
1 tbsp. paprika
1 tsp. salt
1 tsp. freshly ground black pepper

Heat the oil over medium heat, add the red chilis, and cook for 5 to 10 minutes. Let cool. Meanwhile, roast the jalapeño, poblano, and red bell pepper. Remove the skins, and combine with all the other ingredients. Add to the cooled olive oil and chilis, and blend with an immersion blender or in small batches in a food processor or blender until smooth.

ALFREDO SAUCE

This is a bit decadent, and a little goes a long way. I love this on a cool spring night with about an ounce of the sauce over some fresh pasta tossed with veggies right from the garden or farmer's market.

2 tbsp. butter
2 tbsp. flour
1½ c. milk
½ c. cream
⅓ c. parmesan cheese, finely grated
1 tsp. salt
½ tsp. white pepper

In a medium saucepan over medium heat, melt the butter. Add the flour, and whisk together. When you have a soft white paste (or blond roux), add the milk and cream. Continue to heat until the sauce starts to thicken, about 10 minutes. Remove from the heat, whisk in the cheese, and season with salt and white pepper.

Nutrition Facts

Serving Size 2 oz (57g)
Servings Per Container 25

Amount Per Serving	
Calories 160	Calories from Fat 20

	% Daily Value*
Total Fat 2.5g	4%
Saturated Fat 1.5g	7%
Trans Fat 0g	
Cholesterol 5mg	2%
Sodium 140mg	6%
Total Carbohydrate 30g	10%
Dietary Fiber 0g	0%
Sugars 1g	
Protein 6g	

Vitamin A 2%	•	Vitamin C 0%	
Calcium 6%	•	Iron 10%	

* Percent Daily Values are based on a 2,000 calorie diet. Your daily values may be higher or lower depending on your calorie needs.

		Calories	2,000	2,500
Total Fat	Less than		65g	80g
Sat Fat	Less than		20g	25g
Cholesterol	Less than		300mg	300mg
Sodium	Less than		2,400mg	2,400mg
Total Carbohydrate			300g	375g
Dietary Fiber			25g	30g

Calories per gram:
Fat 9 • Carbohydrate 4 • Protein 4

CONTAINS: Milk

BASIC BREAD DOUGH

IF YOU HAVE a stand mixer with dough hook attachment, you do not need a bread machine. I always recommend the first time doing the whole process, kneading included, by hand. There really is no other way to get the "feel" when the dough is right. Once you get this down, it's a snap to make fresh, delicious, homemade bread with very little effort. It takes 10 minutes at the mixer, and then just check the dough. The yeast does all the work. The key to knowing when kneading is done is the "window test." Pinch a portion of the dough ball, and stretch it between your fingers as you hold it up to the light. If it will stretch so you can see the light behind it without breaking and your finger appears as a shadow, it is ready to rise. You can add all sorts of herbs and flavors to this. This makes one regular loaf, two focaccia loaves, or three pizza crusts.

1 packet dry active yeast
⅓ c. hot water
Pinch (approximately ½ tsp.) sugar

16 oz. bread flour
1 tbsp. whole wheat flour
1 c. cold water
2 tsp. salt

Read the directions for the proper temperature to bloom yeast. Place hot water at proper temperature (usually 100 to 110° F) with sugar in a bowl, add the yeast, and allow to bloom for 5 minutes. Place all other dry ingredients in the bowl of a stand mixer. Add the bloomed yeast and mix with dough hook (or knead by hand). Slowly add the water as the dough mixes. Allow to rise, covered, in warm place for 1 to 2 hours, until it is 1½ to 2 times the original size. Punch down, recover, and allow to rise twice the original size. Place into desired form and bake. For bread, bake at 450° F for 20 minutes, and then reduce to 400° F for another 10 minutes.

Nutrition Facts		
Serving Size 14 oz (397g)		
Servings Per Container 2		
Amount Per Serving		
Calories 820	Calories from Fat 40	
		% Daily Value*
Total Fat 4g		7%
Saturated Fat 0g		0%
Trans Fat 0g		
Cholesterol 0mg		0%
Sodium 2320mg		97%
Total Carbohydrate 170g		57%
Dietary Fiber 5g		20%
Sugars 0g		
Protein 30g		
Vitamin A 0%	•	Vitamin C 10%
Calcium 2%	•	Iron 50%

* Percent Daily Values are based on a 2,000 calorie diet. Your daily values may be higher or lower depending on your calorie needs.

	Calories	2,000	2,500
Total Fat	Less than	65g	80g
Sat Fat	Less than	20g	25g
Cholesterol	Less than	300mg	300mg
Sodium	Less than	2,400mg	2,400mg
Total Carbohydrate		300g	375g
Dietary Fiber		25g	30g

Calories per gram:
Fat 9 • Carbohydrate 4 • Protein 4

BASIC PIZZA DOUGH

THIS IS DOUGH specifically for pizza. You can also make pizza from the basic bread dough recipe in this chapter. You can make the dough ahead, store in the refrigerator, and just allow to come up to room temperature before stretching it out. This yields five crusts of twelve inches, or eight ounces, each.

¼ oz. (1 packet) active dry yeast
¼ c. warm water (between 100 and 110° F)
16 oz. bread flour
4 oz. whole wheat flour
4 oz. all-purpose flour
1 tbsp. honey
1 tsp. salt
1½ c. cold water
¼ c. olive oil
Cornmeal for dusting

Add the yeast to ¼ c. of warm water (follow temperature on packet, usually around 100 to 110° F). Using a dough hook in your stand mixer, mix the yeast, bread flour, whole wheat

Nutrition Facts		
Serving Size 6 oz (170g)		
Servings Per Container 5		
Amount Per Serving		
Calories 430	Calories from Fat 70	
		% Daily Value*
Total Fat 8g		12%
Saturated Fat 1g		5%
Trans Fat 0g		
Cholesterol 0mg		0%
Sodium 0mg		0%
Total Carbohydrate 80g		27%
Dietary Fiber 2g		10%
Sugars 3g		
Protein 13g		
Vitamin A 0%	•	Vitamin C 4%
Calcium 0%	•	Iron 20%

* Percent Daily Values are based on a 2,000 calorie diet. Your daily values may be higher or lower depending on your calorie needs.

	Calories	2,000	2,500
Total Fat	Less than	65g	80g
Sat Fat	Less than	20g	25g
Cholesterol	Less than	300mg	300mg
Sodium	Less than	2,400mg	2,400mg
Total Carbohydrate		300g	375g
Dietary Fiber		25g	30g

Calories per gram:
Fat 9 • Carbohydrate 4 • Protein 4

flour, all-purpose flour, honey, salt, and cold water until the dough pulls into a ball and passes the "window" test, which involves pinching off a small piece of dough. You should be able to pull it between your fingers, then hold it up to the light and see through it. This indicates the dough has the proper stretch. Divide the dough into 8 oz. balls (for 12 in. thin crusts). Allow the dough to rise, covered, until doubled in size (1 to 2 hours). Refrigerate or freeze any unused dough. Sprinkle cornmeal on your work surface, and stretch the dough into the desired shape. Cook the dough on a preheated pizza stone at a minimum of 500 or 550° (as hot as you can get it) for about 3 to 5 minutes until it appears golden brown.

BASIC PASTA

FRESH PASTA is one of those unbeatable things. Again, exercise some portion control on the pasta servings. I recommend about four ounces of pasta per person as the main. This recipe gives you another "basic." Once you have this mastered, add spinach, mushrooms, spices, and so on for endless combinations. The fresh pasta tossed with fresh pesto is only outshined by the addition of some fresh grilled garden vegetables and a glass of properly chilled white wine.

Nutrition Facts
Serving Size 4 oz (113g)
Servings Per Container 4

Amount Per Serving	
Calories 300	Calories from Fat 60

	% Daily Value*
Total Fat 6g	10%
Saturated Fat 1g	5%
Trans Fat 0g	
Cholesterol 0mg	0%
Sodium 360mg	15%
Total Carbohydrate 48g	16%
Dietary Fiber 2g	8%
Sugars 0g	
Protein 11g	

Vitamin A 0%	•	Vitamin C 0%
Calcium 2%	•	Iron 2%

* Percent Daily Values are based on a 2,000 calorie diet. Your daily values may be higher or lower depending on your calorie needs.

	Calories	2,000	2,500
Total Fat	Less than	65g	80g
Sat Fat	Less than	20g	25g
Cholesterol	Less than	300mg	300mg
Sodium	Less than	2,400mg	2,400mg
Total Carbohydrate		300g	375g
Dietary Fiber		25g	30g

Calories per gram:
Fat 9 • Carbohydrate 4 • Protein 4

> 9 oz. (roughly 1½ c.) No. 1 durum wheat semolina flour + extra for dusting
> ½ tsp. salt + extra for cooking
> 2 eggs
> 2 tbsp. olive oil + extra for cooking
> 2 tbsp. water + extra for cooking

Combine all the ingredients in a stand mixer, or make a well with the dry ingredients on a working surface, and add the eggs, water, and oil. Gently start the mixer on low, mixing until the dough appears crumbly and binds together when squeezed in your hand. If mixing by hand, add the water to achieve the same consistency. The exact amount of water required may vary by the flour, ambient humidity, and other factors, so you need to go by the look and feel versus specific amounts. Next, knead the dough, if working by hand, or use the dough hook attachment, if using a stand mixer. Knead until the dough takes on a shiny appearance and pulls away from the bowl. Rest at least 1 hour, wrapped, in the refrigerator. Once the dough is rested, use the settings on your pasta rollers or measure out to about ¹⁄₃₂nd of an inch for linguini or fettuccine. Cut the pasta with a sharp knife, or use the pasta cutting attachment for your mixer. Dust the pasta with a little flour to prevent sticking. Bring salted water with a few drops of olive oil added to a boil, add the pasta, reduce to a simmer, and cook for 2 to 3 minutes or until it is al dente. The pasta can be made ahead and will keep for several days in the refrigerator.

BASIC PIZZA SAUCE

THERE IS AN ongoing debate: cook the sauce before you place on the pizza or not. I have made hundreds both ways and experimented with many different sauces. The best I ever had really did come from Italy, and it was simple. Like much of Italian cooking, it was simple, fresh ingredients prepared so they are center stage. That's the way I like it, and I find the simple, uncooked sauce more vivacious after application on the pizza. The key is to make sure you use San Marzano tomatoes, which come from around Naples and have a unique flavor, thought to be due to the volcanic soil.

Nutrition Facts		
Serving Size 1 oz (28g)		
Servings Per Container 34		
Amount Per Serving		
Calories 30	Calories from Fat 15	
		% Daily Value*
Total Fat 2g		3%
Saturated Fat 0.5g		3%
Trans Fat 0g		
Cholesterol 0mg		0%
Sodium 115mg		5%
Total Carbohydrate 3g		1%
Dietary Fiber 1g		3%
Sugars 1g		
Protein 1g		
Vitamin A 4%	•	Vitamin C 4%
Calcium 4%	•	Iron 4%

* Percent Daily Values are based on a 2,000 calorie diet. Your daily values may be higher or lower depending on your calorie needs.

	Calories	2,000	2,500
Total Fat	Less than	65g	80g
Sat Fat	Less than	20g	25g
Cholesterol	Less than	300mg	300mg
Sodium	Less than	2,400mg	2,400mg
Total Carbohydrate		300g	375g
Dietary Fiber		25g	30g

Calories per gram:
Fat 9 • Carbohydrate 4 • Protein 4

    1 can (28 oz.) San Marzano tomatoes
    6 oz. tomato paste
    3 oz. pecorino romano cheese
    ¼ c. olive oil
    2 tsp. sugar
    1 tbsp. salt
    2 tbsp. (about 3 cloves) garlic, finely minced
    1 tbsp. dried oregano
    1 tbsp. dried basil
    1 tbsp. dried thyme

Combine all ingredients in a food processor or blender, and mix. Alternatively, combine in a bowl, and use an immersion blender to mix. Any unused sauce can be frozen if needed.

EXOTIC MUSHROOM DUXELLES

THIS IS A great component to know how to do; although it sounds fancy, it is easy. These are great with some cheese, cream, or otherwise, placed in a wonton wrapper and deep fried. You can fill the phyllo dough and use with spinach for a spanikopita variation. The duxelles is a key component of any Wellington. There are myriad uses.

Nutrition Facts
Serving Size 2 oz (57g)
Servings Per Container 8

Amount Per Serving	
Calories 40	Calories from Fat 0

	% Daily Value*
Total Fat 0g	0%
Saturated Fat 0g	0%
Trans Fat 0g	
Cholesterol 0mg	0%
Sodium 0mg	0%
Total Carbohydrate 10g	3%
Dietary Fiber 2g	7%
Sugars 1g	
Protein 2g	

Vitamin A 2%	•	Vitamin C 6%
Calcium 0%	•	Iron 2%

* Percent Daily Values are based on a 2,000 calorie diet. Your daily values may be higher or lower depending on your calorie needs.

		Calories	2,000	2,500
Total Fat	Less than		65g	80g
Sat Fat	Less than		20g	25g
Cholesterol	Less than		300mg	300mg
Sodium	Less than		2,400mg	2,400mg
Total Carbohydrate			300g	375g
Dietary Fiber			25g	30g

Calories per gram:		
Fat 9 • Carbohydrate 4 • Protein 4		

- ½ c. onion, chopped
- 1 tbsp. shallot, chopped
- Olive oil
- 3 oz. dried exotic mushrooms (reconstituted in vegetable nage or light chicken broth, see recipe in this chapter)
- 8 oz. fresh mushrooms
- ⅓ c. white wine
- ¼ c. parsley, chopped

In a medium saucepan over medium heat, sweat the onion and shallot in some olive oil, about 2 to 3 minutes. Add the exotic and fresh mushrooms and wine. Cook until all the liquid is reduced, about 15 to 20 minutes. Remove from the heat and place into a food processor with the parsley. Pulse until you have a finely minced paste.

FRIED SWEET POTATO PIES

THIS IS A dessert splurge. The reason I like this is it fills that void when you need something crunchy and sweet, yet it sneaks in a little benefit from the sweet potatoes. You can also make the stovetop applesauce and use that as a filling. The basic process is the same for any of these little golden gems. Enjoy it sparingly. They're addictive!

- 4 medium sweet potatoes (approximately 3–4 lbs.)
- 1 tbsp. olive oil
- 1 tbsp. salt, divided
- ½ tsp. freshly ground pepper
- 2 tbsp. Doc's pumpkin pie spice (see recipe in this chapter)
- ½ c. granulated sugar
- 1½ tsp. light corn syrup
- ⅓ c. water, divided

1½ tsp. vanilla extract
1½ packets gelatin (unflavored)
1 egg white
2 packages egg roll wrappers
Vegetable oil for frying
½ c. powdered sugar (optional)
Ice cream (optional)
Caramel sauce (optional; see recipe in this chapter)

<table>
<tr><td colspan="2">Nutrition Facts</td></tr>
<tr><td colspan="2">Serving Size 6 oz (170g)
Servings Per Container 40</td></tr>
<tr><td colspan="2">Amount Per Serving</td></tr>
<tr><td colspan="2">Calories 190   Calories from Fat 30</td></tr>
<tr><td colspan="2" align="right">% Daily Value*</td></tr>
<tr><td>Total Fat 3.5g</td><td>5%</td></tr>
<tr><td>Saturated Fat 0.5g</td><td>3%</td></tr>
<tr><td>Trans Fat 0g</td><td></td></tr>
<tr><td>Cholesterol 0mg</td><td>0%</td></tr>
<tr><td>Sodium 250mg</td><td>10%</td></tr>
<tr><td>Total Carbohydrate 36g</td><td>12%</td></tr>
<tr><td>Dietary Fiber 3g</td><td>12%</td></tr>
<tr><td>Sugars 13g</td><td></td></tr>
<tr><td colspan="2">Protein 5g</td></tr>
<tr><td>Vitamin A 240%</td><td>Vitamin C 4%</td></tr>
<tr><td>Calcium 4%</td><td>Iron 6%</td></tr>
</table>

* Percent Daily Values are based on a 2,000 calorie diet. Your daily values may be higher or lower depending on your calorie needs.

	Calories	2,000	2,500
Total Fat	Less than	65g	80g
Sat Fat	Less than	20g	25g
Cholesterol	Less than	300mg	300mg
Sodium	Less than	2,400mg	2,400mg
Total Carbohydrate		300g	375g
Dietary Fiber		25g	30g

Calories per gram:
Fat 9 • Carbohydrate 4 • Protein 4

CONTAINS: Eggs, Peanuts

Preheat the oven to 425° F. Place the sweet potatoes in a roasting pan, and drizzle with olive oil, 1 tsp. salt, and freshly ground pepper. Roast until tender, about 30 to 45 minutes. Remove from the oven, and scoop the internal contents into a bowl, discarding the skins. Mash the potatoes or place in a food processor with pumpkin pie spice until the sweet potatoes form a smooth paste. Spray a 9" × 13" nonstick cookie sheet with nonstick spray. In a medium saucepan and over medium heat, combine the granulated sugar, corn syrup, and ⅙ c. water. Place a candy thermometer on the pan side so it reaches the liquid but does not touch the bottom of the pan. Stir occasionally until the sugar is dissolved. Once the sugar is dissolved, do not stir any more. Allow this mixture to reach 260° F, the hard-ball stage, and remove immediately from the heat. While the mixture reaches hard-ball stage, in a separate pan, combine the remaining ⅙ c. water, vanilla extract, and gelatin. Stir gently, and allow to bloom for 5 or so minutes. Then, over low heat, gently heat the gelatin so it is liquid in form. Separately, whip the egg white until it forms stiff peaks. Add the sugar solution to the gelatin. In a slow, steady stream, add the liquid ingredients to the egg whites while mixing on low. Once the entire liquid solution is added, whip on high for about 10 minutes. The mixture should turn white and resemble a thick cake batter. Pour the mixture into a bowl with the sweet potatoes, and then pour the entire mixture into the prepared pan, smoothing the top flat. Allow to cool overnight. The filling can be made a day ahead, as it needs to set overnight. You will only need ½ the filling with 1 package of the egg roll wrappers, so you can freeze the rest of the filling or make all the pies and freeze the extra pies. I like to freeze the pies; they keep well, and then you can just drop them in the deep fryer if you need a dessert.

Place the egg roll wrapper in front of you as a diamond shape. Place about 6 oz. of the filling in the middle, slightly toward you, leaving room to the right and left. Fold the bottom of the diamond over the filling, moving away from you, and seal with some water, egg wash, or egg whites. Fold the left and right corners into the middle, and seal. Fold the top over the middle, and seal. Roll away from you so you now have a cylinder. Make sure all ends are sealed. Heat the oil to 375° F. Place the pies in the oil, and cook until golden brown, between 1 and 2 minutes. Upon removal, dust with sugar, and serve on top of a scoop of your favorite ice cream. Drizzle with caramel sauce.

DOC'S PUMPKIN PIE SPICE

FRESH SPICE blends are incredibly superior to store-bought varieties and often much more economical. I like to buy the whole spices and grind them in a spice mill or coffee bean grinder right before use. If you do this, make sure to filter the spice blend through a sieve to remove any big chunks, especially of the cinnamon.

1½ tsp. ground cinnamon
¼ tsp. ground ginger
¼ tsp. ground nutmeg
¼ tsp. ground allspice
⅛ tsp. ground cardamom
⅛ tsp. ground cloves

Combine all ingredients, and mix well. Store in an air-tight container.

CARAMEL SAUCE

1 c. granulated sugar
¼ c. water
1 c. heavy cream

In a small saucepan, combine the sugar and water, and bring the mixture to a boil over medium-high heat. Continue until the mixture becomes a thin syrup with a deep caramel color, about 10 to 15 minutes. Remove from heat, and slowly add the cream in a steady stream, being careful not to allow the mixture to splash. Return the mixture to the stovetop, and boil the sauce until it regains the consistency of a thick syrup, about 2 minutes.

NAAN BREAD

THIS IS MY version of naan bread. I really like adding the fresh herbs, as it gives the bread an incredible vibrancy. You can add whatever you like or can get fresh and seasonally. The bread can be frozen and reheated as needed. This is very hearty bread; one or two pieces and some dhal make a complete and very filling meal.

1 package (¼ oz.) rapid-rise dry yeast
¼ c. sugar
3 tbsp. milk
1 egg, beaten
2 tsp. salt
4 c. bread flour (approximately 22 oz.)
½ c. whole wheat flour (approximately 2.5 oz.)
1 c. warm water
2 tsp. garlic, minced
2 tbsp. onion, finely chopped
2 tbsp. cilantro, finely chopped
1 tbsp. fennel bulb, finely chopped
1 tbsp. olive oil
¼ c. butter, melted

In a large bowl, stir in yeast, sugar, milk, egg, salt, and bread and whole wheat flours to make a soft dough. I do this in a stand mixer with a dough hook. Remember, if you use active yeast, you will need to dissolve the yeast in warm water and let stand about 10 minutes before adding to the flour. Use the stand mixer until the dough forms a ball that pulls away from the sides. The dough will still be slightly sticky. If performing by hand, knead for 8 to 10 minutes on a lightly floured surface, or until smooth. Add garlic, onion, cilantro, and fennel bulb, and knead into the dough, assuring good distribution. Place the dough in a well-oiled bowl, using the olive oil, cover with a damp cloth, and set aside to rise. Let it rise about 1 hour, until the dough has doubled in volume. Punch down the dough. Make small balls of dough of about 2 oz. Place these on a tray, cover with a towel, and allow to rise until doubled in size, about 30 to 45 minutes. Preheat a grill to high heat or an electric nonstick griddle to 400° F. Roll the balls of dough out into thin circles. Before placing the dough on the grill, lightly oil the grill, then cook for

2 to 3 minutes, or until bread is puffy and lightly browned. Brush the uncooked side with butter, and turn over. Brush the cooked side with butter, and cook until browned, another 2 to 4 minutes. Remove from the heat, and serve.

TEMPURA BATTER

ALTHOUGH TEMPURA is often deemed a Japanese food invention, it is not. It is another example of how the Japanese can incorporate a foreign idea, technique, or product and through the will of their society reform it in their image. It was introduced by the Portuguese in the sixteenth century when they were trying to convert the Japanese to Catholicism. The method of batter-dipping fish and vegetables was used on *quattuor tempora*, or Ember Days. These were the days Catholics avoided meat and ate fish and vegetables. People I meet are often intimidated about trying tempura at home, but it is delicious and easy.

¾ c. all-purpose flour (about 3.5 oz.)
¼ c. rice flour (about 1.5 oz.)
1 egg
¾–1 c. cold, nonflavored carbonated water
 (depending on batter consistency)

Nutrition Facts		
Serving Size 38/41 lbs (420g)		
Servings Per Container 1		
Amount Per Serving		
Calories 550	Calories from Fat 60	
		% Daily Value*
Total Fat 6g		**10%**
Saturated Fat 1.5g		**9%**
Trans Fat 0g		
Cholesterol 210mg		**71%**
Sodium 75mg		**3%**
Total Carbohydrate 104g		**35%**
Dietary Fiber 3g		**10%**
Sugars 0g		
Protein 18g		
Vitamin A 4%	•	Vitamin C 0%
Calcium 6%	•	Iron 25%
* Percent Daily Values are based on a 2,000 calorie diet. Your daily values may be higher or lower depending on your calorie needs.		

		Calories	2,000	2,500
Total Fat	Less than		65g	80g
Sat Fat	Less than		20g	25g
Cholesterol	Less than		300mg	300mg
Sodium	Less than		2,400mg	2,400mg
Total Carbohydrate			300g	375g
Dietary Fiber			25g	30g

Calories per gram:
Fat 9 • Carbohydrate 4 • Protein 4

CONTAINS: Eggs

Mix all the batter ingredients together to get to a thin-pancake-batter consistency. The key is to add cold carbonated (nonflavored) water. You may need to add a little additional water to get the batter to the proper consistency. Once you mix, allow the batter to rest 5 minutes before using.

ASIAN DIPPING SAUCE

I love this dipping sauce with tempura-fried vegetables or anything tempura fried. It's great for dumplings, yakitori, or even to drizzle a little on fried rice. It is a collection of flavors that really takes me back to the Orient. Feel free to use a little any time you want to invoke an Asian influence into your dish. For example, this simple sauce drizzled over some sesame-crusted tuna gives it a whole new makeover. You can add diced hot pepper, hot sauce, or some sriracha sauce when you want to heat it up a little.

¼ c. mirin
¼ c. soy sauce
¼ c. sake
1 tbsp. sugar
1 lemon, juiced
1 tsp. garlic, finely chopped
1 tsp. shallot, finely chopped
1 tsp. cilantro, finely chopped

Combine all ingredients, and mix well.

Nutrition Facts

Serving Size 1/2 oz (14g)
Servings Per Container 16

Amount Per Serving

Calories 15	Calories from Fat 0

	% Daily Value*
Total Fat 0g	0%
Saturated Fat 0g	0%
Trans Fat 0g	
Cholesterol 0mg	0%
Sodium 210mg	9%
Total Carbohydrate 4g	1%
Dietary Fiber 0g	0%
Sugars 2g	
Protein 0g	

Vitamin A 0%	•	Vitamin C 0%
Calcium 0%	•	Iron 0%

* Percent Daily Values are based on a 2,000 calorie diet. Your daily values may be higher or lower depending on your calorie needs.

	Calories	2,000	2,500
Total Fat	Less than	65g	80g
Sat Fat	Less than	20g	25g
Cholesterol	Less than	300mg	300mg
Sodium	Less than	2,400mg	2,400mg
Total Carbohydrate		300g	375g
Dietary Fiber		25g	30g

Calories per gram:
Fat 9 • Carbohydrate 4 • Protein 4

CONTAINS: Soy

ROSEMARY RED WINE REDUCTION SAUCE

THIS CONTAINS the elements of a basic red wine reduction sauce, which has a myriad of uses. For the basic, just eliminate the rosemary. If you don't have any veal demi-glace, don't worry. Use one full cup of dark chicken stock, or half a cup of light chicken stock with half a cup of beef stock.

2 tbsp. olive oil
1 shallot, finely chopped
1 tsp. rosemary, chopped
2 garlic cloves, finely chopped
1 c. good red wine, like a zinfandel or pinot noir
¾ c. light chicken stock (see recipe in this chapter)
¼ c. (about 1.5 oz.) veal demi-glace

For the sauce, heat the olive oil in a medium saucepan over medium heat. Add the shallots, and cook for 2 minutes, or until shallots are translucent and soft. Add the rosemary and garlic, and cook for another minute. Add the red wine, and cook until reduced by half. Add the stock and demi-glace. Cook until reduced by half. Pass through a sieve to remove any bits. You should have about 1 c. remaining.

Nutrition Facts

Serving Size 1/2 oz (14g)
Servings Per Container 16

Amount Per Serving	
Calories 10	Calories from Fat 5

	% Daily Value*
Total Fat 0.5g	1%
Saturated Fat 0g	0%
Trans Fat 0g	
Cholesterol 0mg	0%
Sodium 25mg	1%
Total Carbohydrate 1g	0%
Dietary Fiber 0g	0%
Sugars 0g	
Protein 1g	

Vitamin A 0%		Vitamin C 0%	
Calcium 0%		Iron 0%	

* Percent Daily Values are based on a 2,000 calorie diet. Your daily values may be higher or lower depending on your calorie needs.

	Calories	2,000	2,500
Total Fat	Less than	65g	80g
Sat Fat	Less than	20g	25g
Cholesterol	Less than	300mg	300mg
Sodium	Less than	2,400mg	2,400mg
Total Carbohydrate		300g	375g
Dietary Fiber		25g	30g

Calories per gram:
Fat 9 • Carbohydrate 4 • Protein 4

POBLANO SAUCE

THIS IS A delicious, smoky sauce with a gentle heat that you can use on sandwiches and just about anything else. Add some heat with some hot sauce, and "Doc" it up as you like. This is particularly delicious if made with fresh, homemade mayonnaise (see recipe in this chapter).

4 poblano chilis (roast your own if possible)
1 tbsp. garlic, finely chopped
1 c. mayonnaise (see recipe in this chapter)
2 tbsp. lemon juice
Salt
Pepper

Combine the poblanos, garlic, mayonnaise, and lemon juice in a food processor. Season with salt and pepper.

Nutrition Facts

Serving Size 1/2 oz (14g)
Servings Per Container 35

Amount Per Serving	
Calories 50	Calories from Fat 50

	% Daily Value*
Total Fat 6g	9%
Saturated Fat 1g	5%
Trans Fat 0g	
Cholesterol 5mg	1%
Sodium 40mg	2%
Total Carbohydrate 1g	0%
Dietary Fiber 0g	0%
Sugars 0g	
Protein 0g	

Vitamin A 2%		Vitamin C 25%	
Calcium 0%		Iron 0%	

* Percent Daily Values are based on a 2,000 calorie diet. Your daily values may be higher or lower depending on your calorie needs.

	Calories	2,000	2,500
Total Fat	Less than	65g	80g
Sat Fat	Less than	20g	25g
Cholesterol	Less than	300mg	300mg
Sodium	Less than	2,400mg	2,400mg
Total Carbohydrate		300g	375g
Dietary Fiber		25g	30g

Calories per gram:
Fat 9 • Carbohydrate 4 • Protein 4

MAYONNAISE

I RARELY BUY mayo. What I need can be made at home. It's easy, and I can add any flavors I need for the dish: garlic, basil, chipotle, and so on. In addition, it has no preservatives, fillers, and other processing negatives. I also purchase the safflower oil that is high in vitamin E for extra benefits with great taste. If you use olive oil instead of safflower and add garlic, you've just made a fancy aioli. Although you get charged three times more for it in fancy eateries, it's just garlic olive oil mayo. A note of caution: This recipe contains raw eggs, so any persons with compromised immune systems (the very aged, the very young, or pregnant women) should avoid this recipe. Using free-range organic vegetarian-fed chicken eggs also reduces the likelihood of any foodborne illness from salmonella.

1 egg yolk
1 tsp. dry mustard powder
8 oz. safflower oil
½ tsp. salt
½ lemon, juiced
1 tsp. rice wine vinegar

In a bowl with a whisk or in a food processor (using pulse), mix the yolk and mustard powder. Whisking or with the processor on low, slowly drizzle in the oil. Once the liquid has thickened and lightened, you can slowly add the rest of the oil, incorporating as you go. Once it is thickened, add the salt, lemon juice, and rice wine vinegar, and whisk (or blend on pulse) to incorporate. This yields 1 c. mayonnaise.

Nutrition Facts

Serving Size 1 tsp (5g)
Servings Per Container 48

Amount Per Serving

Calories 35	Calories from Fat 35

	% Daily Value*
Total Fat 3.5g	6%
Saturated Fat 0g	0%
Trans Fat 0g	
Cholesterol 5mg	1%
Sodium 65mg	3%
Total Carbohydrate 0g	0%
Dietary Fiber 0g	0%
Sugars 0g	
Protein 0g	

Vitamin A 0%	•	Vitamin C 0%
Calcium 0%	•	Iron 0%

* Percent Daily Values are based on a 2,000 calorie diet. Your daily values may be higher or lower depending on your calorie needs.

	Calories	2,000	2,500
Total Fat	Less than	65g	80g
Sat Fat	Less than	20g	25g
Cholesterol	Less than	300mg	300mg
Sodium	Less than	2,400mg	2,400mg
Total Carbohydrate		300g	375g
Dietary Fiber		25g	30g

Calories per gram:
Fat 9 • Carbohydrate 4 • Protein 4

CONTAINS: Eggs

epilogue
be a buddha

Consume nothing,
No matter where you bought it,
Or who has prepared it,
Not even if I have prepared it,
Unless it agrees with your own taste
And your own common sense.

—Doctor Mike, The Grassroots Gourmet
(and culinary buddha—with all apologies to the Buddha)

notes

CHAPTER 3

1. Cui, Iso, Date, Kikuchi, and Tamakoshi, 2010.
2. House, Eliaszi, Cattran, Churchill, Oliver, Fine, et al., 2010.
3. HealthDay, 2010, n.p.
4. Bolland, Avenell, Baron, Grey, MacLennan, Gamble, et al., 2010.
5. Doheny, 2010.
6. Wilson, O'Hanlon, Prasad, Deighan, Macmillan, Oxborough, et al., 2011.
7. Benito, Gay-Jordi, Serrano-Mollar, Guasch, Shi, Tardif, et al., 2011.
8. Wright, Wang, Kennedy-Stephenson, and Ervin, 2003.
9. Mozes, 2011, n.p.
10. Dongfeng, Chen, Huang, Cao, Chen, Li, et al., 2011.
11. Zhang, Brewer, Schröder, Santos, Grieve, Wang, et al., 2010.
12. Wrangham, 2009.

CHAPTER 4

1. Gadsby, 2004.
2. Adams, 2007.
3. Tolkien, 1981, n.p.
4. Stewart, 1989.

CHAPTER 5

1. Dictionary.com, 2002, n.p.
2. Dongfeng, Chen, Huang, Cao, Chen, Li, et al., 2011.
3. Dietary Guidelines Advisory Committee, 2005.
4. Chen, Caballero, Mitchell, Loria, Lin, Champagne, et al., 2010.
5. Jala, Smits, Johnson, and Chonchol, 2010, p. 1543.
6. Jala, Smits, Johnson, and Chonchol, 2010, p. 1543.
7. Jala, Smits, Johnson, and Chonchol, 2010.
8. Kessler, 2009.
9. Kessler, 2009.
10. Kessler, 2009.
11. Barrett, 2007.
12. Kessler, 2009.
13. Kessler, 2009.
14. Kessler, 2009, p. 18.
15. Schneider, 1989.
16. Kessler, 2009.
17. Kessler, 2009.
18. Butler and Hope, 1995.

CHAPTER 6

1. Stunkard and McLaren-Hume, 1959; Mann, Tomiyama, Westling, Lew, Samuels, and Chatman, 2007.
2. Lewis, McTigue, Burke, Poirier, Eckel, Howard, et al., 2009.
3. Kessler, 2009.
4. National Institutes of Health, 2006.
5. Kessler, 2009.
6. Stevens, McClain, and Truesdale, 2006.
7. Lewis, McTigue, Burke, Poirier, Eckel, Howard, et al., 2009.
8. Jacobs, Newton, and Wang, 2010.
9. Reinberg, 2010, n.p.; referring to Romero-Corral, Sert-Kuniyoshi, Sierra-Johnson, Orban, Gami, Davison, et al., 2010.
10. Grady, 2010, p. A11.
11. Taheri, Lin, Austin, Young, and Mignot, 2004.
12. Ludwig and Currie, 2010.
13. Lewis, McTigue, Burke, Poirier, Eckel, Howard, et al., 2009.
14. Brook, Franklin, Cascio, Hong, Howard, Lipsett, et al., 2004, p. 2364.
15. Brook, Franklin, Cascio, Hong, Howard, Lipsett, et al., 2004, p. 2338.
16. Caspi, Harrington, Moffitt, Milne, and Poulton, 2006, p. 810.

CHAPTER 7

1. North, 2002, n.p.
2. Edelstein, Owesei, and Temkin, 1987.
3. Smith, 2004, p. 212.
4. Lasagna, 1964, n.p.
5. Drayton, 1994.
6. Shun, 1998.

CHAPTER 8

1. Kessler, 2009.
2. Edelman, 2003.
3. Dietary Guidelines Advisory Committee, 2005.
4. Witchel, 2009.
5. Witchel, 2009, p. MM50.
6. Witchel, 2009, p. MM50.
7. Kessler, 2009.
8. Kessler, 2009.
9. Kessler, 2009.
10. National Restaurant Association, 2010.
11. Kessler, 2009.
12. Kessler, 2009.

CHAPTER 9

1. American Heart Association, 2010b.
2. Labensky and Hause, 2003, p. 1178.
3. Dictionary.com, 2011, n.p.
4. American Heart Association, 2009.
5. Kastorini, Milionis, Esposito, Guigliano, Goudevenos, and Panagiotakos, 2011.
6. Salas-Salvadó, Bullo, and Babio, 2010.
7. Nainggolan, 2010, n.p.; referring to Salas-Salvadó, Bullo, and Babio, 2010.
8. Nainggolan, 2010, n.p.; referring to Salas-Salvadó, Bullo, and Babio, 2010.
9. Salas-Salvadó, Bullo, and Babio, 2010.
10. Price, 2000, p. 271.
11. Gadsby, 2004, n.p.
12. Gadsby, 2004, n.p.
13. Gadsby, 2004.
14. Corti, Flammer, Hollenberg, and Luscher, 2009.
15. Franklyn, 1996.

16. Vital Choices, 2006.
17. Micha, Wallace, and Mozaffarian, 2010.
18. Winslow, 2010, n.p.
19. BBC News, 2010, n.p.
20. Siri-Tarino, Sun, Hu, and Krauss, 2010.
21. Geleijnse, Giltay, Schouten, de Goede, Oude, Teitsma-Jansen, et al., 2010.
22. U.S. Government, Food and Drug Administration, 2009.
23. Labensky and Hause, 2003.
24. Agricultural Marketing Service and United States Department of Agriculture, 2002.
25. Trueman, 2008.

CHAPTER 10

1. National Center for Health Statistics, 2006.
2. Kessler, 2009.
3. Kessler, 2009, p. 33.
4. Dictionary.com, 2002.
5. Oz, 2010, n.p.
6. Cahill, 1995, p. 176.
7. Cahill, 1995, p. 177.
8. Knowles, 2009.
9. Knowles, 2009.

CHAPTER 11

1. Stunkard and McClaren-Hume, 1959; National Institutes of Health, 1992; Bild et al., 1992.
2. Kessler, 2009.
3. Santayana, 2011, p. 242.
4. Ackman, 2001; Rich, 2001.
5. Institute of Medicine of the National Academies, 2004.
6. International Foodservice Distributors Association, 2010.
7. Woodward and Armstrong, 1979.
8. Knowles, 2009.
9. Croasmun, 2003; de Graaf, 2008.

CHAPTER 13

1. Mukamal, Chen, Rao, and Breslow, 2010.
2. Mukamal, Chen, Rao, and Breslow, 2010.

3. Ronksley, Brien, Turner, Mukamal, and Ghali, 2011, p. d671.

4. Brien, Ronksley, Turner, Mukamal, and Ghali, 2011, p. d671.

5. Hansel, Thomas, Pannier, Bean, Kontush, Chapman, et al., 2010.

6. Hansel, Thomas, Pannier, Bean, Kontush, Chapman, et al., 2010, p. 567.

7. American Heart Association, 2010b.

8. Harding, 2010.

CHAPTER 14

1. Santayana, 1906, p. 284.

2. Dalai Lama, 2009.

3. American Heart Association, 2010b.

4. Olivos, 2006.

5. Cui, Iso, Date, Kikuchi, and Tamakoshi, 2010.

6. Trans Fat Task Force, 2006, p. 8.

7. Bolland, Avenell, Baron, Grey, MacLennan, Gamble, et al., 2010.

8. Trivedi, 2002.

9. Ding, 2011.

10. Wang-Polagruto, Villablanca, Polagruto, Lee, Holt, Schrader, et al., 2006.

11. Corti, Flammer, Hollenberg, and Luscher, 2009.

12. Corti, Flammer, Hollenberg, and Luscher, 2009.

13. Corti, Flammer, Hollenberg, and Luscher, 2009.

14. Bayard, Chamorro, Motta, and Hollenberg, 2007.

15. De Oliveira e Silva, Seidman, Tian, Hudgins, Sacks, and Breslow, 1996.

16. Halsey, 1996, n.p.

17. Chow, 2008.

18. Song and Kerver, 2000.

19. Kritchevsky, 2004.

20. Renaud and De Lorgeril, 1992.

21. O'Neill, 1991, n.p.

22. O'Neill, 1991, n.p.

23. Erlich, 2008.

24. Weiss, 2008; Robbers and Tyler, 1999.

25. Harding, 2010.

26. Erlich, 2008; Borek, 2006.

27. Childs, King, Dorsett, Ostrander, and Yamanaka, 1990.

28. Childs, Dorsett, Failor, Roidt, and Omenn, 1987.

29. Firstenberg, 2011.

30. Sabate, Oda, and Ros, 2010.

31. Micha, Wallace, and Mozaffarian, 2010; Winslow, 2010.

32. Gadsby, 2004.

33. Gadsby, 2004.

34. Simopoulos, 2002.

35. Cook and Kelly, 2007.

36. Rowe, 2007.

37. Academic Dictionaries and Encyclopedias, 2005.

CHAPTER 15

1. Streib, 2007.

2. Quoted in Streib, 2007, n.p.

CHAPTER 16

1. Labensky and Hause, 2003.

2. Rozin, 1983.

3. Institute of Medicine of the National Academies, 2006.

CHAPTER 17

1. Moghadasian and Frolich, 1999.

2. Engelhard, Gazer, and Paran, 2006.

3. Zheng and Wang, 2001.

4. American Heart Association, 2010a.

5. Storlien, Kraegan, Chisholm, Ford, Bruce, and Pascoe, 1987.

6. Brown, Rosner, Willett, and Sacks, 1999.

CHAPTER 18

1. Tanaka, Sakai, Ikeda, Imaizumi, and Sugano, 1998.

2. Montagne, 2001, p. 837.

CHAPTER 19

1. Escoffier, 1941.

references

Academic Dictionaries and Encyclopedias. (2005). Anandamide. Retrieved August 8, 2010, from *Academic Dictionaries and Encyclopedias* at http://en.academic.ru/dic.nsf/enwiki/63874.

Ackman, D. (2001). How Big Is Porn? Retrieved January 29, 2010, from *Forbes.com* at www.forbes.com/2001/05/25/0524porn.html.

Adams, C. (2007). When One Spouse Dies Does the Surviving Spouse Tend to Follow Soon Afterwards? Retrieved September 1, 2010, from *The Straight Dope* at www.straightdope.com/columns/read/2705/when-one-spouse-dies-does-the-surviving-spouse-tend-to-follow-soon-afterwards.

Agricultural Marketing Service and United States Department of Agriculture. (2002). *USDA Consumer Brochure: Organic Food Standards and Labels: The Facts.* Washington, DC: USDA.

American Heart Association. (2009). Lyon Diet Heart Study. Retrieved June 18, 2009, from *American Heart Association* at www.americanheart.org/presenter.jhtml?identifier=4655.

———. (2010a). Fish and Omega-3 Fatty Acids. Retrieved September 18, 2011, from *American Heart Association* at www.heart.org/HEARTORG/GettingHealthy/NutritionCenter/HealthyDietGoals/Fish-and-Omega-3-Fatty-Acids_UCM_303248_Article.jsp.

———. (2010b). Phytochemicals and Cardiovascular Disease. Retrieved June 1, 2010, from *American Heart Association* at www.americanheart.org/presenter.jhtml?identifier=4722.

Barrett, D. (2007). *Waistland: The (R)evolutionary Science behind Our Weight and Fitness Crises.* W. W. Norton: New York.

Bayard, V., F. Chamorro, J. Motta, and N. K. Hollenberg. (2007). Does Flavanol Intake Influence Mortality from Nitric Oxide–Dependent Processes? Ischemic Heart Disease, Stroke, Diabetes Mellitus, and Cancer in Panama. *International Journal of Medical Sciences*, 4:53–58.

BBC News. (2010). "Sausage Not Steak" Increases Heart Disease Risk: Eating Processed Meat Such as Sausages Increases the Likelihood of Heart Disease, While Red Meat Does Not Seem to Be as Harmful, a Study Suggests. Retrieved September 16, 2011, from *BBC News* at http://news.bbc.co.uk/2/hi/8688104.stm.

Benito, B., G. Gay-Jordi, A. Serrano-Mollar, E. Guasch, Y. Shi, J. C. Tardif, et al. (2011). Cardiac Arrhythmogenic Remodeling in a Rat Model of Long-Term Intensive Exercise Training. *Circulation*, 123:13–22.

Bild, D., et al. (1992). Strategy Development Workshop for Public Education on Weight and Obesity. *Strategy Development Workshop for Public Education on Weight and Obesity.* Bethesda, MD: Office of Prevention, Education, and Control; National Heart, Lung, and Blood Institute; and National Institutes of Health.

Bolland, M. J., A. Avenell, J. A. Baron, A. Grey, G. S. MacLennan, G. D. Gamble, et al. (2010). Effect of Calcium Supplements on Risk of Myocardial Infarction and Cardiovascular Events: Meta-Analysis. *British Medical Journal*, 341:c3691.

Borek, C. (2006). Garlic Reduces Dementia and Heart-Disease Risk. *The Journal of Nutrition*, 136:810S–12S.

Brien, S. J., P. E. Ronksley, B. J. Turner, K. J. Mukamal, and W. A. Ghali. (2011). Effect of Alcohol Consumption on Biological Markers Associated with Risk of Coronary Heart Disease: Systematic Review and Meta-Analysis of Interventional Studies. *British Medical Journal*, 342:d636.

Brook, R. D., B. Franklin, W. Cascio, Y. Hong, G. Howard, M. Lipsett, et al. (2004). Air Pollution and Cardiovascular Disease: A Statement for Healthcare Professionals from the Expert Panel on Population and Prevention Science of the American Heart Association. *Circulation*, 109:2655–71.

Brown, L., B. Rosner, W. W. Willett, and F. M. Sacks. (1999). Cholesterol-Lowering Effects of Dietary Fiber: A Meta-analysis. *American Journal of Clinical Nutrition*, 69(1):30–42.

Butler, G., and T. Hope. (1995). *Managing Your Mind: The Mental Fitness Guide.* New York: Oxford Paperbacks.

Cahill, T. (1995). *How the Irish Saved Civilization: The Untold Story of Ireland's Heroic Role from the Fall of Rome to the Rise of Medieval Europe.* New York: Doubleday.

Caspi, A., H. Harrington, T. Moffitt, B. Milne, and R. Poulton. (2006). Socially Isolated Children 20 Years Later: Risk of Cardiovascular Disease. *Archives of Pediatrics and Adolescent Medicine*, 160(8):805–11.

Chen, L., B. Caballero, D. C. Mitchell, C. Loria, P. H. Lin, C. M. Champagne, et al. (2010). Reducing Consumption of Sugar-Sweetened Beverages Is Associated with Reduced Blood Pressure. *Circulation*, 121:2398–2406.

Childs, M. T., C. S. Dorsett, A. Failor, L. Roidt, and G. S. Omenn. (1987). Effect of Shellfish Consumption on Cholesterol Absorption in Normolipidemic Men. *Metabolism*, 36(1):31–35.

Childs, M. T., I. B. King, C. S. Dorsett, J. G. Ostrander, and W. K. Yamanaka. (1990). Effects of Shellfish Consumption on Lipoproteins in Normolipidemic Men. *American Journal of Clinical Nutrition*, 51(6):1020–27.

Chow, C. K. (2008). *Fatty Acids in Foods and Their Health Implications.* Boca Raton, FL: CRC Press.

Cook, E., and M. Kelly. (2007). Enhanced Production of the Sea Urchin *Paracentrotus Lividus* in Integrated Open-Water Cultivation with Atlantic Salmon *Salmo Salar. Aquaculture,* 273(4):573–85.

Corti, R., A. J. Flammer, N. K. Hollenberg, and T. F. Luscher. (2009). Cocoa and Cardiovascular Health. *Circulation,* 119:1433–41.

Croasmun, J. (2003). Do Vacations Affect Worker Productivity? Retrieved February 3, 2010, from *Ergoweb* at www.ergoweb.com/news/detail.cfm?id=762.

Cui, R., H. Iso, C. Date, S. Kikuchi, and A. Tamakoshi. (2010). Dietary Folate and Vitamin B_6 and B_{12} Intake in Relation to Mortality from Cardiovascular Diseases. *Stroke: Journal of the American Heart Association,* 41:1285–89.

Dalai Lama. (2009). *The Middle Way.* Somerville, MA: Wisdom.

de Graaf, J. (2008). *The Case for a Paid Vacation Law.* Seattle: Take Back Your Time.

De Oliveira e Silva, E. R., C. E. Seidman, J. J. Tian, L. C. Hudgins, F. M. Sacks, and J. L. Breslow. (1996). Effects of Shrimp Consumption on Plasma Lipoproteins. *American Journal of Clinical Nutrition,* (64):712–17.

Dictionary.com. (2002). Addiction. Retrieved August 31, 2010, from *Dictionary.com* at http://dictionary.reference.com/browse/addiction.

———. (2011). Sushi. Retrieved September 16, 2011, from *Dictionary.com* at http://dictionary.reference.com/browse/sushi.

Dietary Guidelines Advisory Committee. (2005). *2005 Dietary Guidelines for Americans.* Washington, DC: U.S. Department of Health and Human Services and the U.S. Department of Agriculture.

Ding, E. L. (2011). *Cocoa Consumption Linked to Lower Risk for High Blood Pressure, Diabetes.* Abstract presented at the American Heart Association's Nutrition, Physical Activity and Metabolism/Cardiovascular Disease Epidemiology and Prevention Meeting, Atlanta, March 22–25.

Doheny, K. (2010). Marathons Affect Heart, but Runners Bounce Back. Retrieved October 25, 2010, from *Healthfinder.gov* at http://healthfinder.gov/News/newsstory.aspx?docid=644825.

Dongfeng, G., J. Chen, J. F. Huang, J. Cao, J. C. Chen, J. Li, et al. (2011). Physical Activity Decreases Salt's Effect on Blood Pressure. *American Heart Association's Nutrition, Physical Activity and Metabolism/Cardiovascular Disease Epidemiology and Prevention 2011 Scientific Sessions.* Atlanta: American Heart Association.

Drayton, A. (1994). *The Physiology of Taste.* New York: Penguin Books.

Edelman, R. M. (2003). Sweet Addiction. Retrieved September 9, 2009, from *Alive.com* at www.alive.com/1512a4a2.php?subject_bread_cramb=77.

Edelstein, L., T. Owesei, and C. L. Temkin. (1987). *Ancient Medicine.* Baltimore: Johns Hopkins University Press.

Engelhard, Y. N., B. Gazer, and E. Paran. (2006). Natural Antioxidants from Tomato Extract Reduce Blood Pressure in Patients with Grade-1 Hypertension: A Double-Blind, Placebo-Controlled Pilot Study. *American Heart Journal,* 151(1):100.

Erlich, S. D. (2008). Garlic. Retrieved June 1, 2010, from *University of Maryland Medical Center* at www.umm.edu/altmed/articles/garlic-000245.htm.

Escoffier, A. (1941). *The Escoffier Cookbook.* New York: Crown.

Firstenberg, J. (2011). Which Shellfish Are High in Cholesterol? Retrieved September 17, 2011, from *eHow Health* at www.ehow.com/about_5268060_shellfish-high-cholesterol.html.

Franklyn, D. (1996). The Healthiest Women in the World. *Health*, 9:57–63.

Gadsby, P. (2004). The Inuit Paradox: How Can People Who Gorge on Fat and Rarely See a Vegetable Be Healthier Than We Are? Retrieved on August 9, 2011, from *Discover Magazine* at http://discovermagazine.com/2004/oct/inuit-paradox.

Geleijnse, J., E. Giltay, E. Schouten, J. de Goede, G. L. Oude, A. Teitsma-Jansen, et al. (2010). Effect of Low Doses of N-3 Fatty Acids on Cardiovascular Diseases in 4,837 Post-Myocardial Infarction Patients: Design and Baseline Characteristics of the Alpha Omega Trial. *American Heart Journal*, 159(4):539–46.e2.

Grady, D. (2010, August 3). Obesity Rates Keep Rising, Troubling Health Officials. *New York Times*, p. A11.

Halsey, E. (1996). Shrimp's High Cholesterol May Not Be So Bad. Retrieved September 17, 2011, from *CNN Interactive* at www.cnn.com/HEALTH/indepth.food/meat/seafood/healthful.shrimp/index.html.

Hansel, B., F. Thomas, B. Pannier, K. Bean, A. Kontush, M. Chapman, et al. (2010). Relationship between Alcohol Intake, Health and Social Status and Cardiovascular Risk Factors in the Urban Paris-Ile-De-France Cohort: Is the Cardioprotective Action of Alcohol a Myth? *European Journal of Clinical Nutrition*, 64:561–68.

Harding, C. (2010). *Foods That Boost Your Good Cholesterol.* Retrieved August 8, 2010, from *Mail Online* at www.dailymail.co.uk/health/article-29998/Foods-boost-good-cholesterol.html.

HealthDay. (2010). High-Dose Vitamin B Risky for Diabetics with Kidney Disease: Study Ties Therapy to Deteriorating Renal Function. Retrieved September 13, 2001, from *U.S. News and World Report* at http://health.usnews.com/health-news/family-health/digestive-disorders/articles/2010/04/27/high-dose-vitamin-b-risky-for-diabetics-with-kidney-disease.

HemOnc Today. (2009). Cigarettes Were Once "Physician" Tested, Approved. Retrieved September 1, 2010, from *HemOnc Today* at www.hemonctoday.com/article.aspx?rid=37712.

House, A. A., M. Eliaszi, D. C. Cattran, D. N. Churchill, M. J. Oliver, A. Fine, et al. (2010). Effect of B-Vitamin Therapy on Progression of Diabetic Nephropathy: A Randomized Controlled Trial. *Journal of the American Medical Association*, 303 (16):1603–9.

Institute of Medicine of the National Academies. (2004). Dietary Supplements: A Framework for Evaluating Safety. Retrieved August 9, 2011, from *Institute of Medicine of the National Academies* at www.iom.edu/Reports/2004/Dietary-Supplements-A-Framework-for-Evaluating-Safety.aspx.

———. (2006). Seafood Choices: Balancing Benefits and Risks. Retrieved February 8, 2010, from *Institute of Medicine of the National Academies* at www.iom.edu/Reports/2006/Seafood-Choices-Balancing-Benefits-and-Risks.aspx.

International Foodservice Distributors Association. (2010). Foodservice Distribution: Connecting the Foodservice Industry. Retrieved February 3, 2010, from *International Foodservice Distributors Association* at www.ifdaonline.org/webarticles/anmviewer.asp?a=622&z=38.

Jacobs, E., C. Newton, and Y. Wang. (2010). Waist Circumference and All-Cause Mortality in a Large U.S. Cohort. *Archives of Internal Medicine*, 170:1293–1301.

Jala, D. I., G. Smits, R. J. Johnson, and M. Chonchol. (2010). Increased Fructose Associates with Elevated Blood Pressure. *Journal of the American Society of Nephrology*, 21:1416–18.

Kastorini, C. M., H. Milionis, K. Esposito, D. Guigliano, J. A. Goudevenos, D. B. Panagiotakos. (2011). The Effect of Mediterranean Diet on Metabolic Syndrome and Its Components: A Meta-Analysis of 50 Studies and 534,906 Individuals. *Journal of the American College of Cardiology*, 57:1299–1313.

Kessler, D. (2009). *The End of Overeating: Taking Control of the Insatiable American Appetite.* New York: Rodale Press.

Knowles, A. (2009). Studies Show Vacation Time Is Vital. Retrieved November 12, 2009, from *The Community Word* at http://thecommunityword.com/online/blog/2009/09/12/studies-show-vacation-time-is-vital.

Kritchevsky, S. B. (2004). A Review of Scientific Research and Recommendations. *Journal of the American College of Nutrition*, 23(6):596S–600S.

Labensky, S. R., and A. M. Hause. (2003). *On Cooking: Techniques from Expert Chefs.* Upper Saddle River, NJ: Prentice-Hall.

Lasagna, L. (1964). The Hippocratic Oath: Modern Version. Retrieved May 31, 2010, from *PBS.org* at www.pbs.org/wgbh/nova/doctors/oath_modern.html.

Lewis, C. A., K. M. McTigue, L. E. Burke, P. Poirier, R. H. Eckel, B. V. Howard, et al. (2009). Mortality, Health Outcomes, and Body Mass Index in the Overweight Range: A Science Advisory from the American Heart Association. *Circulation*, 119:1–9.

Ludwig, D., and J. Currie. (2010). The Association between Pregnancy Weight Gain and Birthweight: A Within-Family Comparison. *The Lancet*, 376(9745):984–90.

Mann, T., A. J. Tomiyama, E. Westling, A. M. Lew, B. Samuels, and J. Chatman. (2007). Medicare's Search for Effective Obesity Treatments: Diets Are Not the Answer. *American Psychologist*, 62(3):220–33.

Micha, R., S. K. Wallace, and D. Mozaffarian. (2010). Red and Processed Meat Consumption and Risk of Incident Coronary Heart Disease, Stroke, and Diabetes Mellitus: A Systematic Review and Meta-Analysis. *Circulation*, 121:2251–52.

Moghadasian, M. H., and J. J. Frolich. (1999). Effects of Dietary Phytosterols on Cholesterol Metabolism and Atherosclerosis: Clinical and Experimental Evidence. *The American Journal of Medicine*, 107(6):588–94.

Montagne, P. (ed.). (2001). *La Rousse Gastronomique.* New York: Clarkson Potter.

Mozes, A. (2011). Exercise May Blunt Salt's Effect on Hypertension: The More Active You Are, the Less a High-Sodium Diet Will Raise Your Blood Pressure, Study Suggests.

Retrieved September 14, 2011, from *HealthDay* at http://health.msn.com/health-topics/ high-blood-pressure/exercise-may-blunt-salts-effect-on-hypertension.

Mukamal, K. J., C. M. Chen, S. R. Rao, and R. J. Breslow. (2010). Alcohol Consumption and Cardiovascular Mortality among U.S. Adults, 1987 to 2002. *Journal of the American College of Cardiology*, 55:1328–35.

Nainggolan, L. (2010). New PREDIMED Data: Mediterranean Diet Halves Incidence of New-Onset Diabetes. Retrieved September 4, 2011, from *Heart.org* at www.theheart.org/ article/1137385.do.

National Center for Health Statistics. (2006). Prevalence of Overweight and Obesity among Adults: 2003–2004. Retrieved June 25, 2009, from *Center for Disease Control* at www.cdc .gov/nchs/products/pubs/pubd/hestats/overweight/overwght_adult_03.htm.

National Institutes of Health. (1992). Methods for Voluntary Weight Loss and Control. *Methods for Voluntary Weight Loss and Control. Technology Assessment Conference Statement.* Bethesda, MD: National Institutes of Health, Office of Medical Applications of Research.

———. (2006). *Clinical Guidelines on the Identification, Evaluation, and Treatment of Overweight and Obesity in Adults: The Evidence Report.* Bethesda, MS: National Institutes of Health and National Heart, Lung, and Blood Intitute in cooperation with the National Institute of Diabetes and Digestive and Kidney Diseases Appendices; September 1998.

National Restaurant Association. (2010). *2010 Restaurant Industry Forecast.* Washington, DC: Author.

North, M. (2002). Greek Medicine. Retrieved May 31, 2010, from *National Library of Medicine, National Institutes of Health* at www.nlm.nih.gov/hmd/greek/greek_oath.html.

Olivos, S. L. (2006). Health Benefits of Avocado Oil. Retrieved June 1, 2010, from *Paltita Avocado Oil* at www.paltita.com/pdf/health_en.pdf.

O'Neill, M. (1991). Can Foie Gras Aid the Heart? A French Scientist Says Yes. Retrieved September 17, 2011, *New York Times* at www.nytimes.com/1991/11/17/world/can-foie-gras-aid -the-heart-a-french-scientist-says-yes.html.

Oz, Mehmet. (2010). Dr. Oz's 25 Greatest Health Tips. Retrieved September 17, 2011, from *Men's Health* at www.menshealth.com/mhlists/essential_health_tips/printer.php.

Price, W. A. (2000). *Nutrition and Physical Degeneration.* La Mesa, CA: Price-Pottenger Nutrition Foundation.

Reinberg, S. (2010). Just a Little Belly Fat Can Damage Blood Vessels: Raises Risk for High Blood Pressure, Other Heart Problems, Study Finds. Retrieved September 15, 2011, from *WomensHealth.gov* at www.womenshealth.gov/news/headlines/641912.cfm.

Renaud, S., and M. De Lorgeril. (1992). Wine, Alcohol, Platelets, and the French Paradox for Coronary Heart Disease. *Lancet*, 339:1523–26.

Rich, F. (2001, May 18). Naked Capitalists: There's No Business Like Porn Business. Retrieved January 25, 2010, from *New York Times Magazine* at www.nytimes.com/2001/05/20/ magazine/20PORN.html?pagewanted=all.

Robbers, J., and V. Tyler. (1999). *Tyler's Herbs of Choice.* New York: Haworth Herbal Press.

Romero-Corral, A., F. H. Sert-Kuniyoshi, J. Sierra-Johnson, M. Orban, A. Gami, D. Davison, et al. (2010). Modest Visceral Fat Gain Causes Endothelial Dysfunction in Healthy Humans. *The Journal of the American College of Cardiology*, 56:662–66.

Ronksley, P. E., S. E. Brien, B. J. Turner, K. J. Mukamal, and W. A. Ghali. (2011). Association of Alcohol Consumption with Selected Cardiovascular Disease Outcomes: A Systematic Review and Meta-Analysis. *British Medical Journal*, 342:d671.

Rowe, A. (2007). Chem Lab: Sea Urchin Eggs Plus Marijuana Equal Amazing New Drugs. Retrieved August 8, 2010, from *Wired Science* at www.wired.com/wiredscience/2007/11/chem-lab-hybrid.

Rozin, E. (1983). *Ethnic Cuisine: The Flavor-Principle Cookbook*. Lexington, MA: S. Greene Press.

Sabate, J., K. Oda, and E. Ros. (2010). Nut Consumption and Blood Lipid Levels: A Pooled Analysis of 25 Intervention Trials. *Archives of Internal Medicine*, 170(9):810–12.

Salas-Salvadó, J., M. Bullo, and N. Babio. (2010). Reduction in the Incidence of Type 2 Diabetes with the Mediterranean Diet: Results of the PREDIMED-Reus Nutrition Intervention Randomized Trial. *Diabetes Care*, 34(1):14–19.

Santayana, G. (1906). *The Life of Reason*. New York: Dover.

———. (2011). *Interpretations of Poetry and Religion*. Charleston, SC: Forgotten Books.

Schneider, L. (1989). Orosensory Self-Stimulation by Sucrose Involves Brain Dopaminergic Mechanisms. *Annals of the New York Academy of Sciences*, 575:307–19.

Shun, Y. (1998). *Teachings in Chinese Buddhism*. Sydney, Australia: Buddha Dharma Education Association.

Simopoulos, A. P. (2002). The Importance of the Ratio of Omega-6/Omega-3 Essential Fatty Acids. *Biomedical: Pharmacotherapy*, 56(8):365–79.

Siri-Tarino, P., Q. Sun, F. B. Hu, and R. M. Krauss. (2010). Meta-Analysis of Prospective Cohort Studies Evaluating the Association of Saturated Fat with Cardiovascular Disease. *American Journal of Clinical Nutritio*, 91(3):535–46.

Smith, R. (2004). Editor's Choice. *British Medical Journal*, 328(7433):212.

Song, W. O., and J. Kerver. (2000). Nutritional Contribution of Eggs to American Diets. *Journal of the American College of Nutrition*, 19(5):556S–62S.

Stevens, J., J. E. McClain, and K. Truesdale. (2006). Commentary: Obesity Claims and Controversies. *International Journal of Epidemiology*, 35:77–78.

Stewart, I. (1989). *Does God Play Dice? The Mathematics of Chaos*. Hoboken, NJ: Blackwell.

Storlien, L. H., E. W. Kraegan, D. J. Chisholm, G. L. Ford, D. G. Bruce, and W. S. Pascoe. (1987). Fish Oil Prevents Insulin Resistance Induced by High-Fat Feeding in Rats. *Science*, 237(4817):885–88.

Streib, L. (2007). World's Fattest Countries. Retrieved July 8, 2009, from *Forbes.com* at www.forbes.com/2007/02/07/worlds-fattest-countries-forbeslife-cx_ls_0208worldfat.html.

Stunkard, A., and M. McLaren-Hume. (1959). The Results of Treatment for Obesity: A Review of the Literature and Report of a Series. *Archives of Internal Medicine*, 103(1):79–85.

Taheri, S., L. Lin, D. Austin, T. Young, and E. Mignot. (2004). Short Sleep Duration Is Associated with Reduced Leptin, Elevated Ghrelin, and Increased Body Mass Index. Retrieved August 21, 2010, from *Public Library of Science Medicine* at www.ncbi.nlm.nih.gov/pmc/articles/PMC535701.

Tanaka, K., T. Sakai, I. Ikeda, K. Imaizumi, and M. Sugano. (1998). Effects of Dietary Shrimp, Squid and Octopus on Serum and Liver Lipid Levels in Mice. Retrieved February 10, 2010, from *PubMed.gov* at www.ncbi.nlm.nih.gov/pubmed/9720219.

Tolkien, J. R. R. (1981). *The Fellowship of the Ring: Being the First Part of the Lord of the Rings.* Boston: Houghton Mifflin.

Trans Fat Task Force. (2006). *TRANSforming the Food Supply: Report of the Trans Fat Task Force Submitted to the Minister of Health.* Ottawa, ON: Ministry of Health.

Trivedi, B. P. (2002). Ancient Chocolate Found in Maya "Teapot." Retrieved August 8, 2010, from *National Geographic News.com* at http://news.nationalgeographic.com/news/2002/07/0717_020717_TVchocolate.html.

Trueman, K. (2008). Time to Mothball the Butterball. Retrieved November 5, 2009, from *Huffington Post* at www.huffingtonpost.com/kerry-trueman/time-to-mothball-the-butt_b_143647.html&cp.

U.S. Government, Food and Drug Administration. (2009). How to Understand and Use the Nutrition Facts Label. Retrieved January 25, 2010, from *U.S. Food and Drug Administration* at www.fda.gov/Food/LabelingNutrition/ConsumerInformation/ucm078889.htm.

Vital Choices. (2006). Farmed Salmon's Diet Yields Unhealthful Cardiovascular Effects. Retrieved August 20, 2010, from *Vital Choices* at http://newsletter.vitalchoice.com/e_article000518607.cfm?x=b6CLG4Q,b1kJpvRw.

Wang-Polagruto, J. F., A. C. Villablanca, J. A. Polagruto, L. Lee, R. R. Holt, H. R. Schrader, et al. (2006). Chronic Consumption of Flavanol-Rich Cocoa Improves Endothelial Function and Decreases Vascular Cell Adhesion Molecule in Hypercholesterolemic Postmenopausal Women. *Journal of Cardiovascular Pharmacology*, (47): S177–86.

Weiss, D. (2008). Garlic. Retrieved June 1, 2010, from *Heartspring.net* at http://heartspring.net/heart_disease_prevention.html.

Wilson, M., R. O'Hanlon, S. Prasad, A. Deighan, P. Macmillan, D. Oxborough, et al. (2011). Diverse Patterns of Myocardial Fibrosis in Lifelong, Veteran Endurance Athletes. *Journal of Applied Physiology*, 110(6):1622–26.

Winslow, R. (2010). A Guilt-Free Hamburger. Retrieved September 16, 2011, from *The Wall Street Journal* at http://online.wsj.com/article/SB10001424052748704314904575250570943835414.html.

Witchel, A. (2009). Putting America's Diet on a Diet. *New York Times Magazine* (October 11):MM50.

Woodward, B., and S. Armstrong. (1979). *The Brethren.* New York: Simon and Schuster.

Wrangham, R. (2009). *Catching Fire: How Cooking Made Us Human.* New York: Basic Books.

Wright, J. D., C. Y. Wang, J. Kennedy-Stephenson, and R. B. Ervin. (2003). *Dietary Intake of Ten Key Nutrients for Public Health*. Hyattsville, MD: U.S. Department of Health and Human Services.

Zhang, M., A. C. Brewer, K. Schröder, C. X. Santos, D. J. Grieve, M. Wang, et al. (2010). NADPH Oxidase-4 Mediates Protection against Chronic Load-Induced Stress in Mouse Hearts by Enhancing Angiogenesis. *Proceedings of the National Academy of Sciences of the United States of America*, 107(42):18121–26.

Zheng, W., and S. Y. Wang. (2001). Antioxidant Activity and Phenolic Compounds in Selected Herbs. *Journal of Agricultural and Food Chemistry*, 49(11):5165–70.

additional resources

THERE ARE a number of great resources available today for anyone interested in learning how to cook better. I recommend watching cooking shows; the Food Network and the Cooking Channel are good places to start. There are many great shows on PBS channels, and I think *America's Test Kitchen* is a gem of information. Emeril Lagasse can make anything look good. And there are other great shows on channels like the Travel Channel. I love Anthony Bourdain and learn a lot by living vicariously through his show. On BBC I love to watch Gordon Ramsay, too; not only do I learn a lot, but it's also gratifying to find someone else who cusses in the kitchen as much as I do. He also always seems to have something on Fox. The BBC shows with Jamie Oliver are quite good, and I love his approach.

The Web is an incredible resource for not only recipes but also basic cooking term definitions and videos on techniques. Our site, www.whatscookingwithdoc.com, has lots of information and links, in addition to the blog *The Rx Pad*. To learn the basics of food chemistry and cooking science, I recommend not only watching Alton Brown but also having his videos as a ready reference. Magazines like *Basil* (free online e-zine), *Bon Appétit*, *Cooks Illustrated*, and *Wine Spectator* are incredibly useful. And every kitchen should have several cookbooks as go-to references (Julia Child's books, any culinary book by Michael Ruhlman, and *La Rousse Gastronomique* are must-haves). For techniques and great recipes, one of my favorites is *How to Cook the Perfect . . .* by Marcus Wareing. He ran Petrus under the Ramsay banner for a while before going out on his own. Not only are the recipes great, but he also gives wonderful tips and techniques. I also use the cookbooks by Emeril Lagasse, Gordon Ramsay, Thomas Keller, Anthony Bourdain, and a slew of less-famous characters. If you can find books from chefs who can demonstrate regional cuisine, like Poppy Tooker from New Orleans (I attended some cooking classes with her, and she was amazing), these can prove invaluable. And I use these books all the time.

BOOKS

Belleme, Jan, and John Belleme. (1986). *Cooking with Japanese Foods: A Guide to the Natural Foods of Japan.* New York: East West Health Books.

Bourdain, Anthony. (2004). *Anthony Bourdain's Les Halles Cookbook.* London: Bloomsbury.

Brown, Alton. (2003). *Alton Brown's Gear for Your Kitchen.* New York: Stewart, Tabori, and Chang.

———. (2003). *I'm Just Here for the Food: Kitchen User's Manual.* New York: Stewart, Tabori, and Chang.

———. (2004). *I'm Just Here for More Food: Food x Mixing + Heat = Baking.* New York: Stewart, Tabori, and Chang.

———. (2006). *I'm Just Here for the Food: Food + Heat = Cooking.* New York: Stewart, Tabori, and Chang.

———. (2008). *Feasting on Asphalt: The River Run.* New York: Stewart, Tabori, and Chang.

———. (2009). *Good Eats: The Early Years.* New York: Stewart, Tabori, and Chang.

Chase, Leah. (2004). *The Dooky Chase Cookbook.* Gretna, LA: Pelican.

Cheng, Rose, and Michele Morris. (1981). *Chinese Cookery.* Tucson, AZ: H. P. Book.

Child, Julia. (2009). *Julia's Kitchen Wisdom: Essential Techniques and Recipes from a Lifetime of Cooking.* New York: Knopf.

Child, Julia, Louisette Bertholle, and Simone Beck. (2001). *Mastering the Art of French Cooking Vols. 1 and 2.* New York: Knopf.

Dornenburg, Andrew, and Karen Page. (2008). *What to Drink with What You Eat.* New York: Bulfinch Press.

Forrestal, Peter, ed. *The Global Encyclopedia of Wine.* South San Francisco, CA: Wine Appreciation Guild.

Fujii, Mari. (2005). *The Enlightened Kitchen: Fresh Vegetable Dishes from the Temples of Japan.* New York: Kodansha.

Ginor, Michael. (1999). *Foie Gras: A Passion.* New York: Wiley.

Immer, Andrea. (2000). *Great Wines Made Simple.* New York: Broadway Books.

———. (2002). *Great Tastes Made Simple.* New York: Broadway Books.

Keller, Thomas. (1999). *The French Laundry Cookbook.* New York: Artisan.

———. (2004). *Bouchon.* New York: Artisan.

———. (2008). *Under Pressure: Cooking Sous Vide.* New York: Artisan.

———. (2009). *Ad Hoc at Home.* New York: Artisan.

Kessler, David. (2009). *The End of Overeating: Taking Control of the Insatiable American Appetite.* Emmaus, PA: Rodale Books.

Konishi, Kiyoko. (1984). *Japanese Cooking for Health and Fitness.* Woodbury, NY: Barron's.

Labensky, Sarah, and Alan Hause. (2003). *On Cooking: Techniques from Expert Chefs.* Upper Saddle River, NJ: Prentice Hall.

Lagasse, Emeril. (1998). *Emeril's TV Dinners.* New York: William Morrow.

———. (1999). *Every Day's a Party: Louisiana Recipes for Celebrating with Family and Friends.* New York: William Morrow.

———. (2004). *Emeril's Potluck: Comfort Food with a Kicked-Up Attitude.* New York: William Morrow.

———. (2005). *Emeril's Delmonico: A New Orleans Restaurant with a Past.* New York: Harper Collins.

———. (2009). *Emeril at the Grill: A Cookbook for All Seasons.* New York: Harperstudio.

Larousse Gastronomique. (2001). New York: Clarkson Potter.

Laube, James. (1999). *Wine Spectator's California Wine.* New York: Wine Spectator Press.

Macquet, Dominque. (2000). *Dominique's Fresh Flavors: Cooking with Latitude in New Orleans.* Berkeley, CA: Ten Speed Press.

Miller, Gloria. (1966). *The Thousand Recipe Chinese Cookbook.* New York: Atheneum.

Nestle, Marion. (2006). *What to Eat.* New York: North Point Press.

Norman, Jill, ed. (2005). *The Cook's Book: Techniques and Tips from the World's Master Chefs.* London: Dorling Kindersley.

Omae, Kinjiro, and Yuzuru Tachibana. (1981). *The Book of Sushi.* Tokyo: Kodansha International.

Ramsay, Gordon. (1999). *Gordon Ramsay's Passion for Seafood.* London: Conran Octopus.

———. (2000). *Gordon Ramsay's Passion for Flavour.* London: Conran Octopus.

———. (2001). *Gordon Ramsay's Just Desserts.* San Diego, CA: Laurel Glen.

———. (2003). *Gordon Ramsay's Secrets.* London: Quadrille.

———. (2004). *Kitchen Heaven.* New York: Penguin Global.

———. (2006). *Sunday Lunch: And Other Recipes from the "F" Word.* London: Quadrille.

Rozin, Elisabeth. (1983). *Ethnic Cuisine: The Flavor-Principle Cook-Book.* Lexington, MA: S. Greene Press.

Ruhlman, Michael. (2001). *The Soul of a Chef: The Pursuit of Perfection.* New York: Penguin.

———. (2005). *Charcuterie: The Craft of Salting, Smoking, and Curing.* New York: W. W. Norton.

———. (2007). *The Elements of Cooking: Translating the Chef's Craft for Every Kitchen.* New York: Scribner.

———. (2007). *The Reach of a Chef: Professional Cooking in the Age of Celebrity.* New York: Penguin.

———. (2009). *The Making of a Chef: Mastering Heat at the Culinary Institute of America.* New York: Henry Holt.

———. (2009). *Ratio: The Simple Codes behind the Craft of Everyday Cooking.* New York: Scribner.

———. (2009). *A Return to Cooking with Eric Ripert.* New York: Artisan.

Sugimoto, Takashi, and Marcia Iwatate. (2002). *Shunju: New Japanese Cuisine.* Singapore: Periplus.

Symon, Michael. (2009). *Michael Symon's Live to Cook: Recipes and Techniques to Rock Your Kitchen.* New York: Clarkson Potter.

Tooker, Poppy. (2009). *Crescent City Farmers Market Cookbook.* New Orleans: Marketumbrella.

Tsuji, Shizuo. (1980). *Japanese Cooking: A Simple Art.* Tokyo: Kodansha International.

Wareing, Marcus. (2007). *How to Cook the Perfect . . .* London: D. K. Publishers.

Zraly, Kevin. (2000). *Windows on the World Complete Wine Course.* New York: Sterling.

MAGAZINES

Bon Appétit. A standard bearer for what is culinary cool. Andrew Knowlton is awesome.

Cook's Illustrated. One of the best resources: useful, unbiased, and reliably delicious. You must subscribe.

Wine Spectator. A standard bearer for the wine world. You always learn something reading this magazine, and the online courses are great.

WEBSITES

www.alaskaharvest.com. Great Alaskan and other seafood.

http://alittlebitofchristo.blogspot.com. Always delicious food and fun with Christo, the Cowboy Warlock.

www.altonbrown.com. He will teach you science *and* good eats. Read and watch everything.

http://anthony-bourdain-blog.travelchannel.com. Keep up with Bourdain; he's a culinary superhero.

www.asianfoodgrocer.com. Excellent resource for hard-to-find Asian items.

www.balsworld.com. Bal Arneson is the spice goddess and delivers all things Indian as only she can.

www.basilmagazine.com. Awesome monthly and free magazine about food and the culinary life.

www.blackwing.com/blog.php. Super source for organic meats.

http://blog.ruhlman.com. You need to be here and make sure you have all his books. One of the best, if not the best, authors on all things culinary. Mandatory.

www.bobbyflay.com. Learn here from the spice master.

www.cameronscookware.com. A great source for smoking chips.

www.channel4.com/food/recipes/chefs/gordon-ramsay/index.html. Great Ramsay recipe source.

www.chefknivestogo.com. Nice resource to find that chef's knife.

www.chowandchatter.com. Excellent website and great resource by Rebecca Subbiah.

http://cookappeal.blogspot.com. Great food and wine site by a poet and chef.

www.dartagnan.com. Great source for hard-to-find items delivered fresh.

www.epicurious.com. A must-have resource site.

www.erobertparker.com. One of my favorite wine resources.

www.foodnetwork.com. A fantastic recipe and inspiration source from your favorite celeb chefs.

www.foodsubs.com. The cook's thesaurus; useful, easy way to look something up.

www.gordonramsay.com. Bourdain's British twin. Check it out, and learn something.

www.localharvest.org. Local, fresh, grassroots cooking ingredients brought to your door.

www.lucascafe.com. Chef Luca Paris's website, a great resource, and radio show.

www.mariobatali.com. Learn here from the emperor of Italian cuisine.

www.mycopia.com. Excellent resource for fresh, hard-to-find mushroom varieties.

www.noramill.com. A great spot for stone-ground products, especially grits and cornmeal.

www.nutritiondata.com. A convenient way to check nutrition data.

www.tasteofbeirut.com. The most amazing food and a tutorial on Middle Eastern cuisine and all things delicious by the incredible Joumana.

www.traditionaloven.com. A great site for measurement conversions.

www.whatscookingwithdoc.com. My website, enough said. Stop by and drop a note!

www.whitneyandsonseafoods.com. Steve and Nancy are my fishmonger buddies and always hook folks up with amazing and fresh Gulf seafood.

www.winespectator.com. A favorite wine site.

index of recipes

index of healthy bytes

about the author

MICHAEL S. FENSTER, MD, F.A.C.C., FSCA&I, PEMBA, is a board-certified interventional cardiologist who has taught and practiced at the university level, achieving appointment as an assistant professor of medicine at the North Eastern Ohio University College of Medicine. He has presented at both the American College of Cardiology and the American Culinary Institute national meetings. His recipes have appeared nationally and internationally. Visit Dr. Fenster online at www.whatscookingwithdoc.com.